Nonpulmonary Critical Care

Guest Editors

JOHN R. McARDLE, MD
MARK D. SIEGEL, MD

CLINICS IN CHEST MEDICINE

www.chestmed.theclinics.com

March 2009 • Volume 30 • Number 1

SAUNDERS an imprint of ELSEVIER, Inc.

W.B. SAUNDERS COMPANY
A Division of Elsevier Inc.

1600 John F. Kennedy Boulevard ● Suite 1800 ● Philadelphia, Pennsylvania 19103

http://www.theclinics.com

CLINICS IN CHEST MEDICINE Volume 30, Number 1
March 2009 ISSN 0272-5231, ISBN-13: 978-1-4377-0460-0, ISBN-10: 1-4377-0460-3

Editor: Sarah E. Barth
Developmental Editor: Donald Mumford

Clinics in Chest Medicine (ISSN 0272-5231) is published quarterly by Elsevier Inc., 360 Park Avenue South, New York, NY 10010-1710. Months of issue are March, June, September, and December. Business and Editorial Offices: 1600 John F. Kennedy Blvd., Suite 1800, Philadelphia, PA 19103-2899. Customer Service Office: 11830 Westline Industrial Drive, St. Louis, MO 63146. Periodicals postage paid at New York, NY and additional mailing offices. Subscription prices are $251.00 per year (domestic individuals), $400.00 per year (domestic institutions), $122.00 per year (domestic students/residents), $275.00 per year (Canadian individuals), $491.00 per year (Canadian institutions), $342.00 per year (international individuals) $491.00 per year (international institutions), and $171.00 per year (international and Canadian students/residents). International air speed delivery is included in all Clinics subscription prices. All prices are subject to change without notice. **POSTMASTER:** Send address changes to *Clinics in Chest Medicine,* 11830 Westline Industrial Drive, St. Louis, MO 63146. Customer Service (orders, claims, online, change of address): Elsevier Periodicals Customer Service, 11830 Westline Industrial Drive, St. Louis, MO 63146. Tel: 1-800-654-2452 (U.S. and Canada). Fax: 314-523-5170. E-mail: journalscustomerservice-usa@elsevier.com (for print support); journalsonlinesupport-usa@elsevier.com (for online support).

Reprints. For copies of 100 or more of articles in this publication, please contact the Commercial Reprints Department, Elsevier Inc., 360 Park Avenue South, New York, NY 10010-1710. Tel.: 212-633-3812; Fax: 212-462-1935; E-mail: reprints@elsevier.com.

Clinics in Chest Medicine is covered in *MEDLINE/PubMed (Index Medicus), Current Contents/Clinical Medicine, EMBASE/ Excerpta Medica, Science Citation Index,* and *ISI/BIOMED.*

Printed and bound by CPI Group (UK) Ltd, Croydon, CR0 4YY

Transferred to Digital Print 2011

Contributors

GUEST EDITORS

JOHN R. McARDLE, MD
Assistant Professor of Medicine, Section
of Pulmonary and Critical Care Medicine,
Department of Medicine, Yale University
School of Medicine, New Haven, Connecticut

MARK D. SIEGEL, MD
Associate Professor of Medicine, Section
of Pulmonary and Critical Care Medicine,
Department of Medicine, Yale University
School of Medicine, New Haven, Connecticut

AUTHORS

DJILLALI ANNANE, MD, PhD
Assistance Publique Hôpitaux de Paris,
Université de Versailles SQY (UniverSud Paris),
Hôpital Raymond Poincaré, Service
de Réanimation, Garches, France

LINDSAY ARNOTT, RN, MHA, CCTC
Transplant Services Manager, Department
of Surgery, Section of Transplant and
Immunology, Yale New Haven Transplantation
Center, New Haven, Connecticut

GHADA BOURJEILY, MD
Assistant Professor of Medicine, Department
of Medicine, Pulmonary and Critical Care,
Women & Infants Hospital, Warren Alpert
Medical School of Brown University,
Providence, Rhode Island

DAVID R. BRUSH, MD
Fellow, Section of Pulmonary and Critical Care
Medicine, Department of Medicine, University
of Chicago Medical Center, Chicago, Illinois

SUSAN T. CROWLEY, MD
Associate Professor of Medicine, Section
of Nephrology, Yale University School of
Medicine, New Haven; Chief, Renal Section,
VA Connecticut Healthcare System, West
Haven, Connecticut

JULIUS CUONG PHAM, MD, PhD
Assistant Professor, Department of
Anesthesiology and Critical Care Medicine;
Department of Emergency Medicine, Johns
Hopkins University, School of Medicine,
Baltimore, Maryland

INNEKE E. DE LAET, MD
Intensive Care Unit, ZiekenhuisNetwerk
Antwerpen, Campus Stuivenberg, Antwerpen,
Belgium

SUKRU EMRE, MD
Professor of Surgery, Department of Surgery;
and Chief, Section of Transplant and
Immunology, Yale New Haven Transplantation
Center, New Haven, Connecticut

CHRISTINE A. GOESCHEL, RN, MPA, MPS
Director of Operations, Quality and Patient
Safety Initiatives, Department of
Anesthesiology and Critical Care Medicine,
Johns Hopkins University, School of Medicine,
Baltimore, Maryland

SHYOKO HONIDEN, MD
Assistant Professor of Medicine, Department
of Medicine; and Division of Pulmonology and
Critical Care, Yale New Haven Transplantation
Center, New Haven, Connecticut

RAMONA O. HOPKINS, PhD
Professor and Chair, Psychology Department, Neuroscience Center, Brigham Young University, Provo; Pulmonary and Critical Care Division, Department of Medicine, LDS Hospital, Salt Lake City; Pulmonary and Critical Care Medicine, Intermountain Medical Center, Murray, Utah

JAMES C. JACKSON, PsyD
Assistant Professor, Division of Allergy/Pulmonary/Critical Care Medicine, Vanderbilt University School of Medicine; Center for Health Services Research, Vanderbilt University School of Medicine, Nashville, Tennessee

JOHN P. KRESS, MD
Associate Professor of Medicine and Director, Medical Intensive Care Unit, Section of Pulmonary and Critical Care Medicine, Department of Medicine, University of Chicago Medical Center, Chicago, Illinois

OLIVIER LESUR, MD, PhD
Service de Soins Intensifs Médicaux, Département de Dédecine, CHU Sherbrooke, Sherbrooke, Québec, Canada

MANU L.N.G. MALBRAIN, MD, PhD
Former President, World Society for the Abdominal Compartment Syndrome; ICU Director, Intensive Care Unit, ZiekenhuisNetwerk Antwerpen, Campus Stuivenberg, Antwerpen, Belgium

JASON B. MARTIN, MD
Clinical Fellow, Division of Allergy, Pulmonary & Critical Care, Vanderbilt University Medical Center, Nashville, Tennessee

PETER W. MARKS, MD, PhD
Associate Professor of Medicine, Section of Hematology, Department of Internal Medicine, Yale University School of Medicine, New Haven, Connecticut

VIRGINIE MAXIME, MD
Assistance Publique Hôpitaux de Paris, Université de Versailles SQY (UniverSud Paris), Hôpital Raymond Poincaré, Service de Réanimation, Garches, France

STEPHAN A. MAYER, MD
Associate Professor of Clinical Neurology and Neurosurgery, Columbia University; Director, Neurological Intensive Care Unit, Milstein Hospital, Columbia University Medical Center, New York, New York

JOHN R. MCARDLE, MD
Assistant Professor of Medicine, Section of Pulmonary and Critical Care Medicine, Department of Medicine, Yale University School of Medicine, New Haven, Connecticut

MARLENE R. MILLER, MD, MSc
Associate Professor, Department of Pediatrics; and Vice Chair of Quality and Safety Initiatives, Johns Hopkins Children's Center, Johns Hopkins University, School of Medicine, Baltimore, Maryland; National Association of Children's Hospitals and Related Institutions, Alexandria, Virginia

MARGARET MILLER, MD
Assistant Professor of Medicine and Obstetrician/Gynecologist, Department of Medicine, Obstetric and Consultative Medicine, Women & Infants Hospital, Warren Alpert Medical School of Brown University, Providence, Rhode Island

ALDO J. PEIXOTO, MD
Associate Professor of Medicine, Section of Nephrology, Yale University School of Medicine, New Haven; Associate Chief, Medical Service, VA Connecticut Healthcare System, West Haven, Connecticut

PETER J. PRONOVOST, MD, PhD
Professor, Department of Anesthesiology and Critical Care Medicine; Department of Surgery; Department of Health Policy and Management, Johns Hopkins University, School of Medicine, Baltimore, Maryland

MICHAEL L. SCHILSKY, MD
Associate Professor of Medicine, Department of Medicine; and Department of Surgery; and Medical Director, Adult Liver Transplant, Section of Transplant and Immunology, Division of Digestive Diseases, Yale New Haven Transplantation Center, New Haven, Connecticut

DAVID B. SEDER, MD
Medical Director of Neurocritical Care, Division of Pulmonary and Critical Care Medicine, Maine Medical Center, Portland, Maine

J. BRYAN SEXTON, PhD
Assistant Professor, Department of Anesthesiology and Critical Care Medicine; Department of Health Policy and Management, Johns Hopkins University, School of Medicine, Baltimore, Maryland

MARK D. SIEGEL, MD
Associate Professor of Medicine, Section of Pulmonary and Critical Care Medicine, Department of Medicine, Yale University School of Medicine, New Haven, Connecticut

ARTHUR P. WHEELER, MD
Associate Professor of Medicine, Division of Allergy, Pulmonary & Critical Care; and Director, Medical Intensive Care Unit, Vanderbilt University Medical Center, Nashville, Tennessee

BRADFORD D. WINTERS, MD, PhD
Assistant Professor, Department of Anesthesiology and Critical Care Medicine, Johns Hopkins University, School of Medicine, Baltimore, Maryland

Contributors

DAVID B. SEDER, MD
Medical Director of Neurocritical Care, Division of Pulmonary and Critical Care Medicine, Maine Medical Center, Portland, Maine

J. BRYAN SEXTON, PhD
Assistant Professor, Department of Anesthesiology and Critical Care Medicine, Department of Health Policy and Management, Johns Hopkins University School of Medicine, Baltimore, Maryland

MARK D. SIEGEL, MD
Associate Professor of Medicine, Section of Pulmonary and Critical Care Medicine, Department of Medicine, Yale University School of Medicine, New Haven, Connecticut

ARTHUR P. WHEELER, MD
Associate Professor of Medicine, Division of Allergy, Pulmonary & Critical Care, and Director, Medical Intensive Care Unit, Vanderbilt University Medical Center, Nashville, Tennessee

BRADFORD D. WINTERS, MD, PhD
Assistant Professor, Department of Anesthesiology and Critical Care Medicine, Johns Hopkins University School of Medicine, Baltimore, Maryland

Contents

> This article reviews the current understanding of sepsis, severe sepsis, and septic shock. The article details definitions and epidemiology pertinent to the sepsis syndrome. A brief discussion of mechanisms of disease is followed a description of organ-specific failures related to sepsis. A concise review of the latest treatment options for each organ dysfunction is provided.

> During disease states, the endocrine axes exhibit different levels of activity according to the severity of illness. These various alterations have been widely investigated. Indeed, evidence indicates that the anterior pituitary is dysfunctional in these states, especially when multiple organ dysfunction syndrome is present, impacting both adrenal and thyroid glands, but also secretion of estrogen, growth hormone, insulin-like growth factor-1, and prolactin. In a majority of these cases, substitutive treatment is not obviously beneficial, inappropriate secretions being considered as adaptive responses to stressful events. The hypothalamic-pituitaryadrenal axis appears to play the most important role in the regulation of inflammation during septic shock. Many factors modulate this axis. Some are well known. Others, such as vasopressin and apelin, are newly ascribed. Therapeutic issues in critically ill patients still remain controversial and are ardently debated, especially with regard to the needs and practical use of corticosteroids in septic shock. This article focuses on actual knowledge, mechanisms, definitions, and therapeutic recommendations, as well as on areas of uncertainty relative to adrenal gland insufficiency in septic shock.

> Acute kidney injury (AKI) is common among critically ill patients and results in increased mortality in this population. This review focuses on the diagnosis and management of AKI. The authors first explore new aspects of diagnosis, including new criteria that take into account even modest changes in renal function, and the development of novel biomarkers to allow earlier identification and better differential diagnosis of AKI. The authors also explore the available data on choice of dialysis modality and dialysis dose for the treatment of AKI, as well as the breakthrough development of the bioartificial kidney. Last, the authors review co-interventions that

life-threatening ischemic strokes is reviewed, emphasizing the care of patients with acute basilar artery occlusion and the malignant middle cerebral artery syndrome. Up-to-date estimates of the long-term outcomes of these syndromes are reviewed.

Coagulation Disorders in the ICU   123

Peter W. Marks

Disorders of hemostasis and thrombosis are frequently encountered in the ICU setting. Understanding the relevance of laboratory findings is essential in providing appropriate therapy. Various blood products and hemostatic agents are available to assist in the control of bleeding, and several different classes of anticoagulants are now available for use. Appropriate use of these agents maximizes therapeutic effect while minimizing complications. Use of fresh frozen plasma, cryoprecipitate, and other hemostatic agents should generally be reserved for those who have active bleeding, those undergoing invasive procedures, and those at high risk for bleeding because of their underlying diagnoses or because of associated hematologic derangements.

Sedation and Analgesia for the Mechanically Ventilated Patient   131

David R. Brush and John P. Kress

Mechanically ventilated patients in the intensive care unit routinely require sedative and analgesic medications to manage pain and anxiety. These medications may have unpredictable effects with long-term use. Strategies that may help to improve patient outcomes include thoughtful selection of medications, use of objective sedation and pain scales, and implementation of protocolized sedation.

Short- and Long-Term Cognitive Outcomes in Intensive Care Unit Survivors   143

Ramona O. Hopkins and James C. Jackson

Evidence increasingly suggests that cognitive impairment is common in intensive care unit survivors, although the nature, severity, and natural history remain unclear. Although the cognitive impairments improve over time in some individuals, they often fail to completely abate. While the functional correlates of these impairments are under-studied, cognitive impairments may adversely impact quality of life, ability to return to work or to work at previously established levels, and ability to function effectively in emotional and interpersonal domains. The potential etiologies of cognitive impairments in intensive care unit survivors are not fully understood and are likely heterogeneous and vary widely across patients. The contributions of these many factors may be particularly significant in patients with pre-existing vulnerabilities for the development of cognitive impairments, such as mild cognitive impairment, dementia, prior traumatic brain injury, or other comorbid disorders, as well as predisposing genetic factors.

Critical Care Outcomes in the Hematologic Transplant Recipient   155

John R. McArdle

Critical illness is a dreaded complication in recipients of hematologic stem cell transplantation, with poor survival described in a number of early series. The perception of futility may impact the approach to therapy. Over the last 20 years, there have been significant advances in the application of intensive care, as well as changes in the management of patients before, during, and after transplantation. These advances and changes may have an impact on this traditionally poor survival. This article discusses the outcomes of critical illness in bone marrow and stem cell transplant recipients, and gives possible reasons for the apparent improvement in outcomes seen in more recent series.

The global health care community has worked tirelessly for nearly a decade to make medical care safer for patients, but it still has limited ability to evaluate whether safety has improved. While there is a universal push to measure safety outcomes, the main barrier has been poor investment in the basic science of patient safety. This science would allow us to comprehend the causes of harm, design and pilot test interventions to reduce harm, and robustly evaluate their impact. This article describes several dilemmas in measuring patient safety, outlines a conceptual model and presents a framework for measuring patient safety, and offers future directions. Future research should seek to create a scientifically sound and feasible safety scorecard and improve performance.

A large proportion of deaths, particularly in the developed world, follows admission to an ICU. Therefore, end-of life decision making is an essential facet of critical care practice. For intensivists, managing death in the critically ill has become a key professional skill. They must be thoroughly familiar with the ethical framework that guides end-of-life decision making. Decisions should generally be made collaboratively by clinicians partnering with patients' families. Treatment choices should be crafted to meet specific, achievable goals. A rational, empathic approach to working with families should encourage appropriate, mutually satisfactory outcomes.

Clinics in Chest Medicine

THE CLINICS ARE NOW AVAILABLE ONLINE!

Access your subscription at:
www.theclinics.com

Preface

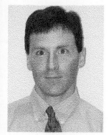 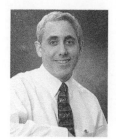

John R. McArdle, MD   Mark D. Siegel, MD
Guest Editors

It has been 5 years since *Clinics in Chest Medicine* devoted an issue to nonpulmonary critical care. Since then, novel scientific discoveries and clinical observations have challenged our approach to critical illness. Previously innovative treatments, such as meticulous glucose control and early goal directed therapy, have evolved into mainstream, if controversial, management paradigms. New insights have fostered awareness of under-appreciated dangers, such as the potential toxicity of blood products and the hidden dangers of abdominal compartment syndrome. The growing power of translational research is helping to explain why some patients succumb to life threatening illness while others survive.

By nature, pulmonologists engaged in critical care are self-reliant. This trait says something about our mindset, but it also reflects a widely held assumption, probably true, that outstanding critical care requires physicians to contribute direction and order to the management of patients who have complex, life-threatening diseases. In turn, this demands leadership skills, insight, knowledge, some wisdom, and endless study.

It is a daunting task for physicians to stay current with pulmonary literature, much less the overwhelming number of publications in other disciplines important to our patients. This issue of *Clinics in Chest Medicine* is devoted to helping chest physicians meet this challenge. We have been fortunate to recruit a panel of highly regarded authors to share their expertise in comprehensive reviews covering a wide variety of topics ranging from the management of specific disease states (such as sepsis, adrenal insufficiency, and abdominal compartment syndrome) to the care of special populations (such as stem cell transplant recipients and pregnant patients). Several articles highlight emerging concepts in the disciplines of neurology, hepatology, hematology, and nephrology, as well as specific topics like sedation, cognitive impairment, quality improvement, and end-of-life decision making.

In assembling this issue, perhaps the only uncertainty was whether a Yankee Fan (McArdle) and a Met Fan (Siegel) could manage to collaborate as effectively as we seem to do each day in the Yale Medical Intensive Care Unit. Once this question was answered successfully, the rest of the project was easy, thanks to our talented contributors; our expert, energetic (and patient) publisher, Sarah Barth; and our wonderfully supportive (and even more patient) wives and children. It is has been a pleasure to edit this issue of *Clinics in Chest Medicine*. We hope our readers find it interesting, enjoyable, provocative, and useful.

John R. McArdle, MD
Section of Pulmonary and Critical Care Medicine
Department of Medicine
Yale University School of Medicine
333 Cedar Street, P.O. Box 208057
New Haven, CT 06073, USA

Mark D. Siegel, MD
Section of Pulmonary and Critical Care Medicine
Department of Medicine
Yale University School of Medicine
333 Cedar Street, LCI 105, P.O. Box 208057
New Haven, CT 06520-8057, USA

E-mail addresses:
john.mcardle@yale.edu (J.R. McArdle)
mark.siegel@yale.edu (M.D. Siegel)

doi:10.1016/j.ccm.2008.12.001

chestmed.theclinics.com

Approach to the Patient with Sepsis

Jason B. Martin, MD[a], Arthur P. Wheeler, MD[a,b],*

KEYWORDS

- Sepsis • Septic shock • Definitions • Management

Sepsis syndrome results from a host reaction to infection, which includes a robust systemic inflammatory response, enhanced coagulation, and impaired fibrinolysis.[1] The relationships among infection, inflammation, and sepsis are well described in professional society consensus statements.[2] The systemic inflammatory response syndrome (SIRS) is defined by the constellation of fever or hypothermia, tachycardia, tachypnea, and leukocytosis, leukopenia, or the presence of immature neutrophils **Table 1**. SIRS can result from numerous conditions but only becomes "sepsis" when infection is etiologic. When sepsis causes at least one organ dysfunction, the syndrome is termed "severe sepsis," and sepsis-induced hypotension that is refractory to fluid challenge defines "septic shock."

While the SIRS criteria are sensitive for septic patients, they are criticized for lacking specificity. Many, if not most, ICU patients have tachypnea and tachycardia, raising doubt as to the diagnostic utility of the SIRS criteria.[3] Although the specificity of SIRS is increased by requiring three of the criteria, or by mandating that one of two required criteria be abnormal temperature or white blood cell count, even two criteria maintain prognostic importance.[4]

EPIDEMIOLOGY AND OUTCOMES

Large epidemiologic studies report an incidence of 1 to 3 cases per 1000 population per year[5] resulting in approximately 750,000 cases annually in the United States. The average sepsis survivor requires 7 to 14 days of intensive care unit (ICU) support with much of this time spent on a ventilator. After ICU discharge, an additional 10- to 14-day hospital stay is typical. Thus, the average hospital length of stay for survivors is 3 to 5 weeks. Hospital charges in excess of tens of thousands of dollars are common for individual patients, resulting in annual US expenditures of nearly $17 billion.[6,7]

Septic patients present typically in their sixth or seventh decade of life,[6,8,9] and the average age of afflicted patients has increased consistently over time.[5,10] For unclear reasons, males are affected more commonly.[6] Although the condition can occur in previously healthy individuals, it is more common in patients with chronic diseases, particularly the immunocompromised. Occurrence rates are higher in those with diabetes mellitus, malignancy, chronic immune suppressive therapy, or human immunodeficiency virus infection. Patients with disrupted skin, especially trauma victims or surgical patients, are also more likely to develop severe sepsis. In the United States, African Americans have higher rates of hospitalization and mortality from sepsis as compared with whites, but the rates of case fatality are similar between the two groups.[11] Despite these observations, sepsis has no definitive age, gender, racial, or geographic boundaries.

Today hospital mortality rates remain unacceptably high; 30% to 40% of patients die despite prompt, comprehensive treatment. Predictors of worse outcomes include advanced age,[10] cancer,[12,13] and a hypothermic presentation.[14]

[a] Division of Allergy, Pulmonary & Critical Care, Vanderbilt University Medical Center, 1161 21st Avenue South, Suite T-1210 MCN, Nashville, TN 37232-2650, USA
[b] Medical Intensive Care Unit, Vanderbilt University Medical Center, 1161 21st Avenue South, Suite T-1210 MCN, Nashville, TN 37232-2650, USA
* Corresponding author. Division of Allergy, Pulmonary & Critical Care, Vanderbilt University Medical Center, 1161 21st Avenue South, Suite T-1210 MCN, Nashville, TN 37232-2650.
E-mail address: art.wheeler@vanderbilt.edu (A.P. Wheeler).

Clin Chest Med 30 (2009) 1–16
doi:10.1016/j.ccm.2008.09.005
0272-5231/08/$ – see front matter © 2009 Elsevier Inc. All rights reserved.

Table 1
Definitions related to sepsis

Term	Definition and Criteria
Infection	Microorganism invasion of a normally sterile site
Bacteremia	Presence of viable microorganisms in the blood
Systemic Inflammatory Response Syndrome (SIRS)	A systemic inflammatory response to a pathologic insult, such as a burn, trauma, pancreatitis, or infection. SIRS requires two or more of the following conditions: • Temperature >38°C or <36°C • Heart rate >90 beats/min • Respiratory rate >20 breaths/min or PaCO2 <32 mm Hg • WBC >12,000/mm^3, <4000 cells/mm^3, or >10% immature (band) forms
Sepsis (= 1 + 3)	The syndrome caused by a systemic inflammatory response secondary to infection
Severe sepsis	Sepsis associated with organ dysfunction. Specific organ dysfunctions include, but are not limited to, hypotension, renal dysfunction, respiratory failure, and altered mental status.
Septic shock (= 5 + 7)	Sepsis with hypotension or hypoperfusion despite adequate fluid resuscitation.
Hypotension, sepsis-induced	A decrease in systolic blood pressure <90 mm Hg, a mean arterial pressure <60 mm Hg, or a reduction of >40 mm Hg from baseline

Data from Bone RC, Balk RA, Cerra FB, et al. American-College of Chest Physicians Society of Critical Care Medicine Consensus Conference—definitions for sepsis and organ failure and guidelines for the use of innovative therapies in sepsis. Crit Care Med 1992;20(6):864–74.

Historically, it was believed specific characteristics of the invading pathogen determined prognosis, but recent investigations have undermined this long-held belief.[15–17] The identity of the infecting organism is of lesser consequence than physiologic derangements provided appropriate, prompt antimicrobial therapy is administered. At the bedside, the best practical predictor of outcome is simply the number of organ systems with sepsis-induced dysfunction.[4,18] Each new organ system failure adds roughly 15% to 20% risk of death to the baseline 10% to 15% mortality rate seen among ICU patients.[5] On average, patients have two or three failing organ systems at the time of diagnosis.[18,19]

In addition to the number of malfunctioning organs, the severity of organ dysfunction also correlates with outcome.[5,20,21] For example, the need for higher or escalating vasoactive medication doses is associated with a worse prognosis than lower dose requirements or no requirement at all.[18] Likewise, increasing levels of renal dysfunction, as measured by either the Risk/Injury/Failure/Loss/End-Stage Renal Disease (RIFLE) or Acute Kidney Injury Network (AKIN) criteria, are also prognostic, including degrees of creatinine elevation heretofore thought to be unimportant.[22,23] Several severity of illness scores have been developed based on assessment of organ functions, including the Acute Physiologic and Chronic Health Evaluation (APACHE) system and the Sequential Organ Failure Assessment (SOFA). These scoring systems are best used as tools to compare severity of illness in large study populations and have less utility as prognostic tools for individual patients.[24]

PRESENTATION AND DIAGNOSIS

Sepsis is diagnosed by history and physical findings, corroborated by laboratory data such as circulating leukocyte count, body fluid examination, and culture. Detecting the syndrome in hospitalized patients is particularly important, as nosocomial sepsis is associated with longer lengths of stay and higher mortality rates as compared with community-acquired sepsis.[25,26] Although there is occasionally some degree of uncertainty, recognition of sepsis usually is not difficult. Most patients will meet at least three SIRS criteria at ICU admission.[27] Minute ventilation is almost always increased, and tachypnea is present in up to 80% of ICU patients. Fever occurs in approximately 60% of patients at admission[27] but may be suppressed in those with advanced age, renal failure, or patients taking anti-inflammatory medications.[14,28] Hypothermia, although uncommon, is an ominous finding associated with mortality rates of up to 60%.[14] The lethality of hypothermia likely is not a consequence of the temperature itself but rather the relationship of hypothermia with underlying chronic diseases, shock, and an exaggerated inflammatory response. Although possible, the diagnosis should be questioned in patients lacking tachypnea or gas exchange abnormalities. Hypoxia is common in septic patients; more than 90% of patients will develop sufficient hypoxemia to require supplemental oxygen, generally correlating with a PaO_2/FiO_2 ratio less than 300. Tachycardia is a cardinal sign of sepsis, and unless patients have intrinsic cardiac disease or are taking nodal blocking medications, tachycardia is nearly universal. Abnormalities in circulating leukocyte count (more than 12,000 cells/mm^3 or fewer than 4000 cells/mm^3) are frequent enough to be considered important diagnostic criteria.

Several serum biomarkers are purported to have diagnostic and/or prognostic value, but none have demonstrated acceptable sensitivity and specificity for routine clinical use. The serum lactate level is suggested to be a marker of global hypoperfusion and tissue hypoxia in sepsis. According to the theory, even *before* patients develop frank hypotension, tissue perfusion is impaired by myocardial depression, relative hypovolemia from a leaky endothelium, increased metabolic demands, and impaired vasoregulatory mechanisms. Consequently, oxygen demand exceeds supply, and anaerobic production of lactate ensues. Not all agree that lactate production is a reliable marker of global hypoxia in sepsis.[29] One alternative explanation asserts that lactate production may be a regional, rather than global, phenomenon. Animal models of polymicrobial sepsis suggest that certain organs, particularly the liver and small intestine, may be more sensitive to impaired oxygen delivery.[30] Regardless of its exact mechanism of production, patients admitted with a sepsis-related diagnosis and elevated serum lactate levels (greater than 4 mmol/L) have an increased mortality rate.[31] Further, septic patients with higher lactate clearance rates after 6 hours of therapy have decreased mortality rates.[32] Procalcitonin and C-reactive protein, both markers of inflammation, have been studied as potential diagnostic tests for sepsis.[33–35] The reported sensitivities and specificities of these tests vary widely, hence neither has achieved widespread acceptance. Measurements of soluble triggering receptor expressed on myeloid cells-1 (sTREM-1), a member of the immunoglobulin superfamily, remains experimental.[36] Interleukin (IL)-6, a cytokine mediator of inflammation, and D-dimer, a marker of coagulation, have substantial sensitivity but lack specificity for the diagnosis.[37,38] Activated protein C (APC) is an endogenous protein that attenuates microvascular thrombosis, and levels of this protein have been shown to be inversely correlated with outcomes.[39] IL-6, APC, and sTREM-1 assays are not readily available, so, despite decades of research, clinicians still yearn for a reliable test to diagnose sepsis.

Body fluid or tissue cultures are widely considered key to the sepsis diagnosis, but current evidence suggests that cultures may not be as pivotal as once thought. While cultures facilitate the diagnosis of infection, not all infected patients develop sepsis, and even fewer, severe sepsis.[40] Interestingly, a clear microbiologic explanation is absent in many patients.[40,41] The likelihood of obtaining an initial positive blood culture increases with disease severity[42] but remains surprisingly low. True positive blood culture rates are reported at about 8.1%,[43] and as many as half of all positive cultures are falsely positive, representing contamination.[44] Avoiding false-positive cultures is important because a positive culture prompts extra diagnostic tests, modifications of antimicrobial therapy, and adds significant costs even when the growth is eventually determined to be a result of contamination.[45] To confound matters further, "true-positive" cultures often do not reflect the sepsis-precipitating infection, as many positive cultures are obtained long after severe sepsis is established and represent insignificant colonization.

PATHOPHYSIOLOGY

Historically, sepsis was considered primarily—or perhaps solely—a disease of unbridled inflammation. One legacy of this view is the widely accepted consensus definition that highlights signs of inflammation as prerequisites to the diagnosis. This paradigm envisioned a multistage inflammatory cascade triggered by microbial invasion into a typically sterile body compartment or fluid. The subsequent proinflammatory state, while considered important to control the spread of local infection or injury, became dysregulated, and inflammation became destructive. In an effort to interrupt this sequence, numerous clinical trials tested the efficacy and safety of anti-inflammatory agents. These trials failed to consistently demonstrate a significant impact on mortality, even when quantitatively down-regulating serum mediators of inflammation (see **Box 1**). The lack of efficacy of anti-inflammatory compounds caused speculation that the pathophysiology of sepsis was more complicated than just uncontrolled inflammation, and discouraged research.

It is now clear that inflammation is just one of many contributors to septic physiology; other factors include enhanced coagulation and impaired fibrinolysis.[1,46] The complex interplay between these pathways is fueled both by endogenous and exogenous factors. Exogenous sepsis triggers are typically protein, lipid, or carbohydrate microbial constituents. The most notorious exogenous microbial component is endotoxin, the integral cell wall component of gram-negative bacteria. Other well-recognized toxins are staphylococcal toxic shock syndrome toxin (TSST-1) and group B streptococcal toxin. Endogenous triggers—such as activated complement proteins, clotting cascade components, or dead host tissue—can also incite the pathophysiologic pathways of sepsis. Neither bacteremia nor endovascular infection is required for the development of sepsis; humoral release of toxic products from localized sites (such as an abscess) or the colon (as with gut translocation) can trigger a septic event.

Abnormal coagulation is nearly universal in severe sepsis.[46,47] The hematologic dysfunction of sepsis is detectable by widely available laboratory assays. Although routine clotting tests (prothrombin and activated partial thromboplastin times) may be near normal, most patients will have elevated fibrin degradation products (fibrin split products and D-dimers) and depleted levels of specific clotting factors (namely, fibrinogen) and anticlotting proteins.[47]

Early in the syndrome, tissue factor expressed by leukocytes and damaged endothelium, together with proinflammatory mediators, stimulate clotting factors V and VII, resulting in the production of thrombin. Initially, the accelerated thrombosis is attenuated by the host's natural anticlotting proteins, namely protein C, protein S, and antithrombin. Over time, clot formation consumes clotting proteins, and anticlotting proteins are depleted as well. Sepsis also selectively impairs host conversion of inactive anticlotting precursors to active anticlotting proteins, and this impairment favors unabated thrombosis. As a second line of defense, fibrinolysis (primarily via plasminogen activation) is normally stimulated to dissolve the clots that threaten to clog the microvascular beds of critical organs. Unfortunately, the fibrinolytic system is also impaired by the production of thrombin, which increases levels of plasminogen activator inhibitor 1 (PAI-1) and thrombin activatable fibrinolysis inhibitor (TAFI). Together, PAI-1 and TAFI combine to stabilize thrombi in microvascular beds, impairing tissue perfusion and contributing to organ failures.

ORGAN FAILURES
Pulmonary Failure

Respiratory failure is common in septic patients with up to 75% requiring mechanical ventilation for an average of 7 to 10 days.[19] Fortunately, fewer than 5% of patients will require chronic mechanical ventilation, and fewer than 10% will require oxygen 30 days after disease onset.[48] The mechanism of respiratory failure is complex and multifactorial. Work of breathing is increased in severe sepsis. Ventilatory demands are increased by hypoxia and compensation for the lactic acidosis of global hypoperfusion. Airflow resistance is increased and lung compliance is reduced.[49] These increased demands occur at a time when ventilatory power is compromised by diaphragmatic dysfunction and reduced respiratory muscle perfusion. This mismatch of supply and demand leads to combined hypoxic and hypercapnic respiratory failure.

Approximately half of all septic patients develop the most severe subset of acute lung injury (ALI), acute respiratory distress syndrome (ARDS). ALI results from a diffuse inflammatory injury to the lung and is characterized clinically by hypoxia and low pulmonary compliance. By consensus definition, ARDS is defined as a PaO_2/FiO_2 (P/F ratio) ratio less than or equal to 200 with bilateral infiltrates on chest radiograph in the absence of left atrial hypertension.[50] ARDS typically occurs early in the course of sepsis, with most afflicted patients manifesting characteristic signs and symptoms within 48 hours. Interestingly, there is only a rough correlation of P/F ratio with mortality until the ratio approaches 150, where the P/F ratio becomes a powerful predictor of death.[51] Paradoxically, the chest radiograph adds little prognostic information after the P/F ratio and lung compliance are considered.

Circulatory Failure

Hypotension sufficient to meet criteria for shock (systolic blood pressure [BP] less than 90, or a fall in systolic BP of more than 40 mm Hg, or mean arterial pressure less than 60 mmHg unresponsive to fluid administration) is present in about 50% of all septic patients at the time of diagnosis.[52] Shock develops in approximately 50% of the remainder within the first few days of illness. As might be expected, of all organ failures, shock typically has the shortest duration, averaging only 1 to 2 days. "Chronic" shock is rare, as many patients die if prompt correction cannot be accomplished. Because pharmacologic elevation of blood pressure usually is achieved rather easily, mean arterial pressure of treated patients with "shock" does not differ from that of patients without shock, making mean arterial pressure a poor prognostic indicator. Clinicians can be lulled into a false sense of security if the quantity of vasopressor therapy administered is not taken into consideration. Data suggest that patients who require even low doses of a vasopressor after adequate volume replacement have a mortality rate approaching 40%, and the need for high doses of a vasoactive drug are associated with nearly a 60% mortality rate.[18]

Severe sepsis blunts myocardial contractility and mimics some aspects of cardiogenic shock. The myocardial depression of sepsis can cause elevated cardiac filling pressure and a low or low-normal cardiac output. One clue to distinguishing between the myocardial depression of sepsis and cardiogenic shock is the systemic vascular resistance (SVR). The SVR tends to be low in volume in resuscitated patients with septic shock and normal to high in pure cardiogenic shock, although there are exceptions to this rule. Also, the lack of focal wall motion abnormalities on echocardiogram may argue against cardiogenic shock, whereas global hypokinesis on echocardiogram might support the diagnosis of sepsis-related myocardial depression.

Renal Failure

Renal dysfunction commonly complicates sepsis. The Acute Kidney Injury Network (AKIN) defines acute kidney injury (AKI) as "an abrupt (within 48 hours) reduction in kidney function defined as an absolute increase in creatinine of either $\geq$ 0.3 mg/dL or a percentage increase of >50% (1.5-fold increase from baseline) or a reduction in urine output (oliguria of < 0.5 mL/kg/hour for > 6 hours)."[22] In a medical ICU study, 56% of patients with severe sepsis met the AKI definition.[53] The AKIN definition predicts hospital mortality, need for renal replacement therapy (RRT), and length of stay. Fortunately, while oliguria and creatinine elevations are common, fewer than 15% of patients with sepsis progress to overt renal failure and receive RRT. Among those who require dialysis, the support is typically transient, as only 10% of critically ill patients with acute kidney injury will require chronic RRT.[54] Patients with premorbid renal impairment are most likely to experience this complication. Interventions that can minimize the incidence of AKI are prompt treatment of hypotension and avoidance of potentially nephrotoxic drugs, especially intravenous contrast and certain antimicrobials.

Metabolic Acidosis

Lactic acidosis is common in patients with severe sepsis but until recently, was considered a late indicator of hypoperfusion. It is now recognized that even in normotensive patients, significantly elevated serum lactate levels (>4 mmol/L) may occur and indicate a need for early and aggressive optimization of oxygen delivery. The pathogenesis of lactic acidosis is controversial and may be a result of low oxygen delivery (DO_2), maldistribution of cardiac output, or mitochondrial dysfunction. Boosting DO_2 to prevent or reverse anaerobic metabolism and lactic acidosis has been extensively studied. Evidence suggests that increasing DO_2 to an arbitrary supra-normal value in *established* sepsis may be ineffective, or even harmful.[55,56] In contrast, *early* and vigorous resuscitation in the setting of elevated lactate or shock may be beneficial.[57]

Coagulation Disorders

The incidence of coagulation disorders varies depending on the defining criteria, but most patients have reduced levels of clotting and anticlotting proteins and elevated clot degradation products.[46] Nearly 100% of sepsis patients have elevated D-dimer levels, and 90% have reduced protein C levels.[58] Likewise, modest thrombocytopenia (platelet counts, 75–100,000/mm),[3] minimal reductions in fibrinogen, and small prolongations of the prothrombin and partial thromboplastin times are common.[47,58] Disseminated intravascular coagulation (DIC) occurs in about a third of severe sepsis cases, and it is a strong predictor of mortality, independent of APACHE II score and age.[59]

Gastrointestinal Failure

Hepatic and bowel functions frequently are impaired in patients with severe sepsis. Gastric motility is reduced as splanchnic blood flow is shunted to other organs. Animal studies suggest that endotoxemia has a direct, but transient effect on gastric emptying.[60] Profound hypotension, especially when prolonged, also can lead to hepatocellular injury—so called "shock liver" characterized by mild increases in hepatic aminotransferases (AST and ALT) with a disproportionate increase in total bilirubin.[61] Although controversial, hypoperfusion may impair the gut mucosa, facilitating bacterial translocation and reduced functional absorptive capacity.[62] Gut ischemia is also largely responsible for the higher incidence of gastrointestinal (GI) bleeding seen in severe sepsis. In the distant past, significant upper GI bleeding occurred in nearly 30% of cases but the practices of early resuscitation and routine use of acid suppression have all but eliminated life-threatening GI bleeding.

Treatment

Sepsis treatment has evolved substantially to a few basic principles: prompt infection source control, culture of pertinent sites, early and appropriate empiric antibiotics, aggressive circulatory support, and noninjurious ventilatory support. For selected patients, recombinant human activated protein C (rhAPC) has been added to the treatment arsenal. Unfortunately, confidence in early studies reporting benefits of glycemic control and corticosteroids in shock has been eroded by subsequent publications. The Surviving Sepsis Campaign (SSC) guidelines, composed on behalf of numerous professional organizations, summarize and grade evidence for sepsis treatment.[63] Although not universally accepted, the guidelines are perhaps the most comprehensive summary of management practices. Several landmark trials provide evidence as to how effective recommended interventions can be when systematically applied.

Infection Control

Drainage of closed space infection, removal of infected foreign bodies, and debridement of devitalized tissue are believed to be important for source control in sepsis, even though no randomized trials support these practices. Because of the circumstantial evidence supporting the use of antimicrobials and strong belief they are effective, there are not, and likely never will be, randomized placebo-controlled trials of antibiotics, or even trials intentionally delaying antimicrobial therapy. Typically, patients with sepsis have blood, urine, and sputum cultured; additional samples, such as wound drainage and ascitic, pleural, and cerebrospinal fluid cultures should be performed as indicated by the clinical scenario. The likelihood of making a culture diagnosis is maximized by obtaining specimens before antibiotics are initiated.

In the absence of definitive data regarding the importance of antimicrobial therapy, it is not surprising that a great deal of emotion is associated with the use of antibiotics. Despite their usefulness, antibiotics alone will never eliminate all severe sepsis. At best, antibiotics kill the offending pathogen; they do not reverse the inflammatory and coagulopathic cascades that likely have been active for hours to days. Nonetheless, the benefits of administering appropriate antibiotics appear to increase with escalating severity of illness and decrease with delays in administration. For instance, among noncritically ill patients with community-acquired pneumonia, faster treatment produces a very small survival benefit.[64] When patients are bacteremic[65] or sufficiently ill to be admitted to an ICU,[66] survival benefits appear larger. Obviously, because these studies are nonrandomized, their results must be interpreted cautiously since it is possible that potentially important covariates were not identified. For example, the reason for "inadequate" coverage is often that patients are infected with highly resistant or unusual organisms as the result of chronic illness, long hospital stays, previous antibiotic exposure, or an immunocompromised state. Despite study limitations, septic shock is probably a special situation where the time to deliver antimicrobial therapy has a powerful association with survival.[67] This report had two key findings: first, half or more of patients with septic shock did not receive antibiotics in the first 6 hours of illness and, second, with each passing hour of delay to antibiotic administration, observed mortality was higher.

Failure to respond to seemingly appropriate antimicrobial therapy may be the result of an undrained closed space infection (eg, empyema, intra-abdominal abscess), presence of a resistant organism(s), insufficient drug levels, or most commonly insufficient time for response after starting therapy. Many clinicians have an overly optimistic view of the speed with which antimicrobials improve physiologic and laboratory abnormalities. For example, among older patients with pneumonia, average time to resolution of fever is 7 days[68] and even in younger patients 4 or more days is often needed for resolution of fever.[69] Radiographic resolution of pneumonia in these studies typically requires weeks. Additional reports indicate that 3 to 4 days may be needed for defervescence of hospitalized patients with what many physicians consider to be a minor problem, urinary tract infection.[70]

Antibiotics should be chosen based on individual patient factors (eg, immunosuppression, allergies, and underlying chronic illnesses), the presumptive site of infection, pattern of local antibiotic resistance, and examination of body fluids/specimens. Unless the etiologic agent is known with a very high degree of certainty, broad-spectrum antibiotic coverage is indicated until culture and sensitivity data are known. The rationale for use of broad-spectrum therapy comes from the observed association of worse outcomes with inappropriate initial antimicrobial therapy.[65,66] Unfortunately, changes in resistance patterns induced by indiscriminate past antibiotic use now frequently necessitate three or sometimes even four antibiotics for empiric coverage. The stark reality is that it is not possible to anticipate or provide empiric therapy for all possible organisms. Within reason, it is best to begin therapy in the critically ill patients with "too broad" a spectrum and then narrow coverage as more clinical data become available. With that caveat, antibiotic coverage should be reassessed on a daily basis and unnecessary drugs should be stopped promptly. Contrary to popular belief, antibiotic therapy is not benign. Use of excessive or unnecessary antibiotics is costly, risks allergic reactions and drug toxicity, and perhaps most importantly, breeds the emergence of highly resistant bacteria that can harm future patients.

Respiratory Support

Most patients with severe sepsis develop some degree of acute lung injury (ALI). In a landmark study of patients largely with sepsis-related ALI, investigators established that use of a 6-mL/kg tidal volume indexed to predicted body weight (PBW) reduced absolute mortality by 9% compared with ventilation with a traditional tidal volume of 12 mL/kg.[71] This practice is commonly known as "low tidal volume" mechanical ventilation; however, the 6-mL/kg tidal volume strategy is actually a *normal* tidal volume; it just happens to be lower than the volumes used traditionally. In the lower volume arm of the study, the tidal volume was adjusted from that used before enrollment to 6 mL/kg PBW but could be reduced as low as 4 mL/kg if needed to maintain plateau pressures below 30 cm water. Data from clinical practice now suggest use of higher tidal volumes in ALI is associated with worse outcomes. Further, patients *without* ALI who are ventilated with higher

tidal volumes, are more likely to develop lung injury.[72] Given that a normal tidal volume strategy does not add cost, or require additional sedation or paralysis, and is simple to implement, it represents a reasonable starting point for ventilation of ALI patients.

Positive end expiratory pressure (PEEP) inhibits atelectasis and attenuates development of ALI in animal models of lung injury, and some nominal level of PEEP ($\sim$5 cm H_2O) should probably be supplied to all patients with sepsis-related ALI. Beyond this minimal recommendation, the selection of PEEP and inspired oxygen concentration should maintain saturations in the 88% to 95% range (or equivalent PaO_2's) while avoiding potentially toxic inspired oxygen concentrations and excessive lung stretch. In a large randomized controlled trial of ALI patients ventilated with 6-mL/kg tidal volume, there was no difference in clinical outcomes between a lower-PEEP versus a higher-PEEP strategy.[48] Those results have now been validated by two additional trials.[73,74] So, in patients with lower tidal volumes, neither higher levels of PEEP nor titration of PEEP to lung compliance have been shown to produce consistently superior outcomes. Ventilation strategies that give a high priority to "recruitment" clearly can improve radiographic images of the lung, and indices of oxygenation, but to date do not translate into improved patient outcomes.[75,76]

Cardiovascular Support

In the setting of severe sepsis, circulatory failure is defined typically as a systolic blood pressure (BP) less than 90 mm Hg, a decrease in normal systolic BP of more than 40 mm Hg unresponsive to fluid challenge (20–30 mL/kg), or a mean arterial pressure below 60 mm Hg. At the onset of the syndrome, most patients with sepsis-induced shock have substantial volume depletion with variable degrees of systemic vascular dilation and myocardial dysfunction. Ventricular filling pressures are usually low because patients have been deprived of oral intake, have increased fluid losses (from sweating, panting, vomiting, or diarrhea), have dilated capacitance vessels, and increased endothelial permeability. The average septic patient needs 4 to 6 L of crystalloid replacement, or a comparable volume-expanding amount of colloid, within the first few hours to optimize ventricular performance.[57] Wide disparities in practice are observed in the fluid volume infused, the rate of administration, or method of monitoring resuscitation adequacy. It seems each physician has a different level of comfort with regard to the amount of fluid infused before instituting invasive monitoring or starting a vasoactive drug. Regardless, when a fluid challenge is used, it is important to use a bolus of sufficient volume to cause a detectable change. A commonly selected "bolus" size, 500 mL, has been shown to make no measurable change in blood pressure, intravascular filling pressures, or cardiac output.[77] Thus, it makes sense use larger fluid challenges (~15 mL/kg of crystalloid). Likewise, it is logical to administer the bolus as rapidly as possible to maximize the hemodynamic effect.

In general, there is no certain difference in efficacy of crystalloid or colloid in the initial resuscitation of septic patients. However, a recent study comparing 10% pentastarch, a low-molecular-weight hydroxyethyl starch (HES 200/0.5), with modified Ringer's lactate demonstrated that pentastarch administration was associated with higher rates of acute renal failure and RRT.[78] One systematic review suggests that crystalloids may be more efficacious in general for resuscitation,[79] whereas a large randomized controlled trial of ICU patients comparing resuscitation with normal saline versus 4% albumin showed no significant differences in pertinent clinical outcomes.[80] A smaller volume of colloid will be required to achieve any given increase in intravascular pressure; however, neither colloid nor crystalloid is confined entirely to the vascular compartment. Although less colloid is required, volume expansion is achieved at substantial cost. Colloid risks allergic reactions and may be priced 20 to 100 times that of an equivalent dose of crystalloid. Because hemodilution accompanies resuscitation with colloid or crystalloid, administration of packed red blood cells is sometimes required to maintain hemoglobin concentrations in an acceptable range.

For patients who are hypotensive after a fluid challenge or who have lactate elevations, use of an explicit hemodynamic protocol can reduce hospital mortality by as much as 16%.[57] This early goal-directed therapy (EGDT) differs in numerous respects from older unsuccessful studies in which attempts were made to boost oxygen delivery later in the course of sepsis.[81] Although the difference in outcomes might simply be the timing of the intervention, it is likely that some or all protocol elements are essential. This strategy uses vasopressors to achieve a mean arterial pressure greater than 65 mm Hg after central venous pressure (CVP) is raised to 8 to 12 mm Hg with fluids. A key distinction between this and other approaches is the measurement of superior vena caval oxygen saturation (ScVO$_2$), targeting a value greater than 70%. This goal is achieved by red blood cell transfusion for anemic patients (hematocrit < 30%) and dobutamine for patients above that threshold.

Application of these rules for a mere 6 hours reduced mortality, the fraction of patients requiring mechanical ventilation and vasopressors, hospital length of stay, and hospital costs.[57]

Like many severe sepsis therapies, controversy and questions surround this treatment. Some question how protocolized administration of packed red blood cells reconciles with earlier data suggesting a lower transfusion target may be acceptable or even beneficial.[82] One plausible explanation would be that septic shock patients are hemodynamically unstable, thus they differ significantly from the stable participants studied in previous transfusion protocols.[83] It is also important to recognize that transfusion was but one part of a complex protocol, and the consequences of applying that protocol without transfusion are unknown. While some practitioners have raised concerns about the risk of transfusion-associated lung injury (TRALI) in this setting, it appears that even if TRALI risk is increased, the net effect of the whole protocol is positive. Another important unanswered question is what is the maximum time window for application of this protocol beyond which benefit wanes? This question is especially important given that studies in which later attempts to modify oxygen delivery may have been harmful. Despite impressive results, this protocol has not been widely adopted,[84] possibly because of the relatively small number of patients studied, or the single-center and nonblinded study design. Other potential reasons for nonimplementation are inadequately staffed emergency departments, the lack of equipment needed to measure central venous pressure or venous saturation, and controversy regarding protocol efficacy.[85]

After resolution of shock, data from the NHLBI Fluid and Catheter Treatment Trial (FACTT) indicate that among patients with ALI, a more conservative approach to fluid management is prudent.[86] Although not exclusively a study of severe sepsis, nearly two thirds of participants met criteria for severe sepsis (pneumonia or sepsis as the ALI risk factor). Application of an explicit hemodynamic management protocol that targets a CVP (< 4 mm Hg) or pulmonary capillary occlusion pressure (< 8 mm Hg) after resolution of shock resulted in a significantly less positive net fluid balance during the first week of treatment. Although the nominally lower mortality (~3%) was not significantly different, fluid conservative patients had more ventilator- and ICU-free days and a reduced duration of mechanical ventilation among survivors. These goals were reached without increased risk of renal insufficiency or hypotension. The tool used to measure the vascular pressure (CVC versus PAC) did not seem to matter, except with regard to complications where PAC-randomized patients had roughly twice as many nonfatal catheter-related complications.[87]

While vasopressors are a mainstay of septic shock management, surprisingly little data are available to guide their use. Small randomized studies suggest norepinephrine is more likely to rapidly achieve a desired blood pressure target than other vasopressors, and do so with less tachycardia.[88] One large cohort observational study, the Sepsis Occurrence in Acutely ill Patients (SOAP) study, suggests that use of dopamine in uncontrolled practice is associated with a higher mortality than use of norepinephrine.[89] Although several studies now suggest that dopamine does not offer significant protection of the kidney at risk from shock or sepsis, it is still ordered by some physicians for that purpose.[90] The past few years have produced numerous reports that some septic shock patients have low vasopressin levels and that fixed dose replacement can reduce or eliminate the need for catecholamines.[91–93] The Vasopressin and Septic Shock Trial (VASST) compared low-dose vasopressin and norepinephrine versus norepinephrine alone, and demonstrated no differences in 28-day or 90-day mortality.[94] However, in an analysis of subgroups defined a priori, a trend toward mortality benefit was observed in patients with lower norepinephrine requirements who were treated with vasopressin.[94] These data are hypothesis generating and suggest more study is needed to clarify the role of vasopressin.

Steroids

Numerous trials using short courses of high-dose corticosteroids in patients with severe sepsis have failed to demonstrate improved survival.[95] In one frequently cited study using lower steroid doses, 300 patients enrolled within 8 hours of shock onset were randomized to receive hydrocortisone plus fludrocortisone or placebo for 7 days.[96] When evaluating all patients, time to death may have been altered somewhat, but there was no significant difference in primary study end points of 28-day, ICU, hospital, or 1-year mortality between treated and placebo recipients. Evaluation of secondary end points found that for patients who failed to increase their total plasma cortisol levels by at least 9 μg/dL after 250 μg ACTH stimulation (so-called "nonresponders"), there was approximately a 10% absolute reduction in adjusted mortality associated with treatment. The "responders" to ACTH stimulation had a nominally higher mortality if treated compared with placebo, although this difference was not statistically significant.[96] This study caused controversy and stimulated additional study. Since benefit appeared to be confined to ACTH nonresponders, perhaps the most pressing unanswered question is whether an ACTH stimulation test is necessary. This is a significant issue in many hospitals where cortisol results are not available for days. Subsequent studies report a poor correlation between free and total cortisol levels, raising doubt as to the soundness of using total cortisol values.[97] Another problem is clinician skepticism that patients with high baseline cortisol values could benefit from even more glucocorticoid merely because they failed to raise plasma cortisol after ACTH. Along those lines, some researchers claim a more relevant provocation may be 1 μg of ACTH.[98,99] Some physicians have also expressed doubt regarding the need to include fludrocortisone because of the volume of fluids that have been administered and the mineralocorticoid effects of hydrocortisone.[100]

Further evidence questioning the effectiveness of corticosteroids in sepsis came from post hoc analysis of the Recombinant Human Activated Protein C Worldwide Evaluation in Severe Sepsis (PROWESS) trial. In this analysis, patients given steroids in a nonrandomized manner as part of usual practice still demonstrated a survival benefit with drotrecogin alpha (activated).[101] Despite these questions, a number of clinicians have adopted glucocorticoid therapy for severe sepsis patients without shock, or with shock of prolonged duration, perhaps based on the recommendations of some authors for broad use.[102]

The Corticosteroid Therapy of Septic Shock (CORTICUS) study was a large, randomized controlled trial comparing hydrocortisone versus placebo in patients with septic shock done in an effort to help clarify the role of corticosteroids.[100] Results of the trial suggest little benefit of corticosteroids in patients with septic shock. In both the "ACTH responders" and the "ACTH nonresponders," there was no significant difference in the primary outcome, 28-day all-cause mortality. Of note, patients in the hydrocortisone group did have faster resolution of shock, but there were more episodes of superinfection, including new sepsis and septic shock.[100] On balance, corticosteroids have a limited use in the management of shock and should probably be limited to those with refractory shock and a history of chronic steroid use and patients proven to have absolute adrenal insufficiency.

Human Recombinant Activated Protein C

Drotrecogin alfa activated, also known as human recombinant activated protein C (rhAPC), is the only sepsis-specific medication proven to have a mortality benefit.[19] rhAPC reduces inflammation, down-regulates coagulation, and inhibits the antithrombolytic actions of PAI-1 and TAFI. The PROWESS trial, a large randomized controlled trial comparing rhAPC to placebo in patients with severe sepsis, demonstrated an absolute mortality reduction of approximately 6% in the treatment group.[19] Long-term follow-up demonstrated a persistent survival benefit 2 to 3 years after treatment.[103] In addition, treated patients had a shorter time on vasopressors and mechanical ventilation compared with placebo.[104]

The treatment effect appears to be time sensitive. A large open-label trial and a multihospital case series found a that patients treated with rhAPC within the first day after developing severe sepsis had a higher survival rate as compared with the second day. Earlier treatment was also associated with a shorter time on ventilator, in the ICU, and in the hospital.[105] A large retrospective analysis of all patients treated in controlled trials in the first 24 hours of sepsis compared with those in the second 24 hours of sepsis supports the observation that earlier is better than later treatment.[106]

The sole toxicity of rhAPC is bleeding, seen in 1.5% to 2.5% more patients than those not treated (a risk comparable in magnitude to anticoagulation with heparin). The risk of serious bleeding can be minimized by avoiding administration to patients with fewer than 30,000 platelets/mm^3, overt hemorrhage, recent stroke, or intracranial or spinal surgery. Avoiding treatment within 12 hours of surgery or trauma, and stopping the drug for 2 hours before performing invasive vascular procedures also minimizes bleeding risk.

In a post hoc subgroup analysis of the PROWESS population, patients with a modified APACHE II score of 25 or higher (ie, those with a "high risk" of death), had an absolute mortality reduction of 13%.[107] As with any subgroup analysis, designating one population with a larger survival benefit than the whole dictates that there must be a complementary group with a lesser benefit. Subsequent study of a heterogeneous group of "low risk" of death patients confirmed that such patients do not experience a survival benefit yet still incur the roughly 1% to 2% increase in serious bleeding risk compared with placebo.[108] Therefore, rhAPC is approved for the treatment of severe sepsis in adult patients at high risk of death.

A major impediment to widespread use of rhAPC has been its substantial cost, approximately $7000 per course of therapy. For many clinicians, the survival benefit, and data suggesting a shorter time on mechanical ventilation, in shock, in the ICU, and in the hospital compared with placebo is not sufficiently compelling to justify the financial costs of rhAPC, despite numerous analyses suggesting cost-effectiveness.[7,109,110]

Glucose Control

Hyperglycemia impairs immune functions[111] and may exert a procoagulant effect, but the role of glucose control in the management of critically ill patients is still evolving. A pivotal study of surgical patients demonstrated that stringent control of glucose (80–110 mg/dL) reduced the risk of death and severe sepsis when compared with more liberal glucose management.[112] Studies to confirm these observations in medical patients have failed to reproduce such results. A follow-up single-center, unblinded trial compared tight glucose control (80–110 mg/dL) to conventional glucose control in 1200 medical ICU patients. In the intention-to-treat population, there was no difference in 28-day mortality between the two groups; however, patients in the intensive insulin therapy arm had less acquired kidney injury, accelerated weaning from mechanical ventilation, and accelerated discharge from the ICU and the hospital.[113] Unfortunately, but perhaps not surprisingly, more hypoglycemia was observed in the tight glucose control group. Analogous to the rhAPC trials, a subgroup analysis identified a group of patients (those requiring >3 days in the ICU) who had a mortality benefit and a complementary group (patients requiring <3 days in the ICU) with a greater mortality in the intervention group. This subgroup analysis is useful for further hypothesis generation.

The Efficacy of Volume Substitution and Insulin Therapy in Severe Sepsis (VISEP) study was a two-by-two factorial trial examining both tight glycemic control and volume substitution strategies in sepsis.[78] With respect to glycemic control, this multicenter trial of septic patients in multidisciplinary intensive care units compared tight glucose control (80–110 mg/dL) with conventional glucose control (180–200 mg/dL). The trial was terminated prematurely secondary to safety concerns. One concern was that the rate of severe hypoglycemia, defined as a glucose level less than 40 mg/dL, was higher in the intensive therapy group than in the conventional therapy group (17.0% versus 4.1%, $P<.001$). Despite effectively lowering serum glucose levels, patients in the intensive glucose control arm had no differences in 28-day mortality or mean score for organ failures.

As these and other studies demonstrate, tight glycemic control is not a trivial undertaking and is associated with risk of hypoglycemia. Strict glycemic control usually requires a continuous insulin infusion with hourly monitoring of blood glucose, and this practice is nursing-intensive. Given the risks of hypoglycemia, lack of demonstrable mortality benefit, and mixed evidence regarding organ failures, the future of tight glycemic control as a pillar of sepsis management in medical patients remains unclear. Further study is needed to define the best population and the best protocol for such therapy.

Therapy of Metabolic Acidosis

Lactic acidosis is common in severe sepsis patients. Fortunately, it is usually a mild and self-limited problem that resolves when intravascular volume deficits are corrected. When lactic acidosis results from low cardiac output and hypotension, it is likely to be improved by increasing arterial pressure. Conversely, when cardiac output and arterial pressure are normal or high, no data convincingly demonstrate a benefit of further increasing output. Survival correlates best with lactate levels and not serum pH. Therefore, buffering an abnormal pH with sodium bicarbonate[114] or dichloroacetate[115] does not improve outcome, unless the underlying reason for lactate generation is corrected simultaneously. Even though experimental data do not support the practice, as a practical matter, many physicians feel compelled to intervene when pH declines below 7.10.

SUPPORT OF THE KIDNEY

The kidneys commonly experience transient dysfunction early in the septic process; more than 40% of patients develop transient oliguria, which is usually reversed by simple fluid administration to correct underlying hypovolemia. For patients with shock, a combination of volume repletion and vasoactive drug administration may be required to raise cardiac output or SVR sufficiently to perfuse the kidneys. Diuretic therapy has not been shown to improve outcome in critically ill patients with acute renal failure.[116] Avoidance of nephrotoxic agents, such as intravenous contrast is prudent, and clinicians should be aware that many antimicrobial agents can adversely affect renal function.

A fraction of patients with sepsis-induced acute kidney injury will require RRT. Intermittent high-flow hemodialysis has been the traditional method for renal replacement in critically ill patients, particularly in the absence of shock. Continuous hemofiltration is growing in popularity. Because it avoids rapid fluid shifts and can be performed by ICU nurses, it has become the preferred method of many nephrologists and intensivists, especially for patients with shock. Despite decades of experience with RRT in critically ill patients, the optimal intensity of RRT—ie, the number of days per week to apply intermittent hemodialysis, or the flow rate to target in continuous hemofiltration—has been controversial. A recent study randomized 1124 critically ill patients to either a more intense, or less intense RRT regimen.[117] The more intense RRT arm had intermittent hemodialysis dosed 6 days per week or continuous hemofiltration rates of 35 mL/kg/h, whereas the less intense RRT arm had intermittent dialysis 3 days per week or continuous hemofiltration rates of 20 mL/kg/h. There was no significant difference between the two groups in the duration of RRT, rate of kidney function recovery, or rate or nonrenal organ failures, and intensive RRT did *not* decrease mortality.[117]

Nutritional Support

As with other critically ill patients, there are two basic "truths" about nutrition. First, prolonged starvation (weeks to months) is fatal, and second, any patient can tolerate a few days without feeding. Almost every other aspect of nutritional support is argued. Even with the disagreements about nutrition, there are some common practices. Nutritional support usually is withheld at least until hemodynamic stability is achieved (1 to 2 days).[118,119] Most practitioners now favor the enteral route of support because it provides more complete nutrition, preserves gut mucosa, and favorably impacts immune function. In addition, enteral nutrition is substantially less expensive than intravenous supplementation and avoids the complications associated with the central venous catheters and hypertonic glucose solutions required for effective parenteral nutrition.

At this time, there is no compelling evidence to suggest that any particular enteral feeding formula or particular balance of components is superior to another for the patient with severe sepsis, but there are compelling phase II data from patients with acute lung injury. Three trials now suggest that an enteral formula enriched with omega-3 fatty acids, antioxidants, and other specialized ingredients may improve outcomes.[120–122] Pending results of a definitive study of specialized tube feeding now under way, current knowledge supports giving a balanced mixture of carbohydrate, protein, and lipid based on the patient's estimated needs. For patients with prolonged (>7 days) gut dysfunction, parenteral nutrition may be indicated.

SUMMARY

Severe sepsis is a common syndrome but because it has variable presentations in patients of all ages and with a wide range of underlying diseases it can be difficult to identify. This problem is compounded by absence of a reliable diagnostic test. Even though there is scientific debate regarding several severe sepsis treatments, an organized approach applied by trained physicians and nurses in which all applicable treatments are applied as rapidly as possible has consistently been shown to reduce mortality and morbidity.

REFERENCES

1. Hotchkiss RS, Karl IE. The pathophysiology and treatment of sepsis. N Engl J Med 2003;348(2): 138–50.
2. Bone RC, Balk RA, Cerra FB, et al. American-College of Chest Physicians Society of Critical Care Medicine Consensus Conference—definitions for sepsis and organ failure and guidelines for the use of innovative therapies in sepsis. Crit Care Med 1992;20(6):864–74.
3. Vincent JL. Dear SIRS, I'm sorry to say that I don't like you. Crit Care Med 1997;25(2):372–4.
4. Brun-Buisson C. The epidemiology of the systemic inflammatory response. Intensive Care Med 2000; 26:S64–74.
5. Martin GS, Mannino DM, Eaton S, et al. The epidemiology of sepsis in the United States from 1979 through 2000. N Engl J Med 2003;348(16): 1546–54.
6. Angus DC, Linde-Zwirble WT, Lidicker J, et al. Epidemiology of severe sepsis in the United States: analysis of incidence, outcome, and associated costs of care. Crit Care Med 2001;29(7):1303–10.
7. Neilson AR, Burchardi H, Chinn C, et al. Cost-effectiveness of drotrecogin alfa (activated) for the treatment of severe sepsis in Germany. J Crit Care 2003;18(4):217–27.
8. Bernard GR, Margolis BD, Shanies HM, et al. Extended evaluation of recombinant human activated protein C United States trial (ENHANCE US)—a single-arm, phase 313, multicenter study of drotrecogin alfa (activated) in severe sepsis. Chest 2004; 125(6):2206–16.
9. Vincent JL, Sakr Y, Ranieri M, et al. Does albumin administration influence outcome? Results of the soap study. Chest 2003;124(4):91S.
10. Martin GS, Mannino DM, Moss M. The effect of age on the development and outcome of adult sepsis. Crit Care Med 2006;34(1):15–21.
11. Dombrovskiy VY, Martin AA, Sunderam J, et al. Occurrence and outcomes sepsis: influence of race. Crit Care Med 2007;35(3):763–8.
12. Regazzoni CJ, Irrazabal C, Luna CM, et al. Cancer patients with septic shock: mortality predictors and neutropenia. Support Care Cancer 2004;12(12): 833–9.
13. Vandijck DM, Benoit DD, Depuydt PO, et al. Impact of recent intravenous chemotherapy on outcome in severe sepsis and septic shock patients with hematological malignancies. Intensive Care Med 2008;34(5):847–55.
14. Clemmer TP, Metz CA, Goris GB, et al. Hypothermia in the sepsis syndrome and clinical outcome. Crit Care Med 1992;20(10):1395–401.
15. Kinasewitz GT, Yan SB, Basson B, et al. Universal changes in biomarkers of coagulation and inflammation occur in patients with severe sepsis, regardless of causative micro-organism. Crit Care 2004;8(2): R82–90.
16. Levi M, van der Poll T. Coagulation in sepsis: all bugs bite equally. Crit Care 2004;8(2):99–101.
17. Opal SM, Garber GE, Larosa SP, et al. Systemic host responses in severe sepsis analyzed by causative microorganism and treatment effects of drotrecogin alfa (activated). Clin Infect Dis 2003; 37(1):50–8.
18. Levy MM, Macias WL, Vincent JL, et al. Early changes in organ function predict eventual survival in severe sepis. Crit Care Med 2005;33(10): 2194–201.
19. Bernard GR, Vincent JL, Laterre P, et al. Efficacy and safety of recombinant human activated protein C for severe sepsis. N Engl J Med 2001;344(10): 699–709.
20. Dhainaut JF, Shorr AF, Macias WL, et al. Dynamic evolution of coagulopathy in the first day of severe sepsis: relationship with mortality and organ failure. Crit Care Med 2005;33(2):341–8.
21. Ferreira FL, Bota DP, Bross A, et al. Serial evaluation of the SOFA score to predict outcome in critically ill patients. JAMA 2001;286(14):1754–8.
22. Mehta RL, Kellum JA, Shah SV, et al. Acute Kidney Injury Network: report of an initiative to improve outcomes in acute kidney injury. Crit Care 2007;11(2): R31.
23. Ricci Z, Cruz D, Ronco C. The RIFLE criteria and mortality in acute kidney injury: a systematic review. Kidney Int 2008;73(5):538–46.
24. Lemeshow S, Klar J, Teres D. Outcome prediction for individual intensive-care patients—useful, misused, or abused. Intensive Care Med 1995;21(9):770–6.
25. Adrie C, Alberti C, Chaix-Couturier C, et al. Epidemiology and economic evaluation of severe sepsis in France: age, severity, infection site, and place if acquisition (community, hospital, or intensive care unit) as determinants of workload and cost. J Crit Care 2005;20(1):46–58.
26. Alberti C, Brun-Buisson C, Burchardi H, et al. Epidemiology of sepsis and infection in ICU patients from an international multicentre cohort study. Intensive Care Med 2002;28(2):108–21.
27. Sprung CL, Sakr Y, Vincent JL, et al. An evaluation of systemic inflammatory response syndrome signs

in the Sepsis Occurrence in Acutely ill Patients (SOAP) study. Intensive Care Med 2006;32(3): 421–7.

28. Bota DP, Ferreira FL, Melot C, et al. Body temperature alterations in the critically ill. Intensive Care Med 2004;30(5):811–6.

29. James JH, Luchette FA, McCarter FD, et al. Lactate is an unreliable indicator of tissue hypoxia in injury or sepsis. Lancet 1999;354(9177):505–8.

30. Yang SL, Chung CS, Ayala A, et al. Differential alterations in cardiovascular responses during the progression of polymicrobial sepsis in the mouse. Shock 2002;17(1):55–60.

31. Shapiro NI, Howell MD, Talmor D, et al. Serum lactate as a predictor of mortality in emergency department patients with infection. Ann Emerg Med 2005;45(5):524–8.

32. Nguyen HB, Rivers EP, Knoblich BP, et al. Early lactate clearance is associated with improved outcome in severe sepsis and septic shock. Crit Care Med 2004;32(8):1637–42.

33. Claeys R, Vinken S, Spapen H, et al. Plasma procalcitonin and C-reactive protein in acute septic shock: clinical and biological correlates. Crit Care Med 2002;30(4):757–62.

34. Ugarte H, Silva E, Mercan D, et al. Procalcitonin used as a marker of infection in the intensive care unit. Crit Care Med 1999;27(3):498–504.

35. Uzzan B, Cohen R, Nicolas P, et al. Procalcitonin as a diagnostic test for sepsis in critically ill adults and after surgery or trauma: a systematic review and meta-analysis. Crit Care Med 2006;34(7): 1996–2003.

36. Gibot S, Cravoisy A, Kolopp-Sarda MN, et al. Time-course of sTREM (soluble triggering receptor expressed on myeloid cells)-1, procalcitonin, and C-reactive protein plasma concentrations during sepsis. Crit Care Med 2005;33(4):792–6.

37. Harbarth S, Holeckova K, Froidevaux C, et al. Diagnostic value of procalcitonin, interleukin-6, and interleukin-8 in critically ill patients admitted with suspected sepsis. Am J Respir Crit Care Med 2001;164(3):396–402.

38. Voves C, Wuillemin WA, Zeerleder S. International Society on Thrombosis and Haemostasis score for overt disseminated intravascular coagulation predicts organ dysfunction and fatality in sepsis patients. Blood Coagul Fibrinolysis 2006;17(6): 445–51.

39. Shorr AF, Bernard GR, Dhainaut JF, et al. Protein C concentrations in severe sepsis: an early directional change in plasma levels predicts outcome. Crit Care 2006;10(3):R92.

40. BrunBuisson C, Doyon F, Carlet J, et al. Bacteremia and severe sepsis in adults: a multicenter prospective survey in ICUs and wards of 24 hospitals. Am J Respir Crit Care Med 1996;154(3):617–24.

41. Kieft H, Hoepelman AIM, Zhou W, et al. The sepsis syndrome in a Dutch University Hospital—clinical observations. Arch Intern Med 1993;153(19): 2241–7.

42. Rangelfrausto MS, Pittet D, Costigan M, et al. The natural-history of the Systemic Inflammatory Response Syndrome (SIRS)—a prospective-study. JAMA 1995;273(2):117–23.

43. Weinstein MP, Reller LB, Murphy JR, et al. The clinical-significance of positive blood cultures—a comprehensive analysis of 500 episodes of bacteremia and fungemia in adults. 1. Laboratory and epidemiologic observations. Rev Infect Dis 1983;5(1):35–53.

44. Weinstein MP, Towns ML, Quartey SM, et al. The clinical significance of positive blood cultures in the 1990s: a prospective comprehensive evaluation of the microbiology, epidemiology, and outcome of bacteremia and fungemia in adults. Clin Infect Dis 1997;24(4):584–602.

45. Weinstein MP. Blood culture contamination: persisting problems and partial progress. J Clin Microbiol 2003;41(6):2275–8.

46. Amaral A, Opal SM, Vincent JL. Coagulation in sepsis. Intensive Care Med 2004;30(6):1032–40.

47. Aird WC. The hematologic system as a marker of organ dysfunction in sepsis. Mayo Clin Proc 2003;78(7):869–81.

48. Brower RG, Lanken PN, MacIntyre N, et al. Higher versus lower positive end-expiratory pressures in patients with the acute respiratory distress syndrome. N Engl J Med 2004;351(4):327–36.

49. Gattinoni L, Bombino M, Pelosi P, et al. Lung structure and function in different stages of severe adult-respiratory-distress-syndrome. JAMA 1994; 271(22):1772–9.

50. Bernard GR, Artigas A, Brigham KL, et al. The American-European Consensus Conference on ARDS. Definitions, mechanisms, relevant outcomes, and clinical trial coordination. Am J Respir Crit Care Med 1994;149(3):818–24.

51. Esteban A, Anzueto A, Frutos F, et al. Characteristics and outcomes in adult patients receiving mechanical ventilation—a 28-day international study. JAMA 2002;287(3):345–55.

52. Bernard GR, Wheeler AP, Russell JA, et al. The effects of ibuprofen on the physiology and survival of patients with sepsis. N Engl J Med 1997;336(13): 912–8.

53. Barrantes F, Tian JM, Vazquez R, et al. Acute kidney injury criteria predict outcomes of critically ill patients. Crit Care Med 2008;36(5):1397–403.

54. Morgera S, Schneider M, Neumayer HH. Long-term outcomes after acute kidney injury. Crit Care Med 2008;36(4):S193–7.

55. Gattinoni L, Brazzi L, Pelosi P, et al. A trial of goal-oriented hemodynamic therapy in critically ill patients. N Engl J Med 1995;333(16):1025–32.

56. Hayes MA, Timmins AC, Yau EHS, et al. Elevation of systemic oxygen delivery in the treatment of critically ill patients. N Engl J Med 1994;330(24): 1717–22.

57. Rivers E, Nguyen B, Havstad S, et al. Early goal-directed therapy in the treatment of severe sepsis and septic shock. N Engl J Med 2001;345(19): 1368–77.

58. Yan SB, Helterbrand JD, Hartman DL, et al. Low levels of protein C are associated with poor outcome in severe sepsis. Chest 2001;120(3):915–22.

59. Dhainaut J, Yan B. Drotrecogin alfa (activated) effects in patients with severe sepsis with or without DIC. Intensive Care Med 2003;29:S88.

60. Cullen JJ, Titler S, Ephgrave KS, et al. Gastric emptying of liquids and postprandial pancreatobiliary secretion are temporarily impaired during endotoxemia. Gastroenterology 1998;114(4):A740.

61. Strassburg CP. Shock liver. Best Pract Res Clin Gastroenterol 2003;17(3):369–81.

62. Johnston JD, Harvey CJ, Menzies IS, et al. Gastrointestinal permeability and absorptive capacity in sepsis. Crit Care Med 1996;24(7):1144–9.

63. Dellinger RP, Levy MM, Carlet JM, et al. Surviving Sepsis Campaign: international guidelines for management of severe sepsis and septic shock: 2008. Crit Care Med 2008;36(1):296–327.

64. Houck PM, Bratzler DW, Nsa W, et al. Timing of antibiotic administration and outcomes for Medicare patients hospitalized with community-acquired pneumonia. Arch Intern Med 2004;164(6):637–44.

65. Leibovici L, Shraga I, Drucker M, et al. The benefit of appropriate empirical antibiotic treatment in patients with bloodstream infection. J Intern Med 1998;244(5):379–86.

66. Kollef MH, Sherman G, Ward S, et al. Inadequate antimicrobial treatment of infections—a risk factor for hospital mortality among critically ill patients. Chest 1999;115(2):462–74.

67. Kumar A, Roberts D, Wood KE, et al. Duration of hypotension before initiation of effective antimicrobial therapy is the critical determinant of survival in human septic shock. Crit Care Med 2006;34(6): 1589–96.

68. Halm EA, Fine MJ, Marrie TJ, et al. Time to clinical stability in patients hospitalized with community-acquired pneumonia—implications for practice guidelines. JAMA 1998;279(18):1452–7.

69. Vidaur L, Planas K, Sierra R, et al. Ventilator-associated pneumonia—impact of organisms on clinical resolution and medical resources utilization. Chest 2008;133(3):625–32.

70. Yee-Cabahug Leilani, Espiritu-Quiza Ma Fidelis. The defervescence period of commonly used antiobiotics for typhoid fever, urinary tract infection and pneumonia in Cebu Velez General Hospital. Philipp J Intern Med 1998;36:283–8.

71. Brower RG, Matthay MA, Morris A, et al. Ventilation with lower tidal volumes as compared with traditional tidal volumes for acute lung injury and the acute respiratory distress syndrome. N Engl J Med 2000;342(18):1301–8.

72. Gajic O, Dara SI, Mendez JL, et al. Ventilator-associated lung injury in patients without acute lung injury at the onset of mechanical ventilation. Crit Care Med 2004;32(9):1817–24.

73. Meade MO, Cook DJ, Guyatt GH, et al. Ventilation strategy using low tidal volumes, recruitment maneuvers, and high positive end-expiratory pressure for acute lung injury and acute respiratory distress syndrome: a randomized controlled trial. JAMA 2008;299(6):637–45.

74. Mercat A, Richard JCM, Vielle B, et al. Positive end-expiratory pressure setting in adults with acute lung injury and acute respiratory distress syndrome—a randomized controlled trial. JAMA 2008;299(6):646–55.

75. Girard TD, Bernard GR. Mechanical ventilation in ARDS—a state-of-the-art review. Chest 2007; 131(3):921–9.

76. Anon. Effects of recruitment maneuvers in patients with acute lung injury and acute respiratory distress syndrome ventilated with high positive end-expiratory pressure. Crit Care Med 2003;31(11): 2592–7.

77. Axler O, Tousignant C, Thompson CR, et al. Small hemodynamic effect of typical rapid volume infusions in critically ill patients. Crit Care Med 1997; 25(6):965–70.

78. Brunkhorst FM, Engel C, Bloos F, et al. Intensive insulin therapy and pentastarch resuscitation in severe sepsis. N Engl J Med 2008;358(2):125–39.

79. Schierhout G, Roberts I. Fluid resuscitation with colloid or crystalloid solutions in critically ill patients: a systematic review of randomised trials. Br Med J 1998;316(7136):961–4.

80. Finfer S, Bellomo R, Boyce N, et al. A comparison of albumin and saline for fluid resuscitation in the intensive care unit. N Engl J Med 2004;350(22):2247–56.

81. Otero RM, Nguyen HB, Huang DT, et al. Early goal-directed therapy in severe sepsis and septic shock revisited—concepts, controversies, and contemporary findings. Chest 2006;130(5):1579–95.

82. Hebert PC, Wells G, Blajchman MA, et al. A multi-center, randomized, controlled clinical trial of transfusion requirements in critical care. N Engl J Med 1999;340(6):409–17.

83. Hebert PC, Tinmouth A, Corwin HL. Controversies in RBC transfusion in the critically ill. Chest 2007; 131(5):1583–90.

84. Jones AE, Kline JA. Use of goal-directed therapy for severe sepsis and septic shock in academic emergency departments. Crit Care Med 2005; 33(8):1888–9.

85. Carlbom DJ, Rubenfeld GD. Barriers to implementing protocol-based sepsis resuscitation in the emergency department—results of a national survey. Crit Care Med 2007;35(11):2525–32.

86. Wiedemann HP, Wheeler AP, Bernard GR, et al. Comparison of two fluid-management strategies in acute lung injury. N Engl J Med 2006;354(24):2564–75.

87. Wheeler AP, Bernard GR, Thompson BT, et al. Pulmonary-artery versus central venous catheter to guide treatment of acute lung injury. N Engl J Med 2006;354(21):2213–24.

88. Müllner M, Urbanek B, Havel C, et al. Vasopressors for shock. Cochrane Database Syst Rev 2004;3:CD003709.

89. Sakr Y, Reinhart K, Vincent JL, et al. Does dopamine administration in shock influence outcome? Results of the Sepsis Occurrence in Acutely Ill Patients (SOAP) study. Crit Care Med 2006;34(3):589–97.

90. Kellum JA, Decker JM. Use of dopamine in acute renal failure: a meta-analysis. Crit Care Med 2001;29(8):1526–31.

91. Holmes CL, Patel BM, Russell JA, et al. Physiology of vasopressin relevant to management of septic shock. Chest 2001;120(3):989–1002.

92. Landry DW, Oliver JA. Mechanisms of disease: the pathogenesis of vasodilatory shock. N Engl J Med 2001;345(8):588–95.

93. Patel BM, Chittock DR, Russell JA, et al. Beneficial effects of short-term vasopressin infusion during severe septic shock. Anesthesiology 2002;96(3):576–82.

94. Russell JA, Walley KR, Singer J, et al. Vasopressin versus norepinephrine infusion in patients with septic shock. N Engl J Med 2008;358(9):877–87.

95. Annane D, Bellissant E, Bollaert PE, et al. Corticosteroids for severe sepsis and septic shock: a systematic review and meta-analysis. Br Med J 2004;329(7464):480–4.

96. Annane D, Sebille V, Charpentier C, et al. Effect of treatment with low doses of hydrocortisone and fludrocortisone on mortality in patients with septic shock. JAMA 2002;288(7):862–71.

97. Hamrahian AH, Oseni TS, Arafah BM. Measurements of serum free cortisol in critically ill patients. N Engl J Med 2004;350(16):1629–38.

98. Oelkers W. The role of high- and low-dose corticotropin tests in the diagnosis of secondary adrenal insufficiency. Eur J Endocrinol 1998;139(6):567–70.

99. Shenker Y, Skatrud JB. Adrenal insufficiency in critically ill patients. Am J Respir Crit Care Med 2001;163(7):1520–3.

100. Sprung CL, Annane D, Keh D, et al. Hydrocortisone therapy for patients with septic shock. N Engl J Med 2008;358(2):111–24.

101. Levy H, Laterre PF, Bates B, et al. Steroid use in PROWESS severe sepsis patients treated with drotrecogin alfa (activated). Crit Care 2005;9(5):R502–7.

102. Minneci PC, Deans KJ, Banks SM, et al. Meta-analysis: the effect of steroids on survival and shock during sepsis depends on the dose. Ann Intern Med 2004;141(1):47–56.

103. Angus DC, Laterre PF, Helterbrand J, et al. The effect of drotrecogin alfa (activated) on long-term survival after severe sepsis. Crit Care Med 2004;32(11):2199–206.

104. Vincent JL, Angus DC, Artigas A, et al. Effects of drotrecogin alfa (activated) on organ dysfunction in the PROWESS trial. Crit Care Med 2003;31(3):834–40.

105. Vincent JL, Bernard GR, Beale R, et al. Drotrecogin alfa (activated) treatment in severe sepsis from the global open-label trial ENHANCE: further evidence for survival and safety and implications for early treatment. Crit Care Med 2005;33(10):2266–77.

106. Vincent JL, O'Brien J, Wheeler A, et al. Use of an integrated clinical trial database to evaluate the effect of timing of drotrecogin alfa (activated) treatment in severe sepsis. Crit Care 2006;10(3):R74.

107. Ely EW, Laterre PF, Angus DC, et al. Drotrecogin alfa (activated) administration across clinically important subgroups of patients with severe sepsis. Crit Care Med 2003;31(1):12–9.

108. Abraham E, Laterre P, Garg R, et al. Drotrecogin alfa (activated) for adults with severe sepsis and a low risk of death. N Engl J Med 2005;353(13):1332–41.

109. Fowler RA, Hill-Popper M, Stasinos J, et al. Cost-effectiveness of recombinant human activated protein C and the influence of severity of illness in the treatment of patients with severe sepsis. J Crit Care 2003;18(3):181–91.

110. Frampton JE, Foster RH. Drotrecogin alfa (activated)—a pharmacoeconomic review of its use in severe sepsis. Pharmacoeconomics 2004;22(7):445–76.

111. Turina M, Fry DE, Polk HC. Acute hyperglycemia and the innate immune system: clinical, cellular, and molecular aspects. Crit Care Med 2005;33(7):1624–33.

112. Van den Berghe G, Wouters P, Weekers F, et al. Intensive insulin therapy in critically ill patients. N Engl J Med 2001;345(19):1359–67.

113. Van den Berghe G, Wilmer A, Hermans G, et al. Intensive insulin therapy in the medical ICU. N Engl J Med 2006;354(5):449–61.

114. Forsythe SM, Schmidt GA. Sodium bicarbonate for the treatment of lactic acidosis. Chest 2000;117(1):260–7.

115. Stacpoole PW, Wright EC, Baumgartner TG, et al. A controlled clinical-trial of dichloroacetate for treatment of lactic-acidosis in adults. N Engl J Med 1992;327(22):1564–9.

116. Mehta RL, Pascual MT, Soroko S, et al. Diuretics, mortality, and nonrecovery of renal function in acute renal failure. JAMA 2002;288(20):2547–53.

117. The VA/NIH Acute Renal Failure Trial Network. Intensity of renal support in critically ill patients with acute kidney injury. N Engl J Med 2008;359(1): 7–20.

118. Krishnan JA, Parce PB, Martinez A, et al. Caloric intake in medical ICU patients—consistency of care with guidelines and relationship to clinical outcomes. Chest 2003;124(1):297–305.

119. Martin CM, Doig GS, Heyland DK, et al. Multicentre, cluster-randomized clinical trial of algorithms for critical-care enteral and parenteral therapy (ACCEPT). Can Med Assoc J 2004; 170(2):197–204.

120. Gadek JE, DeMichele SJ, Karlstad MD, et al. Effect of enteral feeding with eicosapentaenoic acid, gamma-linolenic acid, and antioxidants in patients with acute respiratory distress syndrome. Crit Care Med 1999;27(8):1409–20.

121. Pontes-Arruda A, Aragao AMA, Albuquerque JD. Effects of enteral feeding with eicosapentaenoic acid, gamma-linolenic acid, and antioxidants in mechanically ventilated patients with severe sepsis and septic shock. Crit Care Med 2006;34(9): 2325–33.

122. Singer P, Theilla M, Fisher H, et al. Benefit of an enteral diet enriched with eicosapentaenoic acid and gamma-linolenic acid in ventilated patients with acute lung injury. Crit Care Med 2006;34(4): 1033–8.

Adrenal Insufficiency in Septic Shock

Virginie Maxime, MD[a], Olivier Lesur, MD, PhD[b],
Djillali Annane, MD, PhD[a,*]

KEYWORDS

- Hypothalamic-pituitary-adrenal axis
- Corticosteroids • Vasopressin • Apelin
- Corticotrophin test • Hydrocortisone

Septic shock and related organ dysfunction or failure, common criteria for intensive care unit admission, are major causes of death with a mortality rate of 40% to 60%.[1–3] In the United States, severe sepsis with multiple organ failure causes about the same number of deaths as acute myocardial infarction, lung cancer, or breast cancer.[4] From 75% to over 90% of patients with severe sepsis already exhibit at least two or more organ/system dysfunctions, often during the first 12 hours of admission.[5] As reviewed recently,[6] the stress that results from a severe infection is not only intense but sustained, lowering the chance for a successful host response. This stress response to sepsis is initiated by the release of inflammatory cytokines by immune and structural cells.[7–10] When excessive, these inflammatory cytokines may contribute to the development, number, and severity of organ insults.[11–14] Prevalence of adrenal dysfunction (either "not high enough" or low production of glucocorticoids by the zona fasciculata) in critically ill patients approaches 30% and can be as frequent as 50% to 60% in septic shock.[6,15,16] Surprisingly, adrenal dysfunction was not listed as a potential failing vital organ in the consensus definition of septic shock proposed in 1992.[17] In addition, alteration of the hypothalamic-pituitary-adrenal (HPA) axis network has never been considered per se in the above definition, although often evoked in reports screening the mechanisms of sepsis-induced organ dysfunction.[14]

In this article, actual evidence for adrenal dysfunction/insufficiency in septic shock is provided with a special focus on (1) HPA axis physiology and sepsis and septic shock-induced dysregulation, (2) clinical and biological diagnostic criteria, (3) treatment of adrenal dysfunction/failure/insufficiency, and (4) corticosteroid-related side effects. Areas of uncertainty with regard to diagnostic methodologies and treatment procedures are also addressed through key questions.

HYPOTHALAMIC-PITUITARY-ADRENAL AXIS PHYSIOLOGY

The adrenal glands are composed of two independent zones: (1) the medulla, which is centrally located and produces the powerful endogenous catecholamine vasopressors, epinephrine and norepinephrine; and (2) a surrounding cortical zone, which is divided into glomerulosa, fasciculate, and reticularis regions, from outside to inside (Fig 1). These areas secrete steroid hormones, respectively aldosterone, with mineralocorticoid effects; cortisol, with glucocorticoid effects; and adrenal androgens. Experimental removal of the cortical zone of the adrenal gland is life-threatening[18] and can be cured by pituitary extracts.[19] The basic "backbone" of all steroids is composed of the same sterol nucleus present in cholesterol.

Production of glucocorticoids is stimulated by the adrenocorticotropic hormone (ACTH), which is mainly released by corticotroph cells within the anterior part of the pituitary gland. The

[a] Assistance Publique Hôpitaux de Paris, Université de Versailles SQY (UniverSud Paris), Hôpital Raymond Poincaré, Service de Réanimation, 104 Boulevard Raymond Poincaré, 92380 Garches, France
[b] Service de Soins Intensifs Médicaux, Département de Médecine, CHU Sherbrooke, 3001 12eme Av Nord, Sherbrooke, Québec, Canada
* Corresponding author.
E-mail address: djillali.annane@rpc.aphp.fr (D. Annane).

Clin Chest Med 30 (2009) 17–27
doi:10.1016/j.ccm.2008.10.003

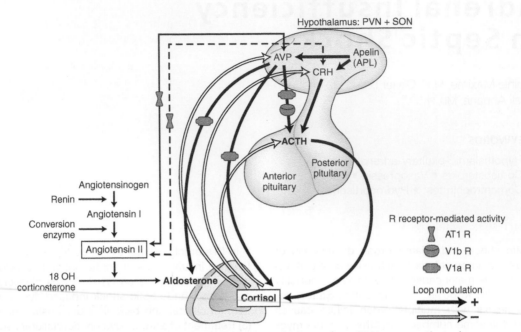

Fig. 1. HPA axis physiology. AVP, vasopressin; PVN, paraventricular nucleus; SON, supraoptic nucleus.

corticotropin-releasing hormone (CRH) triggers ACTH synthesis while glucocorticoids inhibit ACTH and CRH production through a feedback loop. Other factors are also involved in the HPA axis stress-response during sepsis. Indeed, at least in rodents, vasopressin has been shown to increase endogenous adrenal ACTH secretion, through both V1a and b receptors, and to stimulate aldosterone and cortisol secretion through V1a receptors.[20,21] Conversely, cortisol exerts a negative feedback on vasopressin production.[22,23] Vasopressin is produced by the paraventricular and supraoptic nuclei of the hypothalamus and is stored in the posterior pituitary. In addition to its known antidiuretic and vasopressive properties,[24,25] vasopressin has recently been described to exhibit intrinsic anti-inflammatory activity.[26] Angiotensin II is also an HPA axis regulator, acting through its angiotensin II type-1 (AT1) receptor and by the consecutive release of CRH and vasopressin.[27] Hence, vasopressin and angiotensin II are powerful substitutes in increasing ACTH secretion during stress conditions, such as sepsis. In rodents, the physiologic feedback regulation of glucocorticoids decreases during stress through cortisol-driven stimulation of both AT1 and V1b receptors in the paraventricular nucleus and anterior pituitary.[28–30] Apelin, another recently discovered neuropeptide acting on HPA axis regulation, was first described by Tatemoto and colleagues in 1998.[31] Originating from the paraventricular and supraoptic nuclei, apelin acts by releasing CRH (and consequently ACTH)[32,33] and by reducing

plasma vasopressin,[34–36] although related human data are still lacking. In the rodent pituitary gland, apelin is coexpressed with ACTH, where both can potentially co-localize[37] and cross-regulate. These actions require the specific apelin receptor, APJ, to be expressed in the central nervous system, cardiovascular system, hypothalamus, pituitary gland, and adipoinsular axis.[38] APJ shares great homology with the angiotensin II receptor, AT1R, although it does not bind angiotensin II.[39]

The daily production of cortisol is 55 μmol/d, and reaches its physiologic nadir in the morning.[40] Cortisol production follows a circadian cycle and undergoes pulsatile secretion.[41] Esterified cholesterol is the sole storage form of cortisol in the adrenal gland. Ninety percent of circulating cortisol in human serum is bound to proteins, namely corticosteroid-binding globulin (CBG)[42] and albumin, and is therefore inactive. CBG binding is specific and exhibits high affinity in contrast to albumin binding, which is nonspecific with lower affinity.[43,44] Free cortisol is the only active form of the hormone.

Glucocorticoids act on carbohydrate, protein, and lipid metabolism; modulate vascular tone; and have variable mineralocorticoid activity. Moreover, glucocorticoids (1) decrease the synthesis and release of antibodies by lymphocytes, (2) reduce the recruitment of inflammatory cells, and (3) inhibit the production of cyclooxygenase II[45] and phospholipase A2.[46] The binding of free cortisol, with its ubiquitously expressed cytoplasmic receptor, releases heat shock proteins, which are stress molecules sharing important protective abilities.[47] The resulting cortisol-receptor complex translocates into the nucleus, where it modulates gene expression by promoting the production of anti-inflammatory cytokines (eg, interleukin-1 receptor antagonist [IL-1rA], IL-10) and by inhibiting the production of proinflammatory cytokines (IL-1, IL-4, tumor necrosis factor [TNF-α]). In addition, the induction of the nuclear factor κB inhibitor by glucocorticoids further inhibits nuclear factor κB–dependent gene transcription.[48,49] Cortisol also induces macrophage migration inhibitory factor[50] production from macrophages in vitro and in vivo. Conversely, macrophage migration inhibitory factor prevents the inhibitory effects of glucocorticoids on proinflammatory cytokine production by lipopolysaccharide-activated human monocytes.[51]

ADRENAL INSUFFICIENCY IN SEPSIS

Serum cortisol concentrations reflect the severity of illness during sepsis. In abdominal sepsis, cortisol metabolism and synthesis are altered and cortisol clearance is impaired, especially in patients with kidney or liver failure.[52,53] Moreover, adrenocortical cells decrease their sensitivity to ACTH, while their pulsatility as well as their day-night cycle is abrogated. Synthesis and release of CRH and ACTH are stimulated by proinflammatory cytokines, such as IL-6, TNF-α, and IL-1β,[54] and also by vasopressin and noradrenaline.[55] Some investigators have found that, in critically ill patients, concentrations of vasopressin, whether due to endogenous production or exogenous administration, did not correlate with cortisol response to ACTH.[56,57] Others found the opposite—that concentrations of vasopressin did correlate with cortisol response to ACTH.[58]

Serum levels of carrier proteins, notably albumin, may decrease during critical illness and may result in lower than expected concentrations of total serum cortisol and increased free cortisol serum concentrations.[59] At the site of infection, there is increased activity of 11β-hydroxysteroid dehydrogenase type 2, which converts excess active cortisol into inactive cortisone. Indeed, compared with normal subjects, the plasma cortisol/cortisone ratio is significantly elevated in sepsis and trauma patients from day 1 to day 7. Nevertheless, it remains uncertain whether there is a correlation between plasma cortisol/cortisone ratio and severity of illness.[60,61]

ADRENAL INSUFFICIENCY IN SEPTIC SHOCK
Prevalence and Definition

Adrenal insufficiency has been observed in 30% to 70% of septic shock cases, depending on the definition used. It is proposed that a baseline cortisol of less than 10 μg/dL or a delta cortisol of less than 9 μg/dL (250 nmol/L) after a 250-μg ACTH infusion test should prompt intensive care unit physicians to consider that adrenal insufficiency is likely,[62,63] and that so-called "nonresponders" are less responsive to vasopressor therapy and have a higher risk of death.[64]

Mechanisms

Several mechanisms have been proposed to explain sepsis-induced adrenal insufficiency.[65] First, cortisol deficiency may be the result of a defect in synthesis due to adrenal[66] or hypothalamo-hypophysis anatomic damage.[67,68] Indeed, the incidence of ischemia or hemorrhage in the hypothalamus, pituitary gland, or adrenals is about 7% to 10% among septic shock cases, and likely results from weak venous drainage and tremendous increase in arterial blood flow to these glands. During sepsis, hypothalamic inflammation and overexpression of inducible nitric oxide synthase may trigger neuronal apoptosis.[69] Likewise, substance P, superoxide radicals, carbon monoxide, and prostaglandins also accumulate in the hypothalamus or pituitary gland and alter hormone synthesis and pulsatility.

Second, cortisol synthesis can be iatrogenically blunted by drugs that inhibit the last enzymatic step toward cortisol synthesis (eg, etomidate, ketoconazole, fluconazole, phenytoin).[70–72] For instance, a single bolus of etomidate induces adrenal insufficiency for up to 48 hours,[73] and may increase the overall risk of death.[74]

Third, glucocorticoid transport can be altered by decreased CBG availability in early-stage septic shock, increasing the free cortisol fraction. However, CBG is very important in the delivery of cortisol specifically to inflamed tissues. Indeed, elastase produced by activated polymorphonuclear neutrophils at the site of infection may specifically cleave cortisol bound to CBG, allowing free cortisol to enter inflammatory tissues. Therefore, critical illness–induced low CBG may result in less cortisol released at the site of inflammation and may exacerbate tissue resistance to cortisol.

Fourth, there may be a decrease in the number and activity of the glucocorticoid receptors, such a decrease would reduce the ability of cells to respond to cortisol.[65]

A dissociation between ACTH and glucocorticoid levels has been described during critical illness and chronic stress.[75,76] This phenomenon has also been observed in chronically stressed animals and in rodents during long-term voluntary exercise.[77,78] From a practical standpoint, this amounts to an increase in cortisol levels without an accompanying alteration in ACTH. Moreover, there is an intra-adrenal shift toward increased glucocorticoid production to the detriment of mineralocorticoid and androgen production. Several explanations have been proposed for these non-ACTH–driven pathways activated during critical illness or chronic stress: (1) the vast variety of receptors for modulating ACTH-independent adrenal glucocorticoid release (eg, neuropeptides, neurotransmitters, opioids, growth factors, cytokines, adipokines); (2) an extensive intra-adrenal paracrine regulation; and (3) gonadal steroid regulation.[79]

CLINICAL DIAGNOSIS

The clinical diagnosis of adrenal insufficiency lacks specificity during septic shock. Observed symptoms include fever, abdominal pain, persistent hypotension, vomiting, and altered consciousness. Difficulty in weaning off catecholamines is often another indicator. There is not sufficient time to develop skin pigment alterations associated with long-standing adrenal insufficiency. Although rare, the full-blown syndrome of primary adrenal insufficiency can mimic an abdominal surgical emergency with a painful and stiff belly, often associated with high-grade fever and shock.

BIOLOGICAL DIAGNOSIS
Nonspecific Laboratory Findings

Classically, adrenal insufficiency is associated with hyponatremia with excess urinary sodium, hyperkalemia, and hypoglycemia. Hypereosinophilia is usually described, but rarely found. None of these findings are specific during a prolonged stay in critical care.

Specific Laboratory Findings: Hormones

In the intensive care setting, where stress is almost constant, there is no consensus regarding a threshold blood cortisol level beneath which adrenal insufficiency can be clearly defined. The appropriate baseline cortisol level in this condition is also unclear, since many studies have demonstrated a wide range of elevated total plasma cortisol concentrations in stressed patients admitted to intensive care compared with healthy volunteers.

Several dynamic tests are currently available to diagnose adrenal insufficiency. The easiest, fastest, and most reproducible test is the corticotropin test, which consists of measuring cortisol before and 1 hour after HPA axis stimulation with a standardized 250-µg dose of ACTH. A meta-analysis of 20 studies investigating the cortisol response to cosyntropin showed similar results with either a 250- or 1-µg dosage.[80] A recent international task force suggested that in critically ill patients, adrenal insufficiency is best defined by basal cortisol blood levels of less than 10 µg/dL or a cortisol increment of less than 9 µg/dL.[81]

Alternative methods for assessing cortisol are salivary or urinary measurements, which provide an indirect and reliable estimate of free cortisol serum levels. Salivary cortisol is not dependent on serum albumin levels and is easy to collect,[82] whereas urinary cortisol can depend on renal function.[83] Because over 90 % of circulating cortisol is protein-bound, a decrease in albumin levels (which is almost constant during septic shock) can decrease total cortisol levels and renders the specific diagnosis of adrenal insufficiency almost impossible. In contrast, both basal and cosyntropin-stimulated free cortisol are not affected by hypoproteinemia.[59] Free cortisol levels can be measured directly or calculated from CBG levels. However, methods for determination of serum-free cortisol or CBG levels do not permit their use in routine practice in the intensive care unit.[81] The metyrapone and hypoglycemia tests cannot be routinely used in current critical care practice as they are cumbersome and potentially dangerous. Using the overnight metyrapone test, the prevalence of adrenal insufficiency was closed to 60% in patients with severe sepsis.[84]

TREATMENT OF ADRENAL INSUFFICIENCY IN SEPTIC SHOCK

Corticosteroids have been considered as an adjunct therapy for severe infections for more than 60 years. Randomized controlled trials have established the lack of benefit from high doses of corticosteroids given for a short period of time.[85] However, such trials have suggested a favorable benefit-to-risk ratio in the more severe forms of infections.[86] Indeed, since 1998, researchers have consistently demonstrated that a dose of 200 to 300 mg of hydrocortisone (or equivalent) per day given for 5 to 11 days improved hemodynamics, alleviated the symptoms of systemic inflammatory response (by inhibiting inflammatory cells migration and the synthesis and release of most inflammatory mediators), restored the function of failing organs, and may save lives. The recently published Corticus study found similar benefit of an 11-day treatment with hydrocortisone on septic shock morbidity (ie, more rapid shock reversal and more rapid resolution of cardiovascular, respiratory, and liver failures) but did not demonstrate a survival benefit.[74] In comparison with the first phase III trial on low-dose corticosteroids for septic shock,[16] patients included in the Corticus study were less severely ill and treatment generally occurred later. Also, in the Corticus study, abdominal sepsis was dominant over lung sepsis and hydrocortisone was used alone without fludrocortisone (**Table 1**).

In Australia and New Zealand, up to 60% of intensive care physicians use steroids in patients with septic shock. Meanwhile, in Canada up to 75% of intensive care physicians make the same choice (unpublished data, survey release of February 2006).[3] In the Vasopressin in Septic Shock Trial, more than 20% of the randomized patients were already on steroids upon their inclusion in study. Those patients on steroids were started on steroids on average 12 hours from the onset of sepsis.[3] Current recommendations from an international task force of the American College of Critical Care Medicine[81] and the Surviving Sepsis Campaign[87] limit the use of corticosteroids to patients poorly responsive to fluid resuscitation and vasopressor therapy. When used to treat septic shock, corticosteroids should be administrated using hydrocortisone, at a dose of 200 mg/d in four divided doses or as a continuous bolus infusion of 240 mg/d (10 mg/h) for 7 days or more, followed by progressive weaning. Debate over the role of steroids in the treatment of sepsis is still ongoing, however. More studies are needed to reach a consensus in several areas, including which is the best target population, whether an ACTH stimulation test should be used to guide treatment, whether fludrocortisone should be given along with hydrocortisone, and how long treatment should continue.

POTENTIAL SIDE EFFECTS OF GLUCOCORTICOID TREATMENT IN SEPTIC SHOCK

In randomized controlled trials of low-dose corticosteroids, treatment did not increase the risk of superinfection.[86] Likewise, in the Corticus study, treatment with hydrocortisone did not increase the rate of ventilator-associated pneumonia, catheter-related infections, nosocomial bacteremia, urinary tract infections, or wound infections. The observed increase in superinfections, including new episodes of sepsis or septic shock, was mostly driven by new episodes of shock with unproven infection, with an odds ratio of 1.37 (95% CI 1.05–1.79) (ie, one out of four patients in the placebo group; one out of three patients in the corticosteroids group). Treatment with low-dose corticosteroids did not increase the risk of gastroduodenal bleeding[86] (10 trials; n = 1321; odds ratio 1.16; 95% CI 0.82–1.65). Treatment may, however, result in hyperglycemia and hypernatremia. Whether

corticosteroids at a dose of 200 to 300 mg/d for 5 to 11 days may cause critical illness myopathy remains uncertain. Some inception cohort studies suggested that corticosteroid-treated critically ill patients are more likely to develop neuromuscular weakness,[88,89] while others found no link between corticosteroid treatment and neuromuscular weakness.[90,91] In randomized controlled trials, the incidence of neuromuscular weakness was not increased in patients receiving corticosteroid therapy.[16,74]

KEY QUESTIONS

Although many controversies persist regarding the nature of adrenal insufficiency among patients with septic shock, consensus has been achieved in a number of areas, which are illustrated by the response to several frequently asked questions:

What Is the Appropriate Cortisol Level in the ICU?

Response: A basal cortisol level between 10 µg/dL and 44 µg/dL, or an increment of cortisol of more than 9 µg/dL, is associated with better short-term survival than a basal cortisol level of 9 µg/dL or less or above 44 µg/dL, or a cortisol increment of less than 9 µg/dL.[84]

Which Dose of Adrenocorticotropic Hormone Is Best Used for Stimulation Testing: 250 or 1 µg?

Response: Both ACTH tests work almost equally as well. Nevertheless, more evidence supports the use of the 250-µg dose.[81]

Given that Most Circulating Cortisol Is Bound to Cortisol-Binding Globulin and Albumin, Is It More Appropriate to Measure Total or Free Cortisol?

Response: Total cortisol assessment provides an accurate view of actual adrenal function in patients with albumin levels above 25 mg/L. Measurement of free cortisol or CBG (to calculate free cortisol) is more accurate than total cortisol levels in patients with an albumin level of less than 25 mg/L. However, clinicians do not routinely measure either free cortisol or CBG.[59,81]

Should Fludrocortisone Be Given Alongside Hydrocortisone to Patients With Septic Shock?

Response: The question of whether or not to use fludrocortisone in addition to hydrocortisone continues to be debated because it is unclear whether fludrocortisone is absorbed in intensive care unit

Table 1
Main clinical trials on low-dose corticosteroids for severe sepsis or septic shock

Reference	Population	Intervention	Main Results
Bollaert et al[92]	Adults (n = 41) with vasopressor- and ventilator-dependent septic shock	1. Hydrocortisone: 100-mg intravenous bolus every 8 h for 5 d then tapered over 6 d 2. Placebo: treatments have to be initiated after 48 h or more from shock onset	Reduction in shock duration and mortality
Briegel et al[93]	Adults (n = 40) with vasopressor- and ventilator-dependent septic shock	1. Hydrocortisone: 100-mg 30-min intravenous infusion followed by 0.18-mg/kg/h continuous infusion until shock reversal, and then tapered off 2. Placebo: treatments have to be initiated within 72 h from shock onset	Reduction in shock duration
Chawla et al[94]	Adults (n = 44) with vasopressor-dependent septic shock	1. Hydrocortisone (100-mg intravenous bolus every 8 h for 3 d, then tapered over 4 d 2. Placebo: treatments have to be initiated after 72 h or more from shock onset	Reduction in shock duration
Annane et al[16]	Adults (n = 300) with vasopressor- and ventilator-dependent septic shock	1. Hydrocortisone: 50-mg intravenous bolus every 6 h for 7 d plus fludrocortisone 50 µg taken orally every 24 h for 7 d 2. Respective placebos: treatments have to be initiated within 8 h from shock onset	Reduction in shock duration and mortality
Yildiz et al[95]	Adults (n = 40) with sepsis (n = 14), severe sepsis (n = 17), and septic shock (n = 9).	1. Prednisolone: two intravenous bolus, 5 mg at 6 AM and 2.5 mg at 6 PM for 10 d 2. Placebo	Reduction in mortality
Keh et al[96]	Adults (n = 40) with vasopressor dependent septic shock.	1. Hydrocortisone: 100-mg 30-min intravenous infusion followed by 10-mg/h continuous infusion for 3 d 2. Placebo: all participants received hydrocortisone for 3 d preceded or followed by placebo for 3 d	Improvement in hemodynamics; reduction in shock duration, Sepsis-Related Organ Failure Assessment score, and proinflammatory markers

Study	Population	Intervention	Outcome
Confalonieri et al[97]	46 patients with severe community-acquired pneumonia	1. Hydrocortisone: 200-mg intravenous loading bolus followed by a continuous infusion at a rate of 10 mg/h for 7 d then tapered over 4 d 2. Placebo	Prevention of shock and reduction in mortality
Oppert et al[98]	Adults (n = 40) with vasopressor dependent septic shock.	1. Hydrocortisone: 50 mg of intravenous bolus followed by 0.18-mg/kg/h continuous infusion up to cessation of vasopressor for 1 h or more; reduced to a dose of 0.02 mg/kg/h for 24 h; then reduced by 0.02 mg/kg/h every day 2. Placebo	Reduction in shock duration; improvement in hemodynamics and organ function; reduction in proinflammatory mediators
Tandan et al[99]	Adults (n = 28) with septic shock and adrenal insufficiency	1. Hydrocortisone (stated low dose but actual dose and duration not reported) 2. Placebo	Reduction in mortality
Rinaldi et al[100]	Adults (n = 40) with severe sepsis and not receiving a vasopressor support	1. Hydrocortisone: 300 mg/d as a continuous infusion for 6 d and then tapered off 2. Standard therapy	Reduction in proinflammatory mediators and in markers of kidney inflammation
Cicarelli et al[101]	Adults (n = 29) with vasopressor-dependent septic shock	1. Dexamethasone: 0.2 mg/kg intravenous; three doses at intervals of 36 hours	Reduction in shock duration and short-term mortality
Mikami et al[102]	31 patients with severe sepsis due to community-acquired pneumonia	1. Intravenous prednisolone 40 mg for 3 d 2. Standard therapy	Improvement in vital signs and shorter length of stay
Huh et al[103]	82 patients with septic shock and adrenal insufficiency	Hydrocortisone was administered intravenously every 6 h as a 50-mg bolus for 3 d versus 7 d	Reduction in shock duration and mortality
Sprung et al[74]	Adults (n = 499) with septic shock	1. Hydrocortisone: 50 mg every 6 h for 5 d; then 50 mg every 12 h for 3 d; then 50 mg once a day for 3 d 2. Placebo	Reduction in duration of shock and in Sepsis-Related Organ Failure Assessment score; no evidence for survival benefit

patients. Mineralocorticoids play a critical role in arterial blood pressure control in septic shock patients, and the only randomized controlled trial that tested the combination of fludrocortisone and hydrocortisone suggested survival benefits.[16] Given the uncertainty surrounding the benefit of adding fludrocortisone to hydrocortisone, actual recommendations call for the administration of hydrocortisone alone.[81] The efficacy of adding fludrocortisone to hydrocortisone regimen is currently the object of two ongoing trials.

When Hydrocortisone Is Used to Treat Patients With Septic Shock, How Much Should Be Used, for How Long, and by What Route?

Response: Most studies reported using 200 to 300 mg/d of hydrocortisone. Sudden cessation of corticosteroids is deleterious, increasing the risk of rebound inflammation or shock relapse. Therefore, recent international guidelines recommend a 7-day treatment with progressive weaning.[81] While continuous infusion may result in fewer episodes of hyperglycemia, it may also result more frequently in rebound.

SUMMARY

While a growing body of evidence suggests that inappropriate cortisol response to critical illness, such as sepsis, contributes to organ dysfunction and mortality, the question of whether exogenous corticosteroids should be given to these patients remains controversial. While awaiting the results of ongoing clinical trials, physicians may consider giving a dose of 200 to 300 mg/d of hydrocortisone for 5 to 11 days to patients with septic shock poorly responsive to fluid and vasopressor therapy.

REFERENCES

1. Angus DC, Linde-Zwirble WT, Lidicker J, et al. Epidemiology of severe sepsis in the United States: analysis of incidence, outcome, and associated costs of care. Crit Care Med 2001;29(7):1303–10.
2. Schroeder S, Wichers M, Klingmuller D, et al. The hypothalamic-pituitary-adrenal axis of patients with severe sepsis: altered response to corticotropin-releasing hormone. Crit Care Med 2001;29(2):310–6.
3. Russell JA, Walley KR, Singer J, et al. Vasopressin versus norepinephrine infusion in patients with septic shock. N Engl J Med 2008;358(9):877–87.
4. Parrillo JE. Septic shock-vasopressin, norepinephrine, and urgency. N Engl J Med 2008;358(9):954–6.
5. Bernard GR, Wheeler AP, Russell JA, et al. The effects of ibuprofen on the physiology and survival of patients with sepsis. The Ibuprofen in Sepsis Study Group. N Engl J Med 1997;336(13):912–28.
6. Maxime V, Siami S, Annane D. Metabolism modulators in sepsis: the abnormal pituitary response. Crit Care Med 2007;35(9S):S596–601.
7. Betancur C, Borrell J, Guaza C. Cytokine regulation of corticosteroid receptors in the rat hippocampus: effects of interleukin-1, interleukin-6, tumor necrosis factor and lipopolysaccharide. Neuroendocrinology 1995;62(1):47–54.
8. Imura H, Fukata J. Endocrine-paracrine interaction in communication between the immune and endocrine systems. Activation of the hypothalamic-pituitary-adrenal axis in inflammation. Eur J Endocrinol 1994;130(1):32–7.
9. Sternberg EM. Neuroendocrine factors in susceptibility to inflammatory disease: focus on the hypothalamic-pituitary-adrenal axis. Horm Res 1995;43(4):159–61.
10. Elenkov IJ, Chrousos GP. Stress system—organization, physiology and immunoregulation. Neuroimmunomodulation 2006;13(5–6):257–67.
11. Pinsky MR, Vincent JL, Deviere J, et al. Serum cytokine levels in human septic shock. Relation to multiple-system organ failure and mortality. Chest 1993;103(2):565–75.
12. Thijs LG, Hack CE. Time course of cytokine levels in sepsis. Intensive Care Med 1995;21(Suppl 2):S258–63.
13. Loisa P, Rinne T, Kaukinen S. Adrenocortical function and multiple organ failure in severe sepsis. Acta Anaesthesiol Scand 2002;46(2):145–51.
14. Abraham E, Singer M. Mechanisms of sepsis-induced organ dysfunction. Crit Care Med 2007;35(10):2408–16.
15. Marik PE, Zaloga GP. Adrenal insufficiency in the critically ill: a new look at an old problem. Chest 2002;122(5):1784–96.
16. Annane D, Sebille V, Charpentier C, et al. Effect of treatment with low doses of hydrocortisone and fludrocortisone on mortality in patients with septic shock. JAMA 2002;288(7):862–71.
17. Bone RC, Balk RA, Cerra FB, et al. Definitions for sepsis and organ failure and guidelines for the use of innovative therapies in sepsis. The ACCP/SCCM Consensus Conference Committee. American College of Chest Physicians/Society of Critical Care Medicine. Chest 1992;101(6):1644–55.
18. Guillon G, Balestre MN, Chouinard L, et al. Involvement of distinct G-proteins in the action of vasopressin on rat glomerulosa cells. Endocrinology 1990;126(3):1699–708.
19. Brown-Sequard CE. Recherches expérimentales sur la physiologie et la pathologies des capsules

surrenales. C R Hebd Séances Acad Sci (Paris) 1856;43:422–5.

20. Collip JB, Anderson EM, Thomson DL. The adrenotropic hormone of the anterior pituitary lobe. Lancet 1933;2:347–8.

21. Gallo-Payet N, Guillon G. Regulation of adrenocortical function by vasopressin. Horm Metab Res 1998;30(6–7):360–7.

22. Oelkers W. Hyponatremia and inappropriate secretion of vasopressin (antidiuretic hormone) in patients with hypopituitarism. N Engl J Med 1989;321(8):492–6.

23. Papanek PE, Raff H. Chronic physiological increases in cortisol inhibit the vasopressin response to hypertonicity in conscious dogs. Am J Physiol 1994;267(5 Pt 2):R1342–9.

24. Holmes CL, Patel BM, Russel JA, et al. Physiology of vasopressin relevant to management of septic shock. Chest 2001;120(3):989–1002.

25. Mutlu GM, Factor P. Role of vasopressin in the management of septic shock. Intensive Care Med 2004;30(7):1276–91.

26. Antoni FA. Vasopressinergic control of pituitary adrenocorticotropin secretion comes of age. Front Neuroendocrinol 1993;14(2):76–122.

27. Saavedra JM, Benicky J. Brain and peripheral angiotensin II play a major role in stress. Stress 2007;10(2):185–93.

28. Aguilera G, Young WS, Kiss A, et al. Direct regulation of hypothalamic corticotropin-releasing-hormone neurons by angiotensin II. Neuroendocrinology 1995;61(4):437–44.

29. Aguilera G, Kiss A, Luo X. Increased expression of type 1 angiotensin II receptors in the hypothalamic paraventricular nucleus following stress and glucocorticoid administration. J Neuroendocrinol 1995; 7(10):775–83.

30. Castren E, Saavedra JM. Angiotensin II receptors in paraventricular nucleus, subfornical organ, and pituitary gland of hypophysectomized, adrenalectomized, and vasopressin-deficient rats. Proc Natl Acad Sci U S A 1989;86(2):725–9.

31. Tatemoto K, Hosoya M, Habata, et al. Isolation and characterization of a novel endogenous peptide ligand for the human APJ receptor. Biochem Biophys Res Commun 1998;251(2):471–6.

32. Renner U, Pagotto U, Arzt E, et al. Autocrine and paracrine roles of polypeptide growth factors, cytokines and vasogenic substances in normal and tumorous pituitary function and growth: a review. Eur J Endocrinol 1996;135(5):515–32.

33. Schwartz J, Cherny R. Intercellular communication within the anterior pituitary influencing the secretion of hypophysial hormones. Endocr Rev 1992;13(3): 453–75.

34. Kleinz MJ, Davenport AP. Emerging roles of apelin in biology and medicine. Pharmacol Ther 2005; 107(2):198–211.

35. Reaux A, De Mota N, Skultetyova I, et al. Physiological role of a novel neuropeptide, apelin, and its receptor in the rat brain. J Neurochem 2001; 77(4):1085–96.

36. Reaux A, Gallatz K, Palkovits M, et al. Distribution of apelin-synthesizing neurons in the adult rat brain. Neuroscience 2002;113(3):653–62.

37. Reaux-Le Goazigo A, Alvear-Perez R, Zizzari P, et al. Cellular localization of apelin and its receptor in the anterior pituitary: evidence for a direct stimulatory action of apelin on ACTH release. Am J Physiol Endocrinol Metab 2007;292(1):E7–15.

38. Gallo-Payet N, Roussy JF, Chagnon F, Roberge C, Lesur O. Hypothalamic/pituitary/adrenal axis and multiorgan defaillance system in critical illness; a special focus on arginine-vasopressin and apelin. J Organ Dysfunc 4, in press.

39. O'Dowd BF, Heiber M, Chan A, et al. A human gene that shows identity with the gene encoding the angiotensin receptor is located on chromosome 11. Gene 1993;136(1–2):355–60.

40. Cope CL, Black E. The production rate of cortisol in man. Br Med J 1958;1(5078):1020–4.

41. Kraft M, Martin RJ. Chronobiology and chronotherapy in medicine. Dis Mon 1995;41(8):501–75.

42. Daughaday WH. Binding of corticosteroids by plasma proteins. I. Dialysis equilibrium and renal clearance studies. J Clin Invest 1956;355(12): 1428–33.

43. Forest MG, Pugeat M. In: Binding proteins of steroid hormones, vol. 149. London: Edition Libbey Eurotext; 1986.

44. Siiteri PK, Murai JT, Hammond GL, et al. The serum transport of steroid hormones. Recent Prog Horm Res 1982;38:457–510 [review].

45. Santini G, Patrignani P, Sciulli MG, et al. The human pharmacology of monocyte cyclooxygenase 2 inhibition by cortisol and synthetic glucocorticoids. Clin Pharmacol Ther 2001;70(5):475–83.

46. Tajima M, Maruyama S, Ichikawa M, et al. Mechanism of action of an anti-inflammatory steroid on changes in vascular permeability (II). Evaluation of its action as a phospholipase A2 inhibitor. Josai Shika Daigaku Kiyo 1984;13(1):60–7.

47. Anderson RL, Kraft PE, Bensaude O, et al. Binding activity of glucocorticoid receptors after heat shock. Exp cell Res 1991;197(1):100–6.

48. Hart L, Lim S, Adcock I, et al. Effects of inhaled corticosteroid therapy on expression and DNA-binding activity of nuclear factor κB. Am J Respir Crit Care Med 2000;161(1):224–31.

49. Scheinman RI, Cogswell PC, Lofquist AK, et al. Role of transcriptional activation of IkBα in mediation of immunosuppression by glucocorticoids. Science 1995;270(5234):283–6.

50. Yende S, Angus DC, Bucala R. MIF and MODS. J Organ Dysf 4, in press.

51. Calandra T, Bernhagen J, Metz CN, et al. MIF as a glucocorticoid-induced modulator of cytokine production. Nature 1995;377(6544):68–71.

52. Melby JC, Spink WW. Comparative studies on adrenal cortical function and cortisol metabolism in healthy adults and in patients with shock due to infection. J Clin Invest 1958;37(12):1791–8.

53. Koo DJ, Jackman D, Chaudry IH, et al. Adrenal insufficiency during the late stage of polymicrobial sepsis. Crit Care Med 2001;29(3):618–22.

54. McCann SM, De Laurentiis A, Rettori V. Chronology of advances in neuroendocrine immunomodulation. Ann N Y Acad Sci 2006;1088:1–11.

55. Itoi K, Helmreich DL, Lopez-Figueroa MO, et al. Differential regulation of corticotropin-releasing hormone and vasopressin gene transcription in the hypothalamus by norepinephrine. J Neurosci 1999;19(13):5464–72.

56. Dünser MW, Hasibeder WR, Wenzel V, et al. Endocrinologic response to vasopressin infusion in advanced vasodilatory shock. Crit Care Med 2004; 32(6):1266–71.

57. Lauzier F, Levy B, Lamarre P, et al. Vasopressin or norepinephrine in early hyperdynamic septic shock: a randomized clinical trial. Intensive Care Med 2006;32(11):1782–9.

58. Sharshar T, Blanchard A, Paillard M, et al. Circulating vasopressin levels in septic shock. Crit Care Med 2003;31(6):1752–8.

59. Hamrahian AH, Oseni TS, Arafah BM. Measurements of serum free cortisol in critically ill patients. N Engl J Med 2004;350(16):1629–38.

60. Cooper MS, Bujalska I, Rabbitt E, et al. Modulation of 11β-hydroxysteroid deshydrogenase isozymes by proinflammatory cytokines in osteoblasts: an autocrine switch from glucocorticoid inactivation to activation. J Bone Miner Res 2001;16(6):1037–44.

61. Venkatesh B, Cohen J, Hickman I, et al. Evidence of altered cortisol metabolism in critically ill patients: a prospective study. Intensive Care Med 2007;33(10):1746–53.

62. Marik PE. The diagnosis of adrenal insufficiency in the critically ill patient: Does it really matter? Crit Care 2006;10(5):176.

63. Annane D. Time for consensus definition of corticosteroid insufficiency in critically ill patients. Crit Care Med 2003;31(6):1868–9.

64. Annane D, Sébille V, Troché G, et al. A 3-level prognostic classification in septic shock based on cortisol levels and cortisol response to corticotrophin. JAMA 2000;283(8):1038–45.

65. Prigent H, Maxime V, Annane D. Science review: mechanisms of impaired adrenal function in sepsis and molecular actions of glucocorticoids. Crit Care 2004;8(4):243–52.

66. Waterhouse R. Case of suprarenal apoplexy. Lancet 1911;1:577.

67. Case records of the Massachusetts Heneral Hospital (case 15–2001). N Engl J Med 2001;344:1536–42.

68. Cooper MS, Stewart PM. Corticosteroid insufficiency in acutely ill patients. N Engl J Med 2003; 348(8):727–34.

69. Sharshar T, Gray F, Lorin de la Grandmaison G, et al. Apoptosis of neurons in cardiovascular autonomic centres triggered by inductible nitric oxide synthase after death from septic shock. Lancet 2003;362(9398):1799–805.

70. Wagner RL, White PF, Kan PB, et al. Inhibition of adrenal steroidogenesis by the anesthetic etomidate. N Engl J Med 1984;310(22):1415–21.

71. Mohammad Z, Afessa B, Finkielman JD. The incidence of relative adrenal insufficiency in patients with septic shock after the administration of etomidate. Crit Care 2006;10(4):R105.

72. Albert SG, DeLeon MJ, Silverberg AB. Possible association between high-dose fluconazole and adrenal insufficiency in critical ill patients. Crit Care Med 2001;29(3):668–70.

73. Vinclair M, Broux C, Faure P, et al. Duration of adrenal inhibition following a single dose of etomidate in critically ill patients. Intensive Care Med 2008; 34(4):714–9.

74. Sprung CL, Annane D, Keh D, et al. Hydrocortisone therapy for patients with septic shock. N Engl J Med. 2008;358(2):111–24.

75. Pascualy M, Petrie EC, Brodkin K, et al. Hypothalamic pituitary adrenocortical and sympathetic nervous system responses to the cold pressor test in Alzheimer's disease. Biol Psychiatry 2000;48(3): 247–54.

76. Cho YM, Kim SY, Cho BY, et al. Dissociation between plasma adrenocorticotropin and serum cortisol level during the early post operative period after gastrectomy. Horm Res 2000;53(5):246–50.

77. Droste SK, Gesing A, Ulbricht S, et al. Effects of long term voluntary exercise on the mouse hypothalamic-pituitary adrenal axis. Endocrinology 2003;144(7):3012–23.

78. Droste SK, Chandramohan Y, Hill LE, et al. Voluntary exercise impacts on the rat hypothalamic-pituitary adrenal axis mainly at the adrenal level. Neuroendocrinology 2007;86(1):26–37.

79. Bornstein SR, Engeland WC, Ehrhart-Bornstein M, et al. Dissociation of ACTH and glucocorticoids. Trends Endocrinol Metab 2008;19(5):175–80.

80. Dorin RI, Qualls CR, Crapo LM. Diagnosis of adrenal insufficiency. Ann Intern Med 2003;139(3): 194–204.

81. Marik PE, Pastores SM, Annane D, et al. Recommendations for the diagnosis and management of corticosteroid insufficiency in critical ill adult patients: consensus statements from an international task force by the American College of Critical Care Medicine. Crit Care Med 2008;36(6):1937–49.

82. Arafah BM, Nishiyama FJ, Tlaygeh H, et al. Measurement of salivary cortisol concentration in the assessment adrenal function in critical ill subjects: a surrogate marker of the circulating free cortisol. J Clin Endocrinol Metab 2007;92(28):2965–71.

83. Sederberg-Olsen P, Binder C, Kehlet H. Urinary excretion of free cortisol in impaired renal function. Acta Endocrinol 1975;78(1):86–90.

84. Annane D, Maxime V, Ibrahim F, et al. Diagnosis of adrenal insufficiency in severe sepsis and septic shock. Am J Respir Crit Care Med 2006;174(12):1319–26 [Epub 2006 Sep 14].

85. Slotman GJ, Fisher CJ, Bone RC, et al. Detrimental effects of high dose methylprednisolone sodium succinate on serum concentrations of hepatic and renal function indicators in severe sepsis and septic shock. The Methylprednisolone Severe Sepsis Study Group. Crit Care Med;21(2):191–5.

86. Annane D, Bellissant E, Bollaert PE, et al. Corticosteroids for severe sepsis and septic shock: a systematic review and meta-analysis. Br Med J 2004;329(7464):480.

87. Dellinger RP, Levy MM, Carlet JM, et al. Surviving Sepsis Campaign: international guidelines for management of sever sepsis and septic shock. 2008. Crit Care Med 2008;36(1):296–327.

88. De Jonghe B, Sharshar T, Lefaucheur JP, et al. Paresis acquired in the intensive care unit: a prospective multicenter study. JAMA 2002;288(22):2859–67.

89. Herridge MS, Cheung AM, Tansey CM, et al. One-year outcomes in survivors of the acute respiratory distress syndrome. N Engl J Med 2003;348(8):683–93.

90. Van den Berghe G, Schoonheydt K, Becx P, et al. Insulin therapy protects the central and peripheral nervous system of intensive care patients. Neurology 2005;64(8):1348–53.

91. Hermans G, Wilmer A, Meersseman W, et al. Impact of intensive insulin therapy on neuromuscular complications and ventilator dependency in the medical intensive care unit. Am J Respir Crit Care Med 2007;175(5):480–9.

92. Bollaert PE, Charpentier C, Levy B, et al. Reversal of late septic shock with supraphysiologic doses of hydrocortisone. Crit Care Med 1998;26(4):645–50.

93. Briegel J, Forst H, Haller M, et al. Stress doses of hydrocortisone reverse hyperdynamic septic shock: a prospective, randomized, double-blind, single center study. Crit Care Med 1999;27(4):723–32.

94. Chawla K, Kupfer Y, Tessler S. Hydrocortisone reverses refractory septic shock. Crit Care Med 1999;27:A33.

95. Yildiz O, Doganay M, Aygen B, et al. Physiological-dose steroid therapy in sepsis. Crit Care 2002;6(3):251–9.

96. Keh D, Boehnke T, Weber-Cartens S, et al. Immunologic and hemodynamic effects of "low-dose" hydrocortisone in septic shock: a double-blind, randomized, placebo-controlled, crossover study. Am J Respir Crit Care Med 2003;167(4):512–20.

97. Confalonieri M, Urbino R, Potena A, et al. Hydrocortisone infusion for severe community-acquired pneumonia: a preliminary randomized study. Am J Respir Crit Care Med 2005;171(3):242–8.

98. Oppert M, Schindler R, Husung C, et al. Low-dose hydrocortisone improves shock reversal and reduces cytokine levels in early hyperdynamic septic shock. Crit Care Med 2005;33(11):2457–64.

99. Tandan SM, Guleria R, Gupta N. Low dose steroids and adrenocortical insufficiency in septic shock: a double-blind randomised controlled trial from India. Am J Respir Crit Care Med 2005;A24.

100. Rinaldi S, Adembri C, Grechi S, et al. Low-dose hydrocortisone during severe sepsis: effects on microalbuminuria. Crit Care Med 2006;34(9):2334–9.

101. Cicarelli DD, Vieira JE, Besenor FE. Early dexamethasone treatment for septic shock patients: a prospective randomized clinical trial. Sao Paulo Med J 2007;125(4):237–41.

102. Mikami K, Suzuki M, Kitagawa H, et al. Efficacy of corticosteroids in the treatment of community-acquired pneumonia requiring hospitalization. Lung 2007;185(5):249–55.

103. Huh JW, Lim CM, Koh Y, et al. Effect of low doses of hydrocortisone in patient with septic shock and relative adrenal insufficiency: 3 days versus 7 days treatment. Crit Care Med 2007;34:A101.

Acute Kidney Injury in the Intensive Care Unit

Susan T. Crowley, MD[a,b,*], Aldo J. Peixoto, MD[a,b]

KEYWORDS

- Acute kidney injury • Critical care • Dialysis
- Renal replacement therapy • Acute tubular necrosis

Acute kidney injury (AKI) is common in hospitalized patients. The incidence of AKI in the intensive care unit (ICU) varies from 1.5% to 24%,[1] where it is associated with mortality rates as high as 78% (in patients who require dialysis), and as many as one third of survivors may remain on chronic dialysis.[2] In this article, we review recent advances related to AKI in critically ill patients. Our goal is to provide an update on the topic to the initiated reader, focusing on recent developments in the definition of AKI, its diagnosis, and therapeutic options, particularly in the realm of renal replacement therapy (RRT).

THE SPECTRUM OF ACUTE KIDNEY INJURY IN THE ICU

Recent multinational databases have provided good detail on the incidence, spectrum, and outcomes of AKI in ICU patients. Evaluating data from 54 centers in 23 countries, Uchino and colleagues[1] reported on 1738 cases of severe AKI complicating 22,269 ICU admissions in patients aged 12 and older. The criteria for enrollment included a blood urea nitrogen higher than 84 mg/dL and/or oliguria defined as urine output less than 200 mL for 12 hours. Medical patients contributed a larger fraction of AKI cases (59%) than surgical patients (41%), and the overall in-hospital mortality was 60%. A multivariable model was used to analyze the impact of different factors on mortality. It revealed significant associations between mortality and older age (odds ratio [OR] 1.02 [per year]), delayed fulfillment of inclusion criteria (OR 1.02 [per day between admission and inclusion in study]), Simplified Acute Physiologic Score II (OR 1.02 [per point]), mechanical ventilation (OR 2.11), use of vasopressors and/or inotropes (OR 1.95), a hematological medical diagnosis as cause for admission to the ICU (OR 2.7), sepsis (OR 1.36), cardiogenic shock (OR 1.41), hepatorenal syndrome (OR 1.87), admission to a "specific" ICU compared with a general ICU (OR 1.64), and a lower number of ICU beds (OR 0.57 for ICUs with fewer than 10 beds compared with those with more than 30 beds).[1]

The timing of development of AKI in relationship to the admission to the ICU may have relevant prognostic value. An important view of the problem was provided by a large multicenter study in France that analyzed 1086 AKI cases in the ICU setting.[3] The investigators categorized subjects according to the timing of occurrence of AKI: admission through second ICU day (736 cases), third through sixth ICU day (202 cases), or after the seventh day (148 cases). Mortality was lower in those with AKI on admission (61% versus 71% versus 81%), and so was the need for dialysis (51% versus 58% versus 64%), mostly a reflection of the larger number of patients with pre–renal azotemia in the first group.[3] In addition, the burden of comorbid conditions shared by critically ill patients with AKI is remarkable. A multicenter study of 618 cases of AKI in five ICUs in the United States outlined the high prevalence of coexiting chronic diseases (30% chronic kidney disease, 37% coronary artery disease, 29% diabetes, 21% chronic liver disease) and the severity of the acute illness (average 2.9 failed organ systems).[4] This comorbidity is likely to account for the lack of improvements in overall

[a] Section of Nephrology, Yale University School of Medicine, FMP 107, 333 Cedar Street, New Haven, CT, USA
[b] VA Connecticut Healthcare System, 950 Campbell Avenue, West Haven, CT 06516, USA
* Corresponding author. Renal Section (111F), VA Connecticut Healthcare System, 950 Campbell Avenue, West Haven, CT 06516.
E-mail address: susan.crowley@va.gov (S. T. Crowley).

Clin Chest Med 30 (2009) 29–43
doi:10.1016/j.ccm.2008.09.002
0272-5231/08/$ – see front matter. Published by Elsevier Inc.

mortality in AKI over time, despite significant advances in renal and critical care support.

NEW DEFINITIONS OF ACUTE KIDNEY INJURY: RISK, INJURY, FAILURE, LOSS, AND END-STAGE RENAL DISEASE AND ACUTE KIDNEY INJURY NETWORK

There is wide variability in the definition of AKI in clinical studies. To foster uniformity in both research and clinical practice, an expert group (Acute Dialysis Quality Initiative [ADQI]) developed a new classification of AKI that has been increasingly used (risk, injury, failure, loss, and end-stage renal disease [RIFLE] classification, www.adqi. net). The RIFLE classification (**Table 1**) differed from previous approaches by including both biochemical measures of renal function and urine output as components of the definition. Although the use of urine output can be challenged on the grounds that it may decrease in the absence of a change in glomerular filtration rate, we view it as an important measure because the persistence of oliguria following appropriate volume management is a marker of parenchymal injury. The other interesting aspect of this classification is the attribution of time parameters to define "persistent loss of function" (4 weeks or longer) and "end-stage kidney disease" (3 months). These lead to greater uniformity in outcomes assessment in clinical trials, and guide clinicians to two important elements of prognosis: dialysis-requiring AKI that lasts more than 4 weeks is severe and likelihood of recovery is decreased, and its persistence for more than 3 months is rarely associated with enough recovery to remove the patient from dialysis.

The more recent Acute Kidney Injury Network (AKIN) classification is based on the RIFLE system, but has introduced a few relevant modifications (see **Table 1**).[5] First, it uses smaller increments in serum creatinine for the diagnosis of AKI in response to growing data in the literature (see next section). Second, it introduces a time element (48 hours) to diagnosis. This modification has the goal of focusing on truly acute changes in renal function, a factor that is of great relevance to the performance of clinical trials. Last, it eliminates the "LOSS" and "FAILURE" categories. This is an acknowledgment that these categories represent outcomes, and thus should not be listed as part of diagnosis.

These classifications have undergone evaluation of their prognostic value. In a meta-analysis that included patient-level data from more than 71,000 patients in 13 studies, RIFLE criteria displayed a graded association with adverse outcomes.[6] The overall mortality in the study was 6.9% in the group without AKI and 31.2% in the AKI group. RIFLE criteria were associated with increased risk of death and decreased likelihood of renal recovery. Compared with patients with RIFLE R, patients with RIFLE I had 2.2-fold greater odds of ICU mortality. These odds for RIFLE F were 4.9-fold. Renal recovery was also less common among RIFLE I and F patients. Despite wide confidence intervals, all point estimates were statistically significant, and held up in several ICU and non-ICU settings. Overall, we believe they

---

Table 1
The RIFLE and Acute Kidney Injury Network classifications of acute kidney injury

	GFR Criteria	Urine Output Criteria
Risk	Increased SCreat ×1.5 or GFR decrease >25%	UO <0.5 mL/kg/h × 6 h
Injury	Increased SCreat ×2 or GFR decrease >50%	UO <0.5 mL/kg/h × 12 h
Failure	Increased SCreat ×3, GFR decrease >75% or SCreat >4 mg/dL (acute rise >0.5 mg/dL)	UO <0.3 mL/kg/h × 24 h or anuria × 12 h
Loss	Persistent AKI: complete loss of kidney function >4 weeks	
ESKD	End-stage kidney disease: complete loss of kidney function >3 months	
AKIN 1	Increased SCreat by 1.5–2× above baseline or by 0.3 mg/dL	UO <0.5 mL/kg/h × 6 h
AKIN 2	Increased Screat by 2–3× above baseline	UO <0.5 mL/kg/h × 12 h
AKIN 3	Increased SCreat by >3× above baseline or by ≥0.3 mg/dL in patients with baseline SCreat >4 mg/dL	UO <0.3 mL/kg/h × 24 h or anuria for 12 h

Abbreviations: AKI, acute renal failure; GFR, glomerular filtration rate; SCreat, serum creatinine; UO, urine output.

substantiate the prognostic relevance of this classification, although most of these data are based on the creatinine-based component of RIFLE, and there is evidence that the urine output–based criteria are not associated with mortality.[7] As for the AKIN criteria, Barrantes and colleagues recently presented data on 471 patients admitted to a medical ICU over a 1-year period.[8] Patients with a rise in serum creatinine of 0.3 mg/dL or more (or a 50% increase from baseline) within 48 hours, or with a urine output less than 0.5 mL/kg/h for a least 6 hours (AKIN 1) had greater hospital mortality (45.8% versus 16.4%, adjusted odds ratio 3.7, $P < .01$) and hospital length of stay (14 versus 7 days, adjusted odds ratio 3.0, $P < .01$) when compared with patients without AKI. The urine output component of the criteria did not hold a significant association with mortality. Unfortunately, this small observational study did not address whether a graded relationship exists according to AKIN class.

THRESHOLD FOR DEFINITION OF ACUTE KIDNEY INJURY AND PROGNOSIS

The issue of what thresholds to use in the definition of AKI remains a work in progress. Recent evidence indicates that even minor declines in glomerular filtration rate are associated with increased mortality in different populations of hospitalized patients. A meta-analysis of eight studies observed a graded relationship between the amount of elevation of serum creatinine and mortality in AKI.[9] Creatinine elevations of 10% to 24% above baseline resulted in a relative risk of 1.8 (1.3–2.5) for short-term mortality (30 days or less); patients with a rise of 25% to 49% had a relative risk of 3.0 (1.6–5.8), and those with greater than 50% increase had a risk of 6.9 (2.0–24.5).[9] Results were similar regardless of clinical scenario or ICU type. These data, along with those of Barrantes and colleagues,[8] justify the "tighter" criteria proposed in the AKIN classification.

LONG-TERM OUTCOMES OF ACUTE KIDNEY INJURY

The comprehensive impact of AKI on outcomes requires an assessment of not only short-term outcomes but long-term effects on survival, renal recovery, and quality of life as well. Recent examination of the long-term outcome of renal function and patient survival following AKI sustained during an episode of critical illness has yielded disquieting results. In addition to experiencing uniformly high hospital mortality rates, survivors of critical illness complicated by AKI have been reported to sustain excess mortality in the post-hospitalization period as well. Absolute mortality differences between hospital discharge and 1-year post AKI have ranged up to 18% suggesting the possibility of residual mortality risk attributable to the preceding AKI episode.[10,11] The impact of severe AKI on health-related quality of life (HRQOL) has also been recently examined. While not all, most patients surviving AKI who require RRT[12] report impaired QOL, specifically in the domains of physical strength and daily activities for months to years after hospital discharge compared with the general age- and gender-matched population.[13,14]

These findings suggest that the true burden of disease associated with AKI may be seriously underestimated. The 1-year patient survival, renal functional recovery, RRT re-initiation rates, and HRQOL of survivors from the Acute Renal Failure Trial Network (ATN) Study interventional cohort will be forthcoming and should substantially illuminate these underappreciated outcomes. In addition, to further examine the long-term renal consequences of AKI, the National Institutes of Health initiated a U01 grant program in 2007 for ancillary studies in the natural history of AKI.

THE DEVELOPMENT OF BIOMARKERS FOR THE EARLY IDENTIFICATION OF ACUTE KIDNEY INJURY

An exciting recent development is the use of serum and urine biomarkers to identify early renal injury (see Coca and colleagues[15] for a detailed systematic review). The main value of these markers would be to allow for earlier intervention. As of now, knowledge of the likelihood of developing AKI still does not translate into interventions that may abort its development and alter the clinical course (see later in this article). However, the development of novel therapies directed at specific injury pathways may change this in the relatively near future. Previously, late diagnosis may have been a factor hampering the success of tested interventions.

Neutrophil gelatinase–associated lipocalin (NGAL) is a protein expressed in multiple tissues that is up-regulated in proximal tubular cells immediately following ischemic injury.[16] Its value in the evaluation of risk of developing AKI was first shown in 71 children undergoing cardiac surgery for congenital heart disease.[17] In the 20 children who developed clinical AKI, urinary NGAL levels rose within 2 hours of bypass, and preceded any changes in serum creatinine by 34 hours. NGAL levels were unchanged in the 51 children without AKI. Since this groundbreaking study, serum and/or urine NGAL has been shown to identify AKI early in several groups, including adult patients undergoing coronary bypass surgery, AKI in critical care settings, contrast nephropathy, and delayed graft function following renal transplantation.[16]

Interleukin-18 (IL-18) is a proinflammatory cytokine that is activated in proximal renal tubules following injury.[16] In a nested case-control study of 138 patients developing clinical AKI in the ARDS Network study, Parikh and colleagues[18] demonstrated that a rise in urinary IL-18 levels was 73% predictive of the diagnosis of AKI 24 hours before the elevation of serum creatinine.

Cystatin C is a cysteine protease inhibitor that is synthesized and secreted by all nucleated cells; it is freely filtered by the glomerulus and metabolized by proximal tubule cells.[16] It is a better marker of GFR than serum creatinine, and could identify the development of AKI 1 to 2 days before elevation in serum creatinine in one study,[19] although this finding was not corroborated by another study.[20] It is possible that cystatin C levels will allow us to make better estimates of GFR in early AKI, but its value is still uncertain at this time.

Kidney injury molecule 1 (KIM-1) is a transmembrane protein that is overexpressed in dedifferentiated proximal tubular cells following injury.[16] Urine KIM-1 can effectively identify tubular injury following cardiac surgery in both adults and children.[21,22]

Some of the biomarkers listed above have assays that are already commercially available for clinical use. Overall, it appears that several biomarkers, used either alone or in combination, will be useful tools for the early diagnosis of AKI in the near future.

THE DIAGNOSTIC APPROACH TO ACUTE KIDNEY INJURY

The basic diagnostic approach to patients with AKI includes a detailed history and examination, urinalysis, selected urine chemistries, and imaging of the urinary tree. The history should focus on the tempo of loss of function (if known), associated systemic diseases, and symptoms related to the urinary tract (especially those that suggest obstruction). A concise review of systemic diseases associated with renal dysfunction has been recently published.[23] We strongly believe that a review of the medications looking for potentially toxic drugs is essential. **Table 2** presents a list of some medications associated with AKI and illustrates the wide spectrum of possible patterns of injury. The physical examination is directed toward the identification of findings of a systemic disease and a detailed assessment of hemodynamic status. This latter goal often requires invasive

monitoring, especially in the oliguric patient with conflicting clinical findings, where the physical examination has limited accuracy.[24]

Excluding urinary tract obstruction is necessary in all cases. This can be achieved initially with a bladder scan or placement of a bladder catheter to rule out bladder outlet obstruction. It is also possible that a bladder catheter already in place can be obstructed, and this possibility should not be overlooked. In most cases, more detailed evaluation is indicated through radiologic evaluation of the urinary tree, most commonly with an ultrasound.

Microscopic evaluation of the urine sediment from a freshly voided urine sample is essential to the evaluation of AKI. Dysmorphic red blood cells and red blood cell casts suggest glomerulonephritis or vasculitis. Sterile pyuria or white blood cell casts should raise the possibility of interstitial nephritis. "Muddy brown" casts (heavily pigmented casts resulting from tubular cell debris) and/or tubular epithelial cell casts are typically seen in patients with acute tubular necrosis (ATN). Their presence is an important tool in the distinction between ATN and prerenal azotemia, which is characterized by a normal sediment, or by occasional hyaline casts. Eosinophiluria, which is often used to screen for interstitial nephritis, has limited specificity and positive predictive value, since it can be seen in other conditions associated with AKI such as acute glomerulonephritis and atheroembolic renal disease, as well as other common diseases in acutely ill patients, such as pyelonephritis, and prostatitis.[25,26]

Distinguishing between the two most common causes of AKI (prerenal azotemia and ATN) is often difficult, especially because the clinical examination is often misleading in the setting of mild volume depletion or overload.[24] Urinary chemistries are routinely used to help in this distinction. The most discerning test is the fractional excretion of sodium (FENa = U/P Na: U/P creatinine × 100). Values of less than 1% are seen in prerenal azotemia, whereas values greater than 3% are seen in ATN (1%–3% is the diagnostic "gray zone" for this test). A frequent problem in the interpretation of the FENa is the concomitant use of diuretics, which may result in a high FENa despite a low effective circulating volume. To address this problem, investigators have tested the value of the fractional excretion of urea (FEurea = U/P urea nitrogen: U/P creatinine × 100). A prospective study indicated that the FEurea identifies patients who have prerenal azotemia despite the use of diuretics,[27] confirming previous retrospective observations.[28] Cutoff values for FEurea are less than 35% for prerenal azotemia and greater than 50% for ATN. A recent study was unable to corroborate

Table 2
The spectrum of acute kidney injury induced by drugs used in the acute care setting

Type of Renal Injury	Drugs
Induction of volume depletion	Diuretics
Changes in intra-renal hemodynamics that amplify renal sensitivity to hypoperfusion	NSAIDs (including selective COX-2 inhibitors), ACE inhibitors, Angiotensin-2 receptor blockers, renin inhibitors, cyclosporine/tacrolimus, vasopressor agents
Glomerular injury	
Glomerulonephritis	NSAIDs, zoledronate, pamidronate
Microangiopathy	Ticlopidine, clopidogrel, cyclosporine, gemcitabine
Tubular injury	Iodinated contrast, aminoglycosides, amphotericin B, pentamidine, foscarnet, cisplatinum, acetaminophen, cidofovir, adefovir, tenofovir, melphalan, IVIG, hetastarch, mannitol
Interstitial nephritis	NSAIDs, beta-lactams, quinolones, sulfonamides, phenytoin, allopurinol, diuretics (thiazides, loop), indinavir, proton pump inhibitors
Obstruction of the urinary tract	
Crystal deposition (intra-renal obstruction)	Indinavir, sulfadiazine, sulfamethoxazole, methotrexate, high-dose acyclovir
Retroperitoneal fibrosis (ureteral obstruction)	Ergotamine, sotalol, propranolol, bromocriptine (all rare)

Abbreviations: ACE, angiotensin-converting enzyme; COX, cyclooxygenase; IVIG, intravenous immunoglobulin; NSAID, nonsteroidal anti-inflammatory drug.

these observations;[29] however, this latter study used a definition of "transient AKI" (return of serum creatinine to baseline over a 7-day period) as the equivalent of prerenal azotemia, and only 37% of these patients had reached baseline by the third day following the diagnosis of AKI. Therefore, one could certainly argue that many of these patients had some degree of tubular injury that went beyond prerenal azotemia. Therefore, while these data appear to indicate that FEurea is not a good test to distinguish between "transient" and "permanent" AKI, our current interpretation, which is corroborated by our clinical experience, is that the FEurea is valuable to distinguish prerenal azotemia and ATN, especially in patients receiving diuretics.

Biomarkers of tubular injury, some of them discussed in the section above, have been explored to refine this distinction by allowing the detection of lesser degrees of tubular injury.[30] NGAL, IL-18, and KIM-1 may have value in distinguishing ATN from other etiologies of AKI. An important recent paper analyzed the etiology of renal dysfunction in 635 patients seen in an emergency department.[31] It demonstrated that NGAL successfully identified patients with AKI (area under the curve for diagnosis = 0.948). NGAL, alpha-1 microglobulin, N-acetyl glycosamine, and FENa successfully distinguished between ATN and prerenal azotemia, with NGAL having the best discriminating ability. With the exception of the FENa, these markers could also distinguish between ATN and chronic kidney disease. On the other hand, only the FENa could distinguish between prerenal azotemia and chronic kidney disease.[31] Therefore, it appears that the use of new biomarkers may also add to our ability to distinguish between different etiologies of AKI. Ongoing studies are analyzing this issue in greater detail, also addressing the combined use of several proteins to improve specificity.

RISKS ASSOCIATED WITH GADOLINIUM EXPOSURE IN PATIENTS WITH ACUTE KIDNEY INJURY

An issue of great concern to clinical nephrologists is the association between gadolinium exposure and nephrogenic systemic fibrosis, a devastating fibrotic disease, affecting primarily the skin.[32] While this disease was initially described among patients with end-stage kidney disease on dialysis, approximately 10% of cases occur in patients with chronic kidney disease not on dialysis.[33] Of relevance, this disease has been reported in patients with severe AKI.[32,33] Until these issues are resolved, we recommend that patients with AKI do not receive gadolinium. In cases when a magnetic resonance study demands contrast, one should avoid the potentially more toxic agents (gadodiamide [Omniscan] and gadopentetate dimeglumine [Magnevist]),[34] and the patient or surrogate should sign an informed consent form. For patients on dialysis, hemodialysis should be performed immediately following exposure to gadolinium although it should be noted that dialysis has not been shown to diminish the risk of development of nephrogenic systemic fibrosis.[32]

RENAL REPLACEMENT THERAPY IN ACUTE KIDNEY INJURY

The spectrum of choices of RRT for the management of critically ill patients with AKI has grown continuously since the commencement of dialysis for clinical use. Contemporary renal support is now provided via a panoply of intermittent to continuous methods using a host of biocompatible membranes and an increasing spectrum of anticoagulation methodologies, as detailed in an excellent recent systematic review.[35] What will be discussed here are the results of several recent randomized controlled trials (RCTs) specifically examining the effect of "dose" and modality of RRT on outcomes in AKI. The genesis of these trials arose from observations gleaned from several descriptive studies conducted over the past 2 decades.

Dialysis Modality

Ten years ago, the National Kidney Foundation[36] surveyed American nephrologists about their preferences and practice in the management of AKI. It was identified that intermittent hemodialysis (IHD) was the preferred modality for renal support, was used in more than 75% of cases by most nephrologists, while continuous renal replacement therapy (CRRT) and peritoneal dialysis (PD) were used in a minority of treatments (<10%) according most practitioners. More recently, a survey of intensivists and nephrologists practicing at participating sites of the multicenter ATN Study, suggests that IHD remains the most frequently used modality of renal support, estimated to be used in 57% of treatments. However, CRRT is gaining in popularity in the United States and is now reported to account for over a third (36%) of prescribed RRT treatments.[37] The Program to Improve Care in Acute Renal Disease (PICARD) observational study mirrored the new survey results. Among the five participating US tertiary care centers in the PICARD study, IHD was the modality of RRT used in the greatest percentage of patients, but CRRT use had become such commonplace practice that 60% of dialyzed patients had received CRRT for some or all of their renal support.[4] Notably, there was substantial intersite variability in modality preference.

In contrast to the reported US experience, a recent survey of an international multidisciplinary cohort of renal practitioners showed that continuous therapies had become the norm for AKI support outside of the United States.[38] Confirming the international survey results, the multinational prospective epidemiologic Beginning and Ending Supportive Therapy for the Kidney (BEST Kidney) Study of ARF in the ICU reported that CRRT was the initial modality of choice for RRT support in the ICU used in 80% of treatments, distantly followed by IHD (17%).[1]

Preference for CRRT over IHD in the management of more severely ill patients with AKI has been attributed to a presumed survival advantage conveyed by the continuous modality.[39] Several rational theories justifying this presumption have been proffered. For example, in light of CRRT's demonstrated ability to enhance clearance of certain humoral inflammatory cytokines, its use, particularly in high volume, has the potential to restore immunomodulatory balance and improve survival.[40,41] Others have opined that CRRT's presumed survival advantage is related to its greater hemodynamic stability over IHD. However, meta-analyses of earlier trials comparing survival of unselected critically ill patients with AKI assigned to either IHD or CRRT and adjusted for severity of illness have not been able to substantiate the presumed superiority of CRRT.[42,43] Recent prospective evidence has also challenged the advantages of CRRT, particularly with regard to superiority of hemodynamic stability.[44–46] In addition, observational and several prospective RCTs explicitly comparing intermittent and continuous modalities have failed to confirm the expected survival advantage of CRRT.[44,45,47,48]

Reasonable criticisms countering the RCTs that compared modalities have been made. First, the dose of dialysis prescribed in both the IHD and the CRRT arms of earlier studies were below what has subsequently been recommended as a minimally acceptable level, thus prohibiting a fair comparison between adequate IHD and adequate CRRT.[47,49] Second, a relatively high crossover rate between modalities became evident, potentially affecting each study's analytic design.[47] Third, randomization failure occurred in one study resulting in differences in baseline covariates that were independently associated with mortality and biased in favor of IHD.[47] The results of the more recent RCTs comparing modalities in unselected critically ill patient populations have been similarly challenged for high crossover rates, as well as limited trial power and nonstandardization of dialysis protocols.[44,48]

In an attempt to address the limitations of the previous RCTs comparing intermittent and continuous modalities of RRT, a large multicenter study ("Hemodiasafe") was conducted that used standardized dialysis protocols and targeted doses of RRT to meet current recommendations. Hemodynamic stability was optimized for patients treated with IHD through the use of extended time, cool dialysate, sodium modeling, bicarbonate dialysate, and isovolemic initiation of IHD.[45] Again, no difference in 60-day survival (33% versus 32% of CCRT versus IHD) or of renal recovery was found. A low rate (6%) of modality crossover was maintained by the use of policies guiding modality switches and no difference in the incidence of adverse events, including hypotension, was identified.

The premise of CRRT modality superiority was further refuted recently by the PICARD investigators. A subgroup analysis of patients with AKI requiring RRT derived from this multicenter observational study compared survival by initial RRT modality assignment.[50] Despite adjustment for potential confounding variables and modality selection via a propensity score approach, CRRT was in fact associated with increased 60-day mortality as compared with IHD.

How can these negative results be reconciled with the widely accepted premise of the superiority of CRRT? First, earlier studies comparing modalities compared results obtained with more contemporary CRRT to those obtained from historical controls treated with IHD.[47,51] Such comparisons may have erroneously attributed the survival advantage conferred by improvements in nonmodality aspects of care, such as the development of biocompatible membranes and better critical care services, to modality selection instead. Second, developments in IHD technology to improve its effectiveness and tolerability have perhaps been underappreciated. An unexplained improvement in the survival rate of the IHD cohort was noted during the course of the Hemodiasafe Study that was not attributable to changes in patient characteristics or center effects, suggesting that improvements in the standard of care for IHD subjects had occurred.[45] Closer scrutiny revealed that an unrecognized drift toward greater delivery of dialysis had occurred that may have modified the relative benefit of one modality versus another. In fact, an increasing quantity of estimated dialysis dose was also found in the CRRT arm of the Hemodiasafe study, but in the absence of direct measurement of IHD dose, further comparison of relative dose change is not possible. Third, the theoretic advantage of CRRT conferred by its ability to remove cytokines has been questioned. While CRRT has been shown to be capable of removing cytokines, the high cytokine generation rate, particularly during sepsis, may require an impractical increase in effluent volume or in membrane flux to realize a physiologically relevant impact on the inflammatory cascade and to effectively restore immunohomeostasis.[52,53]

The lack of a clear advantage of conventional CRRT over IHD, in conjunction with its increased costs (nearly twofold that of IHD), have led to an expanding interest in hybrid modalities that exploit the best attributes of both intermittent and continuous therapies.[47] Among the recently evolving continuous therapies, continuous high-flux dialysis (CHFD) and/or high volume hemofiltration (HVHF) have the potential to better facilitate removal of middle molecular weight solutes that may be particularly important in the management of sepsis-associated AKI.[53–55] The High Volume in Intensive Care (IVOIRE) study (NCT 00241228) is an ongoing HVHF trial examining 28-day mortality in patients treated with standard (35 mL/kg/h) versus high-volume (70 mL/kg/h) continuous hemofiltration and is scheduled for completion in the near future.

Preliminary studies of hybridized intermittent therapies have also been recently reported. A pilot study comparing the effect of super high-flux/high molecular weight cutoff (HCO) IHD to standard high-flux (HF) IHD in 10 septic patients found that HCO-IHD achieved better diffusive clearance of cytokines and decreased plasma cytokine levels as compared with HF-IHD.[56] Accelerated venovenous hemofiltration (AVVH) is another evolving intermittent therapy, which performs hemofiltration discontinuously, ie, daily but within a compressed time frame. A retrospective review of the experience of one center's use of AVVH demonstrated that large volumes of hemofiltration (36 L) could be delivered in a compressed/intermittent time frame (9 hours), and effectively mitigate the drawback of continuous modalities, which is the need for anticoagulation.[57]

Sustained low-efficiency dialysis (SLED) or extended daily dialysis (EDD) is probably the most familiar hybrid therapy known to intensivists and nephrologists, having been described as a modified form of IHD nearly 20 years ago.[58] Most often delivered by dual-capacity IHD machines, it is typically prescribed from 6 to 12 hours per treatment with modified blood and dialysate flow rates (70–250 and 70–300 mL/min, respectively).[59] Excellent small molecular weight solute clearance and arguably equivalent hemodynamic stability as compared with CRRT have been reported.[60,61] Conceivably, the future of extracorporeal renal support for AKI may be a hybrid of hybrid techniques! Daily SLED using HCO membranes in a diffusive fashion or delivery of HVHF over a compressed period could potentially achieve excellent small and middle molecular weight solute clearance, without anticoagulation and without sacrificing hemodynamic tolerability. Because there is limited information on the combined clinical use of these hybrid therapies, the precise role of these various modalities in the management of AKI remains to be defined.

In summary, no consensus concerning the choice of RRT modality for the treatment of AKI exists. Although CRRT is gaining in popularity in the United States and worldwide, practice patterns vary substantially by region. No evidence currently supports the superiority of one continuous modality over another, or of continuous over intermittent treatment. Choice of RRT modality, therefore, should most properly remain determined by the preference and experience of the prescribing physician, and the technologic, fiscal, and nursing resources available to deliver RRT. An ongoing multicenter international observational ICU study, the Dose Response Multicenter International (Do-Re-Mi) trial, is designed to further elaborate on current RRT practice patterns and how RRT is chosen and administered.[62] Hybrid therapies hold promise for combining the best of all extracorporeal modalities.

Dialysis Dose

Historically, trials examining the impact of renal support in critical illness have focused on modulation of "dose" of treatment. In the early years of RRT, comparisons were made between historical cohorts of patients with AKI who were initiated on RRT and maintained at advanced degrees of azotemia (BUN >200 mg/dL) and those treated and maintained at more modest levels of azotemia (BUN 100–150 mg/dL).[63–65] Because mortality was drastically reduced by earlier initiation and greater reduction of azotemia, the timing of initiation and dose of RRT required was adjusted to maintain the patient at progressively lower levels of BUN.[66–68]

More recently, instead of prescribing RRT to achieve an absolute BUN level, quantification of dialysis dose has used the concept of urea clearance, exported from the field of chronic hemodialysis. For IHD it is described by a unit-less parameter: KT/V_{urea}. Arguably, the physiology of the patient with AKI nullifies several of the mathematical assumptions underlying the calculation of KT/V_{urea}, however in the absence of a more representative measure of dialysis dose, KT/V_{urea} has been used by default. When considering dose for intermittent modalities, frequency of treatment must also be considered. In CRRT, the measurement of dose of renal support is different, but simpler than in IHD. In CRRT, because of the low blood and dialysate flow rates used, the ultrafiltrate generated is isotonic to blood with respect to urea nitrogen. Therefore, effluent volume is used as a surrogate for urea clearance. Obviously, direct comparison of urea removal measured by effluent volume in CRRT to KT/V_{urea} measured in IHD is limited.

In the past decade, five single-center clinical trials involving critically ill patients with AKI requiring renal support have examined the effect of dose, quantified by KT/V_{urea} or effluent volume, on mortality.[69–73]

The first and only IHD trial compared daily versus alternate day IHD and reported a mortality benefit conferred by daily treatment.[69] This trial has been criticized on several accounts, including nonrandom treatment assignment, the floating end point of "14 days after the last session of dialysis," the limited representativeness of the enrolled population, and suboptimal per treatment dialysis dose, leading to the more limited conclusion that suboptimal delivery of dialysis results in suboptimal outcomes. Importantly, this study did highlight the exceptional difficulty in achieving solute clearance in the critically ill noting an average KT/V_{urea} of less than 1 in both treatment arms despite a minimum prescribed dose equal to 1.2.

Four other studies have examined the effect of differing weight-based doses of CRRT on outcomes. The first study suggested that CRRT effluent volume of 35 mL/kg/h was superior to 20 mL/kg/h with respect to survival 15 days after discontinuation of therapy and that no incremental benefit was achieved from prescribing a higher effluent volume (ie, > 35 mL/kg/h).[70] Similarly, another investigation reported improved 28-day survival by augmenting CVVH of 25 mL/kg/h by an additional 18 mL/kg/h of dialysate suggesting that additional small solute clearance was important in modifying outcomes.[72]

Other trials, however, have come to the opposite conclusion. A two-center randomized controlled trial comparing outcome of critically ill oliguric patients treated with "high-" (45 mL/kg/h) versus "low-" (20 mL/kg/h) volume CVVH found no difference in 28-day mortality between groups.[71] Although criticized for being potentially underpowered, this study's results were confirmed recently by other investigators who found no difference in 30-day survival between patients treated with CVVHDF at 35 versus 20 mL/kg/h.[73]

The only multicenter trial designed to examine the effect of dose or "intensity" of renal support on mortality in the critically ill with AKI was recently published.[74] The Acute Renal Failure Trial Network (ATN) Study was a very large trial that uniquely used integrated strategies of renal support mirroring customary practice rather than restricting RRT to a single modality, which would have limited the generalizability of its results.[4,75] Also distinct in study design was the per-treatment IHD delivered dose, set at a target KT/V_{urea} of 1.2, which was higher than in other comparable studies. Hemodynamically stable patients (Cardiovascular SOFA ≤ 2) were treated with IHD, whereas hemodynamically unstable patients (Cardiovascular SOFA > 2) were assigned to CVVHDF or SLED based on local practice. Subjects were randomized to either of the two interventional arms: the intensive management strategy (IMS) consisted of six times weekly IHD or SLED or CVVHDF at 35 mL/kg/h; the less intensive management strategy (LIMS) consisted of thrice-weekly IHD or SLED or CVVHDF at 20 mL/kg/h. No significant difference in hospital- or 60-day survival was found, nor of any other secondary end point including recovery of renal function or rate of nonrenal organ failure.

The results of the ATN Study should not be misconstrued to mean that "dose" does not matter. Instead they suggest that dose of RRT beyond a delivered KT/V_{urea} of 1.2 thrice weekly for patients managed with IHD or SLED, and beyond a total effluent flow rate of 20 mL/kg/h for patients managed with CVVHDF is not helpful in reducing overall mortality nor is it associated with improved renal recovery in survivors.[74]

Ongoing clinical trials that may contribute additional understanding of the impact of RRT dose on patient outcomes include the Randomized Evaluation of Normal versus Augmented Level of renal replacement therapy in ICU (RENAL) Study (NCT 00221013), a large multicenter RCT being conducted in Australia of CVVHDF in severe AKI in ICU comparing 90-day mortality of patients treated with an "augmented" effluent flow rate of 40 mL/kg/h versus patients treated with a "normal" flow rate of 25 mL/kg/h. Approximately one third of the prespecified total trial population (N = 1500) has been enrolled and trial completion is anticipated in late 2008.

Another multicenter trial, the IVOIRE study (NCT 00241228), is under way in France. It is a prospective RCT comparing outcomes of patients treated with high-volume (70 mL/kg/h) to "standard" volume (35 mL/kg/h) CVVH in patients with septic shock and AKI. Initiated in 2005, enrollment of a total of 460 patients is expected by the end of 2008.

Surprisingly, despite the body of trials examining dose of RRT support, all survey and observational studies of RRT support published to date convey quite clearly that the concept of "dose" in RRT in the ICU has been largely ignored or at least not fully adopted by practicing clinicians.[36–38,62] Reluctance to adopt any targeted "dosing" of RRT may stem from the belief that toxicity of AKI is only partially related to small solute clearance, and thus prescription focused only on its modification should not be expected to yield substantial improvement in outcomes. Urea clearance, regardless of how great it is or by which modality of renal support it is achieved, tells us nothing about middle molecular weight or cytokine clearance or other aspects of the uremic state that may also be important in influencing outcomes. An excellent review of uremic retention solutes and their toxicity has been recently published.[76] Non-urea small molecular weight solute, as well as middle and large molecular weight solutes may not be differentially impacted or may even be negatively impacted by prescriptions of RRT that further enhance urea clearance. Also, AKI is a state of extreme inflammation, and RRT of any modality may be associated with exacerbation rather than amelioration of the state of inflammation.[77] It is reasonably possible, therefore, that any benefit derived from enhanced urea clearance by RRT, beyond a minimum threshold, is offset by the counteracting increase in the inflammatory state induced by increasing exposure to RRT.

It is becoming evident that achievement of further improvement in outcomes of critically ill patients with AKI will require alternate strategies of care beyond RRT modality selection or increasing the dose of RRT beyond a minimum threshold. Recent trials examining unifactorial treatment of complex disease illustrate the limitations of this approach.[78,79] AKI is a pathophysiologically complex disease that likely requires a multifaceted approach if treatment is to be successful. More comprehensive strategies of RRT and facilitated recovery from AKI are fortunately on the horizon.[80]

SELECT PHARMACOLOGIC INTERVENTIONS AND FUTURE DIRECTIONS

Prior pharmacotherapeutic trials of AKI have been disappointing. Reasons for the failure of the multitude of agents that have been trialed are detailed in a concise review.[81] More recent appreciation of AKI as a multisystem disorder triggered by widespread stereotypical molecular responses to injury has caused a reconsideration of the strategic approach toward AKI and its treatment. Interventional strategies that target pathways involved in the early systemic response to AKI, or broad treatment strategies to address its protean systemic manifestations are being actively explored.

Of the emerging pharmacologic agents for the treatment of AKI, two that are currently in use as co-interventions in critical illness are intensive insulin therapy (IIT) and erythropoietin (EPO).

Intensive Insulin Therapy and Glycemic Management in Acute Kidney Injury

Hyperglycemia has emerged as an important predictor of outcomes of critical illness, including the outcome of renal failure.[82–87] The effect of the treatment of hyperglycemia on outcomes, including the development of AKI, has thus been of great interest to investigators and has been a focus of recent studies.

One such study was a large observational trial of a mixed ICU patient population in which a historical ICU cohort was compared with a contemporary one of consecutively admitted patients who were treated with insulin to achieve moderate glycemic control (serum glucose < 140 mg/dL). This study demonstrated that glycemic control achieved with insulin treatment resulted in a startling reduction in hospital mortality (from 29.3% to 10.8%) and in the incidence of acute renal failure (by 75%) defined as an increase of serum creatinine by 1 mg/dL or a doubling of serum creatinine.[84]

The landmark study that put glycemic control on the map was a multicenter RCT using an insulin-based protocol in the treatment of patients admitted to a surgical ICU in Leuven, Belgium.[85] IIT to reduce serum glucose to less than 110 mg/dL, was associated with a significant reduction in ICU mortality (from 8% to 4.6%) and in the incidence of acute renal failure requiring RRT (8.2% to 4.8%, $P = .007$).

A subsequent prospective RCT broadening the application of IIT to the MICU population was unable to demonstrate a similar reduction in mortality or need for RRT, but did demonstrate a significant reduction in newly acquired kidney injury, from 8.9% to 5.9% ($P = .04$) defined as either a doubling of ICU admission serum creatinine or a peak serum creatinine greater than 2.5 mg/dL.[86]

A more recent secondary analysis of pooled data from the two RCTs comparing conventional therapy to IIT scrutinized the effect of IIT on the development of renal outcomes.[88] Overall, nearly 20% of the combined patient cohorts developed AKI, defined as a combined end point of patients classified with renal dysfunction according to modified (m) RIFLE criteria of m-RIFLE-F, I or F, or oliguria or need for RRT. Interestingly, while IIT significantly reduced the incidence of RIFLE-I/F from 7.6% to 4.5% ($P = .0006$), there was no effect of IIT on the incidence of the most severe renal outcomes (ie, need for RRT or oliguria), except in the surgical subset of patients where it was associated with a reduced need for RRT (4.0% versus 7.4% , $P = .003$) and a lower incidence of oliguria (2.6% versus 5.6%, $P = .003$) . The lower acuity of illness and premorbid disease in the surgical cohort as compared with the medical counterpart has led to the conclusion that IIT's beneficial effect is likely one of primary prevention of AKI rather than secondary reversal of established renal injury.

How IIT and glycemic control may affect renal outcomes in critical illness is complex and incompletely understood. Indirectly, dysglycemia may adversely impact renal function via accentuation of complications such as sepsis-associated AKI.[88] Directly, hyperglycemia may contribute to renal injury via accentuation of the acute inflammatory response and oxidative stress of critical illness.[87,89,90] IIT on the other hand, may prevent renal injury through favorable effects on serum lipids, which can act as scavengers of endotoxins.[91] IIT may also reduce renal injury via modulation of aberrant endothelial activation (ICAM and E-selectin) and deranged endothelial nitric oxide synthesis.[88]

IIT currently remains a controversial co-intervention in the management of patients with critical illness. Earlier recommendations for glucose management in the ICU[92] were heavily influenced by the Leuven trial[85,92]; however, aspects of the landmark study's design as well as its generalizability to all critically ill have recently been challenged.[93] In addition, two European RCTs (VISEP NCT 00135473 and GLUCONTROL, NCT 00220987) examining intensive glycemic control in the critically ill with and without septic shock were prematurely terminated because of safety concerns.[94]

Currently a large multicenter randomized trial (NICE-SUGAR; NCT 00220987) is under way to re-affirm or refute the Leuven study's findings in a heterogeneous critically ill population, and renal outcome as defined by the need for RRT is a predetermined secondary end point. Until the results of theses trials are available, prudence in the use of IIT and liberalization of glycemic control has been advocated.

Erythropoietin

Erythropoietin (EPO) is a hematopoietic cytokine that has been used in the management of the anemia of chronic kidney disease for 20 years. Recent studies have shown however that EPO's effects extend well beyond erythropoiesis. Erythropoietin receptors have been identified in a wide variety of tissues including neurons, endothelial cells, cardiac myocytes, vascular smooth muscle cells, mesangial cells, and renal proximal tubular cells.[95] In addition, EPO has been shown to result in a host of hematopoietic-independent cytoprotective effects in experimental models of neuronal, cardiac, hepatic, and acute renal ischemia: modulation of mitogenesis, vascular repair, oxidative stress, inflammation, and apoptosis have all been described.[96,97] Numerous in vitro and in vivo AKI models reported to date have examined EPO use as a preconditioning treatment to prevent AKI, but there is also a rationale for EPO's use as an accelerant in the recovery from ischemic injury through its vascular and anti-inflammatory effects.[97] As an initial exploration into the potential role of EPO as a renoprotective strategy in the critically ill, an open-label, randomized controlled trial has been initiated (NCT 00676234). This single-center study of medical and surgical ICU patients "at risk for AKI" will examine the effect of EPO, administered as either a single dose of 20,000 units or 40,000 units, on the short-term incidence of AKI as measured by a battery of standard and novel biomarkers of renal injury.

Tempering enthusiasm for the use of EPO are recent reports of an increased risk of adverse outcomes including increased cardiovascular morbidity and mortality in clinical trials investigating optimal EPO treatment of CKD patients.[98,99] A newly engineered desialated form of EPO mitigates the adverse effects associated with erythropoiesis. Known as asialo-EPO, this derivative has normal EPO receptor affinity but an extremely short half-life, which reduces its erythropoietic properties while retaining its cytoprotective effects.[95] Parenteral injection of asialo-EPO has been shown to reduce contrast-associated ischemic renal injury in an in vivo rat model without adverse effect on hematocrit.[95] Mechanistic investigations have recently shown that the asialo-EPO attenuates contrast-associated renal tubular cell apoptosis via modulation of the signal-transductive JAK2/STAT5 pathway with beneficial downstream effects on stress-responsive protein (eg, HSP70) expression and capsase-3 activation.[95] A comprehensive characterization of asialo-EPO's renoprotective effects as well as its clinical safety and optimal dosage in the prevention and facilitated recovery of AKI are exciting forefronts of investigation.

Bioartificial Kidney

Currently available RRT is essentially designed to facilitate solute and water clearance. This approach hardly mimics the expansive metabolic and endocrinological functions of the human kidney and may explain the limited impact that RRT has had on survival in patients with AKI. A visionary strategy toward the treatment of AKI that addresses these previously overlooked functions of the kidney is the bioartificial kidney. Also known as the renal tubular assist device (RAD), the bioartificial kidney consists of a hemofiltration cartridge lined with nonautologous human renal tubule cells along the inner surface of hollow fibers within the device. Preclinical studies of the device showed that the cells within were able to perform renal transport and endocrine and metabolic functions.[100,101] Subsequent large animal studies using the RAD in series with a conventional hemofilter in the treatment of sepsis-associated AKI demonstrated a substantial reduction in multiorgan dysfunction.[102] Initial results of phase I/II trials using the RAD in conjunction with CRRT in critically ill patients with AKI have demonstrated a near halving of mortality.[103,104] Notwithstanding the valid criticisms of the preliminary studies pertaining to design and analysis, the initial clinical results are nothing short of remarkable.[105] Although substantial hurdles remain before the RAD might be a routine therapeutic intervention in the treatment of AKI, the revolutionary design of the device and its early trial results offer prophetic evidence that genuine biological mimicry is at hand and that we might soon be able to positively impact the health of critically ill patients with AKI in a meaningful way.

Summary

In conclusion, AKI is a common illness in the hospitalized population and is associated with significant mortality. New diagnostic criteria using small changes in creatinine and urine output have been developed to facilitate diagnosis and aide in prognosis as well. A host of biomarkers are in development that will allow for effective interdiction of AKI and earlier intervention with pharmacotherapies such as IIT and modified erythropoietin to prevent and facilitate renal recovery. Renal replacement therapy for AKI is evolving toward a hybridized modality approach to exploit the benefits of different modalities. Recently completed studies suggest that excessive solute removal does not yield incremental benefit, thus we must reevaluate how to optimize the replacement of renal function beyond simply escalating dose. A more comprehensive approximation of the normal human kidney may be available shortly in the form of the bioartificial kidney.

REFERENCES

1. Uchino S, Kellum JA, Bellomo R, ot al. Acute renal failure in critically ill patients: a multinational, multicenter study. JAMA 2005;294(7):813–8.
2. Liano F, Junco E, Pascual J, et al. The spectrum of acute renal failure in the intensive care unit compared with that seen in other settings. The Madrid Acute Renal Failure Study Group. Kidney Int Suppl 1998;66:S16–24.
3. Guerin C, Girard R, Selli JM, et al. Initial versus delayed acute renal failure in the intensive care unit. A multicenter prospective epidemiological study. Rhone-Alpes Area Study Group on Acute Renal Failure. Am J Respir Crit Care Med 2000; 161(3 Pt 1):872–9.
4. Mehta RL, Pascual MT, Soroko S, et al. Spectrum of acute renal failure in the intensive care unit: the PICARD experience. Kidney Int 2004;66(4): 1613–21.
5. Mehta RL, Kellum JA, Shah SV, et al. Acute Kidney Injury Network: report of an initiative to improve outcomes in acute kidney injury. Crit Care 2007;11(2): R31.
6. Ricci Z, Cruz D, Ronco C. The RIFLE criteria and mortality in acute kidney injury: a systematic review. Kidney Int 2008;73(5):538–46.
7. Cruz DN, Bolgan I, Perazella MA, et al. North East Italian Prospective Hospital Renal Outcome Survey on Acute Kidney Injury (NEiPHROS-AKI): targeting the problem with the RIFLE Criteria. Clin J Am Soc Nephrol 2007;2(3):418–25.
8. Barrantes F, Tian J, Vazquez R, et al. Acute kidney injury criteria predict outcomes of critically ill patients. Crit Care Med 2008;36(5):1397–403.
9. Coca SG, Peixoto AJ, Garg AX, et al. The prognostic importance of a small acute decrement in kidney function in hospitalized patients: a systematic review and meta-analysis. Am J Kidney Dis 2007; 50(5):712–20.
10. Bagshaw SM, Laupland KB, Doig CJ, et al. Prognosis for long-term survival and renal recovery in critically ill patients with severe acute renal failure: a population-based study. Crit Care 2005;9(6): R700–9.
11. Oeyen S, Vandijck D, Benoit D, et al. Long-term outcome after acute kidney injury in critically-ill patients. Acta Clin Belg Suppl 2007;(2):337–40.
12. Morgera S, Kraft AK, Siebert G, et al. Long-term outcomes in acute renal failure patients treated with continuous renal replacement therapies. Am J Kidney Dis 2002;40(2):275–9.
13. Ahlstrom A, Tallgren M, Peltonen S, et al. Survival and quality of life of patients requiring acute renal replacement therapy. Intensive Care Med 2005; 31(9):1222–8.
14. Gopal I, Bhonagiri S, Ronco C, et al. Out of hospital outcome and quality of life in survivors of combined acute multiple organ and renal failure treated with continuous venovenous hemofiltration/hemodiafiltration. Intensive Care Med 1997;23(7):766–72.
15. Coca SG, Yalavarthy R, Concato J, et al. Biomarkers for the diagnosis and risk stratification of acute kidney injury: a systematic review. Kidney Int 2008;73(9):1008–16.
16. Parikh CR, Devarajan P. New biomarkers of acute kidney injury. Crit Care Med 2008;36(4 Suppl): S159–65.
17. Mishra J, Dent C, Tarabishi R, et al. Neutrophil gelatinase-associated lipocalin (NGAL) as a biomarker for acute renal injury after cardiac surgery. Lancet 2005;365(9466):1231–8.
18. Parikh CR, Abraham E, Ancukiewicz M, et al. Urine IL-18 is an early diagnostic marker for acute kidney injury and predicts mortality in the intensive care unit. J Am Soc Nephrol 2005;16(10):3046–52.
19. Herget-Rosenthal S, Marggraf G, Husing J, et al. Early detection of acute renal failure by serum cystatin C. Kidney Int 2004;66(3):1115–22.
20. Ahlstrom A, Tallgren M, Peltonen S, et al. Evolution and predictive power of serum cystatin C in acute renal failure. Clin Nephrol 2004;62(5):344–50.
21. Han WK, Waikar SS, Johnson A, et al. Urinary biomarkers in the early diagnosis of acute kidney injury. Kidney Int 2008;73(7):863–9.
22. Liangos O, Perianayagam MC, Vaidya VS, et al. Urinary N-acetyl-beta-(D)-glucosaminidase activity and kidney injury molecule-1 level are associated with adverse outcomes in acute renal failure. J Am Soc Nephrol 2007;18(3):904–12.
23. Rajashekar A, Perazella MA, Crowley S. Systemic diseases with renal manifestations. Prim Care 2008;35(2):297–328, vi–vii.
24. Peixoto AJ. Birth, death, and resurrection of the physical examination: clinical and academic perspectives on bedside diagnosis. Yale J Biol Med 2001;74(4):221–8.

25. Ruffing KA, Hoppes P, Blend D, et al. Eosinophils in urine revisited. Clin Nephrol 1994;41(3):163–6.

26. Nolan CR 3rd, Anger MS, Kelleher SP. Eosinophiluria—a new method of detection and definition of the clinical spectrum. N Engl J Med 1986; 315(24):1516–9.

27. Carvounis CP, Nisar S, Guro-Razuman S. Significance of the fractional excretion of urea in the differential diagnosis of acute renal failure. Kidney Int 2002;62(6):2223–9.

28. Kaplan AA, Kohn OF. Fractional excretion of urea as a guide to renal dysfunction. Am J Nephrol 1992;12(1–2):49–54.

29. Pepin MN, Bouchard J, Legault L, et al. Diagnostic performance of fractional excretion of urea and fractional excretion of sodium in the evaluations of patients with acute kidney injury with or without diuretic treatment. Am J Kidney Dis 2007;50(4): 566–73.

30. Han WK, Bonventre JV. Biologic markers for the early detection of acute kidney injury. Curr Opin Crit Care 2004;10(6):476–82.

31. Nickolas TL, O'Rourke MJ, Yang J, et al. Sensitivity and specificity of a single emergency department measurement of urinary neutrophil gelatinase-associated lipocalin for diagnosing acute kidney injury. Ann Intern Med 2008;148(11):810–9.

32. Knopp EA, Cowper SE. Nephrogenic systemic fibrosis: early recognition and treatment. Semin Dial 2008;21(2):123–8.

33. Abu-Alfa A. The impact of NSF on the care of patients with kidney disease. J Am Coll Radiol 2008; 5(1):45–52.

34. Reilly RF. Risk for nephrogenic systemic fibrosis with gadoteridol (ProHance) in patients who are on long-term hemodialysis. Clin J Am Soc Nephrol 2008;3(3):747–51.

35. Pannu N, Klarenbach S, Wiebe N, et al. Alberta Kidney Disease N: Renal replacement therapy in patients with acute renal failure: a systematic review. JAMA 2008;299(7):793–805.

36. Mehta RL, Letteri JM. Current status of renal replacement therapy for acute renal failure. A survey of US nephrologists. The National Kidney Foundation Council on Dialysis. Am J Nephrol 1999; 19(3):377–82.

37. Overberger P, Pesacreta M, Palevsky PM, et al. Management of renal replacement therapy in acute kidney injury: a survey of practitioner prescribing practices. Clin J Am Soc Nephrol 2007;2(4):623–30.

38. Ricci Z, Ronco C, D'Amico G, et al. Practice patterns in the management of acute renal failure in the critically ill patient: an international survey. Nephrol Dial Transplant 2006;21(3):690–6.

39. Chang JW, Yang WS, Seo JW, et al. Continuous venovenous hemodiafiltration versus hemodialysis as renal replacement therapy in patients with acute renal failure in the intensive care unit. Scand J Urol Nephrol 2004;38(5):417–21.

40. Kellum JA, Johnson JP, Kramer D, et al. Diffusive vs. convective therapy: effects on mediators of inflammation in patients with severe systemic inflammatory response syndrome. Crit Care Med 1998;26(12):1995–2000.

41. Piccinni P, Dan M, Barbacini S, et al. Early isovolaemic haemofiltration in oliguric patients with septic shock. Intensive Care Med 2006;32(1):80–6.

42. Tonelli M, Manns B, Feller-Kopman D. Acute renal failure in the intensive care unit: a systematic review of the impact of dialytic modality on mortality and renal recovery. Am J Kidney Dis 2002;40(5): 875–85.

43. Kellum JA, Angus DC, Johnson JP, et al. Continuous versus intermittent renal replacement therapy: a meta-analysis. Intensive Care Med 2002;28(1): 29–37.

44. Uehlinger DE, Jakob SM, Ferrari P, et al. Comparison of continuous and intermittent renal replacement therapy for acute renal failure. Nephrol Dial Transplant 2005;20(8):1630–7.

45. Vinsonneau C, Camus C, Combes A, et al. Continuous venovenous haernodiafiltration versus intermittent haemodialysis for acute renal failure in patients with multiple-organ dysfunction syndrome: a multicentre randomised trial. Lancet 2006; 368(9533):379–85.

46. Misset B, Timsit JF, Chevret S, et al. A randomized cross-over comparison of the hemodynamic response to intermittent hemodialysis and continuous hemofiltration in ICU patients with acute renal failure. Intensive Care Med 1996;22(8):742–6.

47. Mehta RL, McDonald B, Gabbai FB, et al. A randomized clinical trial of continuous versus intermittent dialysis for acute renal failure. Kidney Int 2001; 60(3):1154–63.

48. Augustine JJ, Sandy D, Seifert TH, et al. A randomized controlled trial comparing intermittent with continuous dialysis in patients with ARF. Am J Kidney Dis 2004;44(6):1000–7.

49. Kellum JA, Mehta RL, Angus DC, et al. The first international consensus conference on continuous renal replacement therapy. Kidney Int 2002;62(5): 1855–63.

50. Cho KC, Himmelfarb J, Paganini E, et al. Survival by dialysis modality in critically ill patients with acute kidney injury. J Am Soc Nephrol 2006; 17(11):3132–8.

51. Bellomo R, Farmer M, Wright C, et al. Treatment of sepsis-associated severe acute renal failure with continuous hemodiafiltration: clinical experience and comparison with conventional dialysis. Blood Purif 1995;13(5):246–54.

52. De Vriese AS, Colardyn FA, Philippe JJ, et al. Cytokine removal during continuous hemofiltration in

septic patients. J Am Soc Nephrol 1999;10(4): 846–53.

53. Ronco C, Kellum JA, Bellomo R, et al. Potential interventions in sepsis-related acute kidney injury. Clin J Am Soc Nephrol 2008;3(2):531–44.

54. Lonnemann G, Bechstein M, Linnenweber S, et al. Tumor necrosis factor-alpha during continuous high-flux hemodialysis in sepsis with acute renal failure. Kidney Int Suppl 1999;56(72):S84–7.

55. Brunet S, Leblanc M, Geadah D, et al. Diffusive and convective solute clearances during continuous renal replacement therapy at various dialysate and ultrafiltration flow rates. Am J Kidney Dis 1999; 34(3):486–92.

56. Haase M, Bellomo R, Baldwin I, et al. Hemodialysis membrane with a high-molecular-weight cutoff and cytokine levels in sepsis complicated by acute renal failure: a phase 1 randomized trial. Am J Kidney Dis 2007;50(2):296–304.

57. Gashti CN, Salcedo S, Robinson V, et al. Accelerated venovenous hemofiltration: early technical and clinical experience. Am J Kidney Dis 2008; 51(5):804–10.

58. Tam PY, Huraib S, Mahan B, et al. Slow continuous hemodialysis for the management of complicated acute renal failure in an intensive care unit. Clin Nephrol 1988;30(2):79–85.

59. Fliser D, Kielstein JT. Technology insight: treatment of renal failure in the intensive care unit with extended dialysis. Nat Clin Pract Nephrol 2006;2(1): 32–9.

60. Marshall MR, Golper TA, Shaver MJ, et al. Sustained low-efficiency dialysis for critically ill patients requiring renal replacement therapy. [erratum appears in Kidney Int 2001;60(4):1629]. Kidney Int 2001;60(2):777–85.

61. Kumar VA, Craig M, Depner TA, et al. Extended daily dialysis: a new approach to renal replacement for acute renal failure in the intensive care unit. Am J Kidney Dis 2000;36(2):294–300.

62. Kindgen-Milles D, Journois D, Fumagalli R, et al. Study protocol: the DOse REsponse Multicentre International collaborative initiative (DO-RE-MI). Crit Care 2005;9(4):R396–406.

63. Teschan PE, Baxter CR, O'Brien TF, et al. Prophylactic hemodialysis in the treatment of acute renal failure. Annals of Internal Medicine, 53:992–1016, 1960. J Am Soc Nephrol 1998; 9(12):2384–97.

64. Teschan PE, Baxter CR, O'Brien TF, et al. Prophylactic hemodialysis in the treatment of acute renal failure. Ann Intern Med 1960;53:992–1016.

65. Fischer RP, Griffen WO Jr, Reiser M, et al. Early dialysis in the treatment of acute renal failure. Surg Gynecol Obstet 1966;123(5):1019–23.

66. Kleinknecht D, Jungers P, Chanard J, et al. Uremic and non-uremic complications in acute renal failure: evaluation of early and frequent dialysis on prognosis. Kidney Int 1972;1(3):190–6.

67. Conger JD. A controlled evaluation of prophylactic dialysis in post-traumatic acute renal failure. J Trauma 1975;15(12):1056–63.

68. Gillum DM, Dixon BS, Yanover MJ, et al. The role of intensive dialysis in acute renal failure. Clin Nephrol 1986;25(5):249–55.

69. Schiffl H, Lang SM, Fischer R. Daily hemodialysis and the outcome of acute renal failure. N Engl J Med 2002;346(5):305–10.

70. Ronco C, Bellomo R, Homel P, et al. Effects of different doses in continuous veno-venous haemofiltration on outcomes of acute renal failure: a prospective randomised trial. Lancet 2000; 356(9223):26–30.

71. Bouman CSC, Oudemans-Van Straaten HM, Tijssen JGP, et al. Effects of early high-volume continuous venovenous hemofiltration on survival and recovery of renal function in intensive care patients with acute renal failure: a prospective, randomized trial. Crit Care Med 2002;30(10):2205–11.

72. Saudan P, Niederberger M, De Seigneux S, et al. Adding a dialysis dose to continuous hemofiltration increases survival in patients with acute renal failure [see comment]. Kidney Int 2006;70(7): 1312–7.

73. Tolwani AJ, Campbell RC, Stofan BS, et al. Standard versus high-dose CVVHDF for ICU-related acute renal failure. J Am Soc Nephrol 2008;19(6): 1233–8.

74. Network VNARFT, Palevsky PM, Zhang JH, et al. Intensity of renal support in critically ill patients with acute kidney injury. N Engl J Med 2008;359(1): 7–20.

75. Palevsky PM, O'Connor T, Zhang JH, et al. Design of the VA/NIH Acute Renal Failure Trial Network (ATN) Study: intensive versus conventional renal support in acute renal failure. Clin Trials 2005; 2(5):423–35.

76. Vanholder R, Baurmeister U, Brunet P, et al. A bench to bedside view of uremic toxins. J Am Soc Nephrol 2008;19(5):863–70.

77. Himmelfarb J, McMonagle E, Freedman S, et al. Oxidative stress is increased in critically ill patients with acute renal failure. J Am Soc Nephrol 2004; 15(9):2449–56.

78. Chiche J-D, Angus DC. Testing protocols in the intensive care unit: complex trials of complex interventions for complex patients [comment]. JAMA 2008;299(6):693–5.

79. Krumholz HM, Lee TH. Redefining quality—implications of recent clinical trials. N Engl J Med 2008;358(24):2537–9.

80. Humes HD. Cell therapy: leveraging nature's therapeutic potential [comment]. J Am Soc Nephrol 2003;14(8):2211–3.

81. Jo SK, Rosner MH, Okusa MD. Pharmacologic treatment of acute kidney injury: why drugs haven't worked and what is on the horizon. Clin J Am Soc Nephrol 2007;2(2):356–65.

82. Gandhi GY, Nuttall GA, Abel MD, et al. Intraoperative hyperglycemia and perioperative outcomes in cardiac surgery patients. Mayo Clin Proc 2005; 80(7):862–6.

83. Krinsley JS. Association between hyperglycemia and increased hospital mortality in a heterogeneous population of critically ill patients. Mayo Clin Proc 2003;78(12):1471–8.

84. Krinsley JS. Effect of an intensive glucose management protocol on the mortality of critically ill adult patients. [see comment] [erratum appears in Mayo Clin Proc. 2005 Aug;80(8):1101]. Mayo Clin Proc 2004;79(8):992–1000.

85. van den Berghe G, Wouters P, Weekers F, et al. Intensive insulin therapy in the critically ill patients. N Engl J Med 2001;345(19):1359–67.

86. Van den Berghe G, Wilmer A, Hermans G, et al. Intensive insulin therapy in the medical ICU. N Engl J Med 2006;354(5):449–61.

87. Basi S, Pupim LB, Simmons EM, et al. Insulin resistance in critically ill patients with acute renal failure. Am J Physiol Renal Physiol 2005;289(2):F259–64.

88. Schetz M, Vanhorebeek I, Wouters PJ, et al. Tight blood glucose control is renoprotective in critically ill patients. J Am Soc Nephrol 2008;19(3):571–8.

89. Collier B, Dossett LA, May AK, et al. Glucose control and the inflammatory response. Nutr Clin Pract 2008;23(1):3–15.

90. Sarafidis PA, Ruilope LM. Insulin resistance, hyperinsulinemia, and renal injury: mechanisms and implications. Am J Nephrol 2006;26(3):232–44.

91. Mesotten D, Swinnen JV, Vanderhoydonc F, et al. Contribution of circulating lipids to the improved outcome of critical illness by glycemic control with intensive insulin therapy. J Clin Endocrinol Metabol 2004;89(1):219–26.

92. Garber AJ, Moghissi ES, Bransome ED Jr, et al. American College of Endocrinology position statement on inpatient diabetes and metabolic control. Endocr Pract 2004;10(1):77–82.

93. Bellomo R, Egi M. Glycemic control in the intensive care unit: why we should wait for NICE-SUGAR. [comment]. Mayo Clin Proc 2005;80(12):1546–8.

94. Marik PE, Varon J. Intensive insulin therapy in the ICU: is it now time to jump off the bandwagon? Resuscitation 2007;74(1):191–3.

95. Yokomaku Y, Sugimoto T, Kume S, et al. Asialoerythropoietin prevents contrast-induced nephropathy. J Am Soc Nephrol 2008;19(2):321–8.

96. Hochhauser E, Pappo O, Ribakovsky E, et al. Recombinant human erythropoietin attenuates hepatic injury induced by ischemia/reperfusion in an isolated mouse liver model. Apoptosis 2008;13(1): 77–86.

97. Sturiale A, Campo S, Crasci E, et al. Experimental models of acute renal failure and erythropoietin: what evidence of a direct effect? Ren Fail 2007; 29(3):379–86.

98. Besarab A, Bolton WK, Browne JK, et al. The effects of normal as compared with low hematocrit values in patients with cardiac disease who are receiving hemodialysis and epoetin. N Engl J Med 1998;339(9):584–90.

99. Drueke TB, Locatelli F, Clyne N, et al. Normalization of hemoglobin level in patients with chronic kidney disease and anemia. N Engl J Med 2006;355(20): 2071–84.

100. Humes HD, Buffington DA, MacKay SM, et al. Replacement of renal function in uremic animals with a tissue-engineered kidney. Nat Biotechnol 1999;17(5):451–5.

101. Humes HD, MacKay SM, Funke AJ, et al. Tissue engineering of a bioartificial renal tubule assist device: in vitro transport and metabolic characteristics. Kidney Int 1999;55(6):2502–14.

102. Humes HD, Buffington DA, Lou L, et al. Cell therapy with a tissue-engineered kidney reduces the multiple-organ consequences of septic shock. Crit Care Med 2003;31(10):2421–8.

103. Humes HD, Weitzel WF, Bartlett RH, et al. Initial clinical results of the bioartificial kidney containing human cells in ICU patients with acute renal failure. Kidney Int 2004;66(4):1578–88.

104. Tumlin J, Wali R, Williams W, et al. Efficacy and safety of renal tubule cell therapy for acute renal failure. J Am Soc Nephrol 2008;19(5): 1034–40.

105. Chertow GM, Waikar SS. Toward the promise of renal replacement therapy. J Am Soc Nephrol 2008; 19(5):839–40.

Intra-Abdominal Hypertension: Evolving Concepts

Manu L.N.G. Malbrain, MD, PhD*, Inneke E. De laet, MD

KEYWORDS

- Abdominal pressure • Abdominal hypertension
- Abdominal compartment syndrome
- Measurement • Diagnosis • Pathophysiology
- Organ support • Treatment

A compartment syndrome (CS) exists when increased pressure in a closed anatomic space threatens the viability of enclosed tissue.[1] Within the body there are four types of compartments, the head, the chest, the abdomen, and the extremities, but when a compartment syndrome occurs in the abdominal cavity the impact on end-organ function both within and outside of the cavity can be devastating (**Table 1**). Intra-abdominal hypertension (IAH) is a graded phenomenon and can evolve to the end-stage abdominal compartment syndrome (ACS), which is an all or nothing phenomenon. The ACS is not a disease and as such it can have many causes and it can develop within many disease processes. The development of IAH is of extreme importance in the care of critically ill patients, because of the impact of increased intra-abdominal pressure (IAP) on end-organ function. Recent animal and human data suggest that the adverse effects of elevated IAP can occur at much lower levels than previously thought and even before the development of clinically overt ACS. This review gives a concise overview of the definitions, epidemiology, pathophysiology, and management of IAH and ACS.

DEFINITIONS

The term ACS was first used by Fietsam and colleagues[2] in the late 1980s to describe the pathophysiologic alterations resulting from IAH secondary to aortic aneurysm surgery: "In four patients that received more than 25 L of fluid resuscitation increased IAP developed after aneurysm repair. It was manifested by increased ventilatory pressure, increased central venous pressure, and decreased urinary output. This set of findings constitutes an *abdominal compartment syndrome* caused by massive interstitial and retroperitoneal swelling… Opening the abdominal incision was associated with dramatic improvements…."

The World Society on Abdominal Compartment Syndrome (WSACS, www.wsacs.org) was founded in 2004 to serve as a peer-reviewed forum and educational resource for all health care providers as well as industry who have an interest in IAH and ACS. Recently the first consensus definitions on IAH and ACS have been published.[1,3] **Table 2** summarizes these consensus definitions: a sustained increase in IAP equal to or above 12 mm Hg defines IAH where ACS is defined by a sustained IAP above 20 mm Hg with new-onset or progressive organ failure.

RECOGNITION OF ABDOMINAL COMPARTMENT SYNDROME
Clinical Awareness

Despite an escalation of the medical literature on the subject, there still appears to be an underrecognition of the syndrome. The results of several surveys on the physician's knowledge of IAH and ACS have recently been published.[4,5] The bottom line is that there is still a general lack of clinical

Intensive Care Unit, ZiekenhuisNetwerk Antwerpen, Campus Stuivenberg, Lange Beeldekensstraat 267, B-2060 Antwerpen 6, Belgium

* Corresponding author.

E-mail address: manu.malbrain@skynet.be (M.L.N.G. Malbrain).

Clin Chest Med 30 (2009) 45–70

doi:10.1016/j.ccm.2008.09.003

Table 1
The four compartments

	Head	Chest	Abdomen	Extremities
Syndrome	Cerebral herniation	Thoracic compartment syndrome	Abdominal compartment syndrome	Extremity compartment syndrome
Potential implication	Brain death	Cardiopulmonary collapse	Multiple organ dysfunction	Extremity loss
Primary physiologic parameter	Intracranial pressure (ICP)	Intrathoracic pressure (ITP)	Intra-abdominal pressure (IAP)	Extremity compartment pressures (CP)
Secondary parameter	Cerebral perfusion pressure (CPP)	Peak/mean airway pressure	Abdominal perfusion pressure (APP)	Peripheral arterial perfusion pressure
Fluid	Cerebrospinal fluid (CSF)	Pleural fluid	Ascites	Interstitial fluid
Enclosure	Skull	Rib cage	Abdominal cage	Muscle fascia
Therapeutic intervention	Lower ICP: CSF drainage; Increase CPP: vasopressors, fluids	Lower ITP: Escharotomy, chest tube	Lower IAP: ascites drainage; Increase APP: vasopressors, fluids	Lower CP
Resuscitative plan	Open compartment Decompressive craniectomy	Open compartment Decompressive sternotomy	Open compartment Decompressive laparotomy	Open compartment Decompressive fasciotomy
Importance	Adaptation of ventilatory support essential	Recognition of syndrome can be life saving	Prevention of bacterial translocation and MODS can be life saving	Recognition can be limb saving

Abbreviations: APP, abdominal perfusion pressure; CP, compartment pressure; CPP, cerebral perfusion pressure; CSF, cerebrospinal fluid; IAP, intra-abdominal pressure; ICP, intracranial pressure; ITP, intrathoracic pressure; MODS, multiple organ dysfunction syndrome.
Adapted from Cheatham M. Compartment syndrome. The four compartment syndromes. 2008. Available at: http://www.surgicalcriticalcare.net/Lectures/compartment_syndrome.pdf; with permission.

Table 2
Consensus definitions

Definition 1	IAP is the steady-state pressure concealed within the abdominal cavity.
Definition 2	APP = MAP − IAP
Definition 3	FG = GFP − PTP = MAP − 2 * IAP
Definition 4	IAP should be expressed in mm Hg and measured at end-expiration in the complete supine position after ensuring that abdominal muscle contractions are absent and with the transducer zeroed at the level of the mid-axillary line.
Definition 5	The reference standard for intermittent IAP measurement is via the bladder with a maximal instillation volume of 25 mL of sterile saline.
Definition 6	Normal IAP is approximately 5–7 mm Hg in critically ill adults.
Definition 7	IAH is defined by a sustained or repeated pathologic elevation of IAP ≥ 12 mmHg.
Definition 8	IAH is graded as follows: Grade I: IAP 12–15 mm Hg Grade II: IAP 16–20 mm Hg Grade III: IAP 21–25 mm Hg Grade IV: IAP > 25 mm Hg
Definition 9	ACS is defined as a sustained IAP > 20 mm Hg (with or without an APP < 60 mm Hg) that is associated with new organ dysfunction / failure.
Definition 10	Primary ACS is a condition associated with injury or disease in the abdomino-pelvic region that frequently requires early surgical or interventional radiological intervention.
Definition 11	Secondary ACS refers to conditions that do not originate from the abdomino-pelvic region.
Definition 12	Recurrent ACS refers to the condition in which ACS redevelops following previous surgical or medical treatment of primary or secondary ACS.

Abbreviations: ACS, abdominal compartment syndrome, APP, abdominal perfusion pressure; FG, filtration gradient; GFP, glomerular filtration pressure; IAH, intra-abdominal hypertension; IAP, intra-abdominal pressure; MAP, mean arterial pressure; PTP, proximal tubular pressure.
  Adapted from Malbrain ML, Cheatham ML, Kirkpatrick A, et al. Results from the International Conference of Experts on Intra-abdominal Hypertension and Abdominal Compartment Syndrome. I. Definitions. Intensive Care Med 2006;32: 1722–32; with permission.

awareness and many ICUs never measure the IAP. No consensus exists on optimal timing of measurement or decompression. In a recent editorial, Ivatury[6] states that: "One potential exegesis of this widespread under-appreciation of these syndromes may be related to our rapidly evolving understanding of their patho-physiology. Our knowledge is no longer restricted to experimentally sound (isolated IAH) concepts, but is elevated to a true clinical phenomenon (IAH as a 'second-hit' after ischemia-reperfusion)."

Etiology

The ACS can be diagnosed when there is increased IAP with evidence of end-organ dysfunction. Although multiple causes of acute cardiopulmonary, renal, hepatosplanchnic, or neurologic deterioration exist in the ICU, it is important that we recognize IAP as being an independent risk factor for this organ function deterioration. Hence, the timely recognition of the underlying risk factors and predisposing conditions that lead to IAH and ACS is extremely important. Indications for IAP monitoring should be based on the presence/absence of these risk factors. Many conditions are reported in association with IAH/ACS, and they can be classified into four categories: first, conditions that decrease abdominal wall compliance; second, conditions that increase intraluminal contents; third, conditions related to abdominal collections of fluid, air, or blood; and finally, conditions related to capillary leak and fluid resuscitation. **Box 1** lists some of the clinical conditions related to these four categories.

Hence, it becomes clear that ACS can develop both in nonsurgical and surgical patients. An algorithm for the assessment of IAH is proposed in **Fig. 1**.

DIAGNOSIS
Clinical and Radiologic Examination

The abdominal perimeter or girth cannot be used as a surrogate for IAP because it only poorly

Box 1
Risk factors for the development of IAH and ACS

Related to diminished abdominal wall compliance

- Mechanical ventilation, especially fighting with the ventilator and the use of accessory muscles
- Use of positive end expiratory pressure (PEEP) or the presence of auto-PEEP
- Basal pneumonia
- High body mass index
- Pneumoperitoneum
- Abdominal (vascular) surgery, especially with tight abdominal closures
- Pneumatic anti-shock garments
- Prone and other body positioning
- Abdominal wall bleeding or rectus sheath hematomas
- Correction of large hernias, gastroschisis, or omphalocele
- Burns with abdominal eschars

Related to increased intra-abdominal contents

- Gastroparesis
- Gastric distention
- Ileus
- Volvulus
- Colonic pseudo-obstruction
- Abdominal tumor
- Retroperitoneal/ abdominal wall hematoma
- Enteral feeding
- Intra-abdominal or retroperitoneal tumor
- Damage control laparotomy

Related to abdominal collections of fluid, air, or blood

- Liver dysfunction with ascites
- Abdominal infection (eg, pancreatitis, peritonitis, abscess)
- Hemoperitoneum
- Pneumoperitoneum
- Laparoscopy with excessive inflation pressures
- Major trauma
- Peritoneal dialysis

Related to capillary leak and fluid resuscitation

- Acidosis[a] (pH below 7.2)
- Hypothermia[a] (core temperature below 33°C)
- Coagulopathy[a] (platelet count below 50,000/mm³ OR an activated partial thromboplastin time [APTT] more than 2 times normal OR a prothrombin time [PTT] below 50% OR an international standardized ratio [INR] more than 1.5)
- Polytransfusion/trauma (>10 units of packed red cells/24 hours)
- Sepsis (as defined by the American–European Consensus Conference definitions)
- Severe sepsis or bacteremia
- Septic shock

- Massive fluid resuscitation (>5 L of colloid or >10 L of crystalloid/24 hours with capillary leak and positive fluid balance)
- Major burns

[a] The combination of acidosis, hypothermia, and coagulopathy has been described in the literature as the deadly triad.[186,187]

correlates with it. Studies have shown that clinical IAP estimation is also far from accurate with a sensitivity and positive predictive value of around 40% to 60%.[7,8] Radiologic investigation with plain radiography of the chest or abdomen, abdominal ultrasound, or CT scan is also insensitive to the presence of increased IAP.

Measurement of Intra-Abdominal Pressure

Because the abdomen and its contents can be considered as relatively noncompressive and primarily fluid in character, behaving in accordance with Pascal's law, the IAP measured at one point may be assumed to represent the IAP throughout the abdomen.[9,10] The IAP is therefore defined as the steady-state pressure concealed within the abdominal cavity, IAP increases with inspiration (diaphragmatic contraction) and decreases with expiration (diaphragmatic relaxation).

In the strictest sense, normal IAP ranges from 0 to 5 mm Hg.[11] Certain physiologic conditions, however, such as morbid obesity,[12,13] ovarian tumors, cirrhosis, or pregnancy, may be associated with chronic IAP elevations of 10 to 15 mm Hg to which the patient has adapted with an absence of significant pathophysiology. In contrast, children commonly demonstrate low IAP values.[14] The clinical importance of any IAP must be assessed in view of the baseline steady-state IAP for the individual patient.

The key to recognizing ACS in a critically ill patient is the demonstration of elevated IAP: "measuring is knowing!"[15] IAP can be directly measured with an intraperitoneal catheter attached to a pressure transducer. During CO_2-insufflation in laparoscopic surgery IAP is measured directly via the Verres needle.

Different indirect methods for estimating IAP are used clinically because direct measurements are considered to be too invasive.[9,16] These techniques include rectal, uteral, gastric, inferior vena caval, and urinary bladder pressure measurement. Only gastric and bladder pressures are used clinically. Over the years, bladder pressure has been forwarded as the gold-standard indirect method. The bladder technique has achieved the most widespread adoption

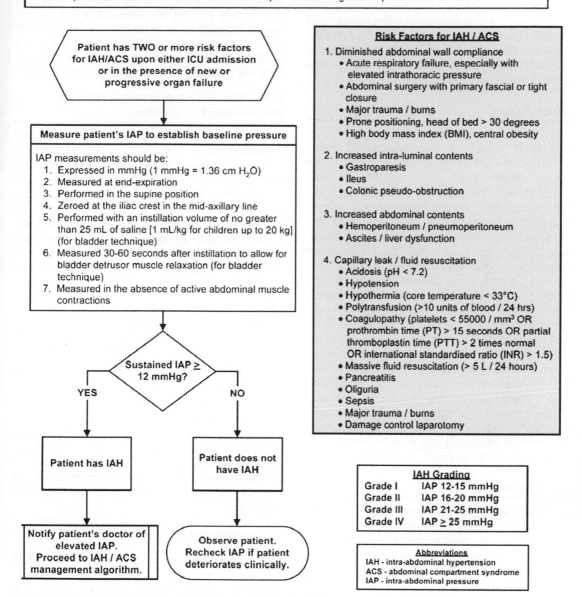

• Patients should be screened for IAH/ACS risk factors upon ICU admission and with new or progressive organ failure.
• If two or more risk factors are present, a baseline IAP measurement should be obtained.
• If IAH is present, serial IAP measurements should be performed throughout the patient's critical illness.

Patient has TWO or more risk factors for IAH/ACS upon either ICU admission or in the presence of new or progressive organ failure

Measure patient's IAP to establish baseline pressure

IAP measurements should be:
1. Expressed in mmHg (1 mmHg = 1.36 cm H_2O)
2. Measured at end-expiration
3. Performed in the supine position
4. Zeroed at the iliac crest in the mid-axillary line
5. Performed with an instillation volume of no greater than 25 mL of saline [1 mL/kg for children up to 20 kg] (for bladder technique)
6. Measured 30-60 seconds after instillation to allow for bladder detrusor muscle relaxation (for bladder technique)
7. Measured in the absence of active abdominal muscle contractions

Sustained IAP ≥ 12 mmHg?

YES

NO

Patient has IAH

Patient does not have IAH

Notify patient's doctor of elevated IAP. Proceed to IAH / ACS management algorithm.

Observe patient. Recheck IAP if patient deteriorates clinically.

Risk Factors for IAH / ACS

1. Diminished abdominal wall compliance
   • Acute respiratory failure, especially with elevated intrathoracic pressure
   • Abdominal surgery with primary fascial or tight closure
   • Major trauma / burns
   • Prone positioning, head of bed > 30 degrees
   • High body mass index (BMI), central obesity

2. Increased intra-luminal contents
   • Gastroparesis
   • Ileus
   • Colonic pseudo-obstruction

3. Increased abdominal contents
   • Hemoperitoneum / pneumoperitoneum
   • Ascites / liver dysfunction

4. Capillary leak / fluid resuscitation
   • Acidosis (pH < 7.2)
   • Hypotension
   • Hypothermia (core temperature < 33°C)
   • Polytransfusion (>10 units of blood / 24 hrs)
   • Coagulopathy (platelets < 55000 / mm³ OR prothrombin time (PT) > 15 seconds OR partial thromboplastin time (PTT) > 2 times normal OR international standardised ratio (INR) > 1.5)
   • Massive fluid resuscitation (> 5 L / 24 hours)
   • Pancreatitis
   • Oliguria
   • Sepsis
   • Major trauma / burns
   • Damage control laparotomy

IAH Grading	
Grade I	IAP 12-15 mmHg
Grade II	IAP 16-20 mmHg
Grade III	IAP 21-25 mmHg
Grade IV	IAP ≥ 25 mmHg

Abbreviations
IAH - intra-abdominal hypertension
ACS - abdominal compartment syndrome
IAP - intra-abdominal pressure

Fig. 1. Intra-abdominal hypertension (IAH) assessment algorithm.

worldwide because of its simplicity and minimal cost.[9,10] However, considerable variation is noted between the different techniques used, and recent data suggest to instill minimal volumes (10–25 mL) into the bladder for priming.[17–20]

Recently, new measurement kits, either via a FoleyManometer (Holtech Medical, Copenhagen, Denmark, at www.holtech-medical.com), Abdo Pressure (Unomedical, Birkersd, Denmark, at www.unomedical.com) or an AbViser-valve (Wolfe Tory Medical, Salt Lake City, Utah, at www.

wolfetory.com) have become commercially available.

Continuous Intra-Abdominal Pressure Measurement

The IAP can also be measured via a balloon-tipped stomach catheter (Spiegelberg, Hamburg, Germany, at www.spiegelberg.de and Pulsion Medical Systems, Munich, Germany, at www.pulsion.com).[10] This avoids the problems associated with the creation of a hydrostatic fluid column and allows continuous IAP and APP measurement.[21]

Several other methods for continuous IAP measurement via the stomach, peritoneal cavity (using air-chamber or piezoresistive membranes), and bladder have been validated.[16,22–24] Although these techniques seem promising, further clinical validation needs to be done before their general use can be recommended.

Which Patient?

Although the prevalence and incidence of IAH in critically ill patients is considerable,[25,26] routine IAP measurement in all patients admitted to the ICU is currently rarely performed, and probably not indicated. The ACS can be diagnosed when there is increased IAP with evidence of end-organ dysfunction. While multiple causes of acute cardiopulmonary, renal, hepatosplanchnic, or neurologic deterioration exist in the ICU, it is important that we recognize the IAP as being an independent risk factor for this organ function deterioration. The WSACS has provided a list with risk factors associated with IAH and ACS and if two or more risk factors are present, baseline routine IAP monitoring is advised (**Box 1**).[3,27] Massive volume resuscitation after a "first hit" for any reason (eg, burns, trauma, pancreatitis, hemorrhagic shock) can lead to increased IAP, particularly postoperatively or in a septic patient. The "second hit" probably results from the effects of "capillary leak," shock with ischemia-reperfusion injury and the release of cytokines combined with massive increases in total extracellular volume.[15]

What Technique?

According to the WSACS consensus guidelines, IAP should be measured at end-expiration in the complete supine position after ensuring that abdominal muscle contractions are absent and with the transducer zeroed at the level of the midaxillary line at the iliac crest after an instillation volume of maximal 20 to 25 mL.[1] An intermittent technique may be used for screening, whereas in some patients, a continuous technique may be preferable, eg, when the APP is used as a resuscitation end point, or in patients with impending ACS requiring urgent abdominal decompression.

What Frequency?

When an intermittent method is used, measurements should be obtained at least every 4 to 6 hours, and in patients with evolving organ dysfunction, this frequency should be increased up to hourly measurements.

When to Stop Intra-Abdominal Pressure Measurement?

IAP measurement can be discontinued when the risk factors for IAH are resolved or the patient has no signs of acute organ dysfunction, and IAP values have been below 10 to 12 mm Hg for 24 to 48 hours. In case of recurrent organ dysfunction, IAP measurement should be reconsidered.

What About Intra-Abdominal Pressure Measurement in Children?

Some studies have been performed regarding IAP measurement in children.[14,28] The transvesical route can be used safely in children, but obviously, the instillation volume is important in this population. Davis and colleagues[14] found that 1 mL/kg produces reliable IAP values when compared with higher volumes. Normal IAP values are lower in children up to 40 kg body weight (3–5 mm Hg) and the thresholds defining IAH (9 mm Hg) and ACS (16 mm Hg) are also lower compared with adults.

What About Intra-Abdominal Pressure Measurement in Awake Patients?

IAP measurement is most often performed in sedated patients, where muscle contractions are absent. When measuring IAP in awake patients, specific attention should be made that no muscle contractions are present, eg, during forced expiration in a patient who has chronic obstructive pulmonary disease with auto-PEEP. Adequate pain medication should be administered, especially after abdominal surgery, as even putting the patient in supine position may induce abdominal pain and muscle contractions, leading to elevated IAP readings.

PATHOPHYSIOLOGIC IMPLICATIONS

IAH affects multiple organ systems in a graded fashion. To better understand the clinical presentation and management of disorders of IAH, one must understand the physiologic derangements within each organ system separately.[15] It is beyond the scope of this review to give a concise and complete review of the pathophysiologic implications of raised IAP on end-organ function within and outside the abdominal cavity.[29,30] We will discuss only some key messages related to each organ that will affect daily clinical practice; these are summarized in **Fig. 2**.

Neurologic Function

Acute IAH may cause an increase in intracranial pressure (ICP) because of augmentation in pleural

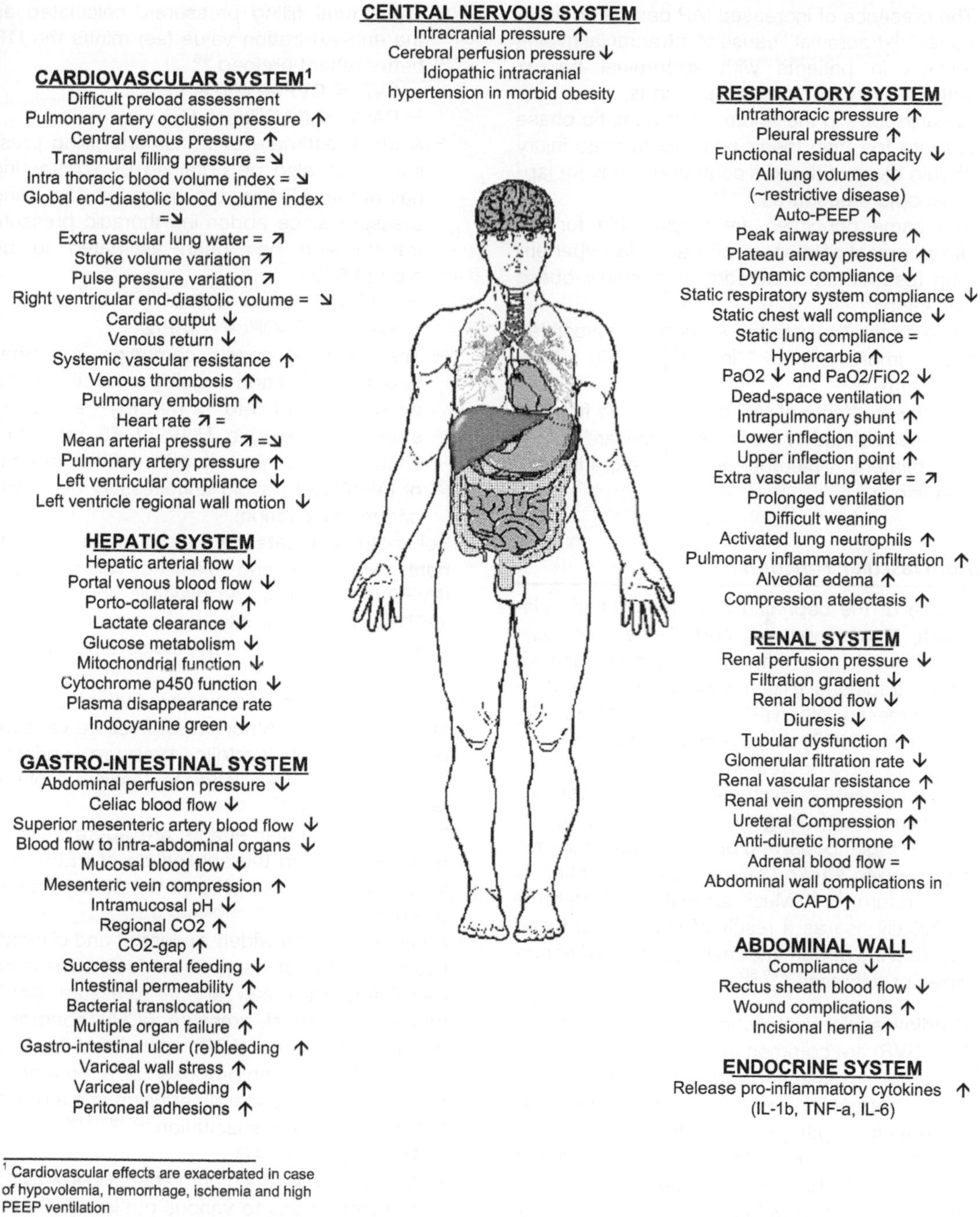

CENTRAL NERVOUS SYSTEM
Intracranial pressure ↑
Cerebral perfusion pressure ↓
Idiopathic intracranial
hypertension in morbid obesity

CARDIOVASCULAR SYSTEM[1]
Difficult preload assessment
Pulmonary artery occlusion pressure ↑
Central venous pressure ↑
Transmural filling pressure = ↘
Intra thoracic blood volume index = ↘
Global end-diastolic blood volume index
= ↘
Extra vascular lung water = ↗
Stroke volume variation ↗
Pulse pressure variation ↗
Right ventricular end-diastolic volume = ↘
Cardiac output ↓
Venous return ↓
Systemic vascular resistance ↑
Venous thrombosis ↑
Pulmonary embolism ↑
Heart rate ↗ =
Mean arterial pressure ↗ = ↘
Pulmonary artery pressure ↑
Left ventricular compliance ↓
Left ventricle regional wall motion ↓

RESPIRATORY SYSTEM
Intrathoracic pressure ↑
Pleural pressure ↑
Functional residual capacity ↓
All lung volumes ↓
(~restrictive disease)
Auto-PEEP ↑
Peak airway pressure ↑
Plateau airway pressure ↑
Dynamic compliance ↓
Static respiratory system compliance ↓
Static chest wall compliance ↓
Static lung compliance =
Hypercarbia ↑
PaO_2 ↓ and PaO_2/FiO_2 ↓
Dead-space ventilation ↑
Intrapulmonary shunt ↑
Lower inflection point ↓
Upper inflection point ↑
Extra vascular lung water = ↗
Prolonged ventilation
Difficult weaning
Activated lung neutrophils ↑
Pulmonary inflammatory infiltration ↑
Alveolar edema ↑
Compression atelectasis ↑

HEPATIC SYSTEM
Hepatic arterial flow ↓
Portal venous blood flow ↓
Porto-collateral flow ↑
Lactate clearance ↓
Glucose metabolism ↓
Mitochondrial function ↓
Cytochrome p450 function ↓
Plasma disappearance rate
Indocyanine green ↓

RENAL SYSTEM
Renal perfusion pressure ↓
Filtration gradient ↓
Renal blood flow ↓
Diuresis ↓
Tubular dysfunction ↑
Glomerular filtration rate ↓
Renal vascular resistance ↑
Renal vein compression ↑
Ureteral Compression ↑
Anti-diuretic hormone ↑
Adrenal blood flow =
Abdominal wall complications in
CAPD ↑

GASTRO-INTESTINAL SYSTEM
Abdominal perfusion pressure ↓
Celiac blood flow ↓
Superior mesenteric artery blood flow ↓
Blood flow to intra-abdominal organs ↓
Mucosal blood flow ↓
Mesenteric vein compression ↑
Intramucosal pH ↓
Regional CO_2 ↑
CO_2-gap ↑
Success enteral feeding ↓
Intestinal permeability ↑
Bacterial translocation ↑
Multiple organ failure ↑
Gastro-intestinal ulcer (re)bleeding ↑
Variceal wall stress ↑
Variceal (re)bleeding ↑
Peritoneal adhesions ↑

ABDOMINAL WALL
Compliance ↓
Rectus sheath blood flow ↓
Wound complications ↑
Incisional hernia ↑

ENDOCRINE SYSTEM
Release pro-inflammatory cytokines ↑
(IL-1b, TNF-a, IL-6)

[1] Cardiovascular effects are exacerbated in case
of hypovolemia, hemorrhage, ischemia and high
PEEP ventilation

Fig. 2. Pathophysiology of intra-abdominal hypertension.

pressure. Cerebral perfusion pressure (CPP) will decrease owing to a functional obstruction of cerebral venous outflow caused by the increased intrathoracic pressure (ITP) owing to the cephalad displacement of the diaphragm in combination with a reduced systemic blood pressure as a result of decreased preload and cardiac output (CO). Cerebral blood flow and jugular bulb saturation will decrease. The effects of IAP on the central nervous system (CNS) have not been extensively studied to date, and remain a challenging area for laboratory and clinical investigators.[31–38]

– Because of the interactions between IAP, ITP, and ICP, accurate monitoring of IAP in head trauma victims with associated abdominal lesions is worthwhile.

- The presence of increased IAP can be an additional "extracranial" cause of intracranial hypertension in patients with abdominal trauma without overt craniocerebral lesions.
- Laparoscopy in the acute posttraumatic phase is more foe than friend and recent head injury should be considered a contraindication for laparoscopic procedures.[39–41]
- The same principles are responsible for the development of idiopathic intracranial hypertension (pseudotumor cerebri) in morbidly obese patients.[35,42,43]
- Weight loss by bariatric surgery is associated with improvements in ICP and CNS symptoms.[42,44]
- The direct effects of IAH on neurologic function has been ablated by sternotomy, pericardiotomy, or bilateral pleurotomy in experimental conditions.[37]

Cardiovascular Function

Because of the cephalad movement of the diaphragm, pleural pressure and ITP will increase. This will result in a difficult preload assessment because traditional filling pressures will be erroneously increased. When IAP rises above 10 mm Hg, cardiac output (CO) drops because of an increase in afterload and a decrease in preload and left ventricular compliance. Systemic vascular resistance (SVR) increases (owing to mechanical compression of vascular beds) and preload is reduced (owing to drop in stroke volume and a reduction of venous return).[45–48] Mean arterial blood pressure may initially rise as a result of shunting of blood away from the abdominal cavity but thereafter normalizes or decreases.[49,50]

- Cardiovascular dysfunction and failure (low CO, high SVR) are common in IAH or ACS.
- Accurate assessment and optimization of preload, contractility, and afterload is essential to restore end-organ perfusion and function.
- Our understanding of traditional hemodynamic monitoring techniques and parameters, however, must be reevaluated in IAH/ACS, since pressure-based estimates of intravascular volume as pulmonary artery occlusion pressure (PAOP) and central venous pressure (CVP) are erroneously increased.
  - The clinician must be aware of the interactions between ITP, IAP, PEEP, and intracardiac filling pressures.
  - Misinterpretation of the patient's minute-to-minute cardiac status may result in the institution of inappropriate and potentially detrimental therapy.

- Transmural filling pressures, calculated as the end-expiration value (ee) minus the ITP better reflect preload.[46]
  - CVP = CVPee − ITP
  - PAOP = PAOPee − ITP
- A quick estimate of transmural filling pressures can also be obtained by subtracting half of the IAP from the end-expiratory filling pressure since abdomino-thoracic pressure transmission has been estimated to be around 50%.
  - CVP = CVPee − IAP/2
  - PAOP = PAOPee − IAP/2
- The surviving sepsis campaign guidelines targeting initial and ongoing resuscitation toward a CVP of 8 to 12 mm Hg[51] and other studies targeting a MAP of 65 mm Hg[52] should be interpreted with caution in case of IAH/ACS to avoid unnecessary over- and underresuscitation!
- Volumetric estimates of preload status, such as right ventricular end diastolic volume index (RVEDVI) or global end diastolic volume index (GEDVI), are especially useful because of the changing ventricular compliance and elevated ITP.[48,53–56]
- Functional hemodynamic parameters such as stroke volume (SVV) or pulse pressure variation (PPV) but not systolic pressure variation (SPV) should be used to assess volume responsiveness.[57]
- The cardiovascular effects are aggravated by hypovolemia and the application of PEEP,[58–62] whereas hypervolemia has a temporary protective effect.[37]
- Analogous to the widely accepted and clinically used concept of cerebral perfusion pressure, calculated as mean arterial pressure (MAP) minus intracranial pressure (ICP), abdominal perfusion pressure (APP), calculated as MAP minus IAP, has been proposed as a more accurate predictor of visceral perfusion and a potential end point for resuscitation.[33,49,63,64]
  - APP = MAP − IAP
  - APP, by considering both arterial inflow (MAP) and restrictions to venous outflow (IAP), has been demonstrated to be statistically superior to either parameter alone in predicting patient survival from IAH and ACS.[49]
  - A target APP of at least 60 mm Hg has been demonstrated to correlate with improved survival from IAH and ACS.

Pulmonary Function

The interactions between the abdominal and the thoracic compartment pose a specific challenge to the ICU physicians.[65] Both compartments are linked via the diaphragm and on average a 50% (range 25%–80%) transmission of IAP to the ITP has been noted in previous animal and human studies.[48] Patients with primary ACS will often develop a secondary ARDS and will require a different ventilatory strategy and more specific treatment than a patient with primary ARDS.[66,67] The major problem lies in the reduction of the functional residual capacity (FRC). Together with the alterations caused by secondary ARDS, this will lead to the so-called "baby-lungs." Some key issues to remember are the following:

- IAH decreases total respiratory system compliance by a decrease in chest wall compliance, while lung compliance remains unchanged.[68,69]
- Best PEEP should be set to counteract IAP while in the same time avoiding over-inflation of already well-aerated lung regions.[70]
  - Best PEEP = IAP
- The ARDS consensus definitions should take into account PEEP and IAP values.
- During lung protective ventilation, the plateau pressures should be limited to transmural plateau pressures below 35 cmH$_2$O.
  - Pplat = Pplat − IAP/2
- The PAOP criterion in ARDS consensus definitions is futile in the case of IAH and should be adapted (most patients with IAH and secondary ARDS will have a PAOP above 18 mm Hg).
- IAH increases lung edema; therefore monitoring of extravascular lung water index (EVLWI) seems warranted.[71]
- The combination of capillary leak, positive fluid balance, and raised IAP put the patient at exponential risk for lung edema.
- Body position affects IAP.
  - Putting an obese patient in the upright position can cause ACS.[72]
  - The abdomen should hang freely during prone positioning.[73]
  - The reverse Trendelenburg position may improve respiratory mechanics, however it can decrease splanchnic perfusion.[74]
- Consideration of neuromuscular blockade should balance the potentially beneficial effects on abdominal muscle tone resulting in decreased IAP and improved APP against the potentially detrimental effect on lung mechanics resulting in atelectasis and super-infection.[75]
- The presence of IAH will lead to pulmonary hypertension via increased ITP with direct compression on lung parenchyma and vessels and via the diminished left and right ventricular compliance.

- The effect of IAP on parenchymal compression is exacerbated in cases of hemorrhagic shock or hypotension.

Hepatic Function

The liver appears to be particularly susceptible to injury in the presence of elevated IAP. Animal and human studies have shown impairment of hepatic cell function and liver perfusion even with only moderately elevated IAP of 10 mm Hg.[76,77] Furthermore, acute liver failure, decompensated chronic liver disease, and liver transplantation are frequently complicated by IAH and the ACS.[78,79]

- Close monitoring and early recognition of IAH, followed by aggressive treatment may confer an outcome benefit in patients with liver disease.
- In the management of these patients it might be useful to measure the plasma disappearance rate (PDR) for indocyanine green (ICG), as this correlates not only with liver function and perfusion but also with IAP.[73,80]
- Since cytochrome P450 function may be altered in case of IAH/ACS, medication doses should be adapted accordingly.
- Within the capsule of the liver itself, local hematoma formation may have an adverse affect on tissue perfusion causing a local hepatic compartment syndrome.
- With increasing IAP there is decreased hepatic arterial flow, decreased venous portal flow, and increase in the portacollateral circulation. In turn, physiologic effects include
  - decreased lactate clearance
  - altered glucose metabolism
  - altered mitochondrial function

Renal Function

IAH has been associated with renal impairment for over 150 years.[81] It is only recently however that a clinically recognized relationship has been found.[82,83] An increasing number of large clinical studies have identified that IAH ($\geq$ 15 mm Hg) is independently associated with renal impairment and increased mortality.[84,85] The etiology of these changes is not entirely well established; however, it may be multifactorial: reduced renal perfusion, reduced cardiac output, and increased systemic vascular resistance and alterations in humoral and neurogenic factors. Elevated IAP significantly decreases renal venous and arterial blood flow leading to renal dysfunction and failure.[86] Oliguria develops at an IAP of 15 mm Hg and anuria at 30 mm Hg in the presence of normovolemia and at lower levels of IAP in the patient with hypovolemia or sepsis.[87,88] Renal perfusion pressure (RPP) and renal filtration gradient (FG) have been proposed as key factors in the development of IAP-induced renal failure.

- RPP = MAP − IAP
- FG = GFP − PTP = (MAP − IAP) − IAP = MAP − 2*IAP
  - Where GFP = glomerular filtration pressure
  - And PTP = proximal tubular pressure

Thus, changes in IAP have a greater impact on renal function and urine production than will changes in MAP. It should not be surprising, therefore, that decreased renal function, as evidenced by development of oliguria, is one of the first visible signs of IAH. Conversely, therefore, it behooves us as clinicians to be cognizant that elevated IAP and its effect on renal function is often the first sign of impending ACS. Other key points to remember are

- The prerenal azotemia seen in IAH is unresponsive to volume expansion to a normal CO, dopaminergic agents, or loop diuretics.[2,89]
- Renal function may be improved by paracentesis of ascitic fluid and reduction in the IAP.[90]
- Prompt reduction of IAP has dramatic beneficial effect on urine output in patients with primary and secondary ACS after trauma.[91–96]
- Within the capsule of the kidney itself, local hematoma formation may have an adverse affect on tissue perfusion causing a local renal compartment syndrome.[97,98]

Gastrointestinal Function

IAH has profound effects on splanchnic organs, causing diminished perfusion, mucosal acidosis, and setting the stage for multiple organ failure.[99] The pathologic changes are more pronounced after sequential insults of ischemia-reperfusion and IAH. It appears that IAH and ACS may serve as the second insult in the two-hit phenomenon of the causation of multiple-organ dysfunction syndrome.[100,101] Recent clinical studies have demonstrated a temporal relationship between ACS and subsequent multiple organ failure (MOF).[99,102,103] In animals, ACS provokes cytokine release and neutrophil migration, resulting in remote organ failure. In humans, ACS results in splanchnic hypoperfusion that may occur in the absence of hypotension or decreased cardiac output. This ischemia and reperfusion injury to the gut serves as a second insult in a two-hit model of MOF where the lymph flow conducts gut-derived proinflammatory cytokines to remote organs.

- IAP inversely correlates with intramucosal (pHi) or regional CO_2.[104–106]

- IAP inversely correlates with indocyanine green plasma disappearance rate (ICG-PDR).[80]
- IAH triggers a vicious cycle leading to intestinal edema, ischemia, bacterial translocation, and finally MOF.[107–109]
- Maintenance of adequate perfusion pressure (APP > 60–65 mm Hg) is mandatory.[63]
- The back pressure at the venous side is even more important to the pressure-flow relations.

Abdominal Wall and Endocrine Function

Increased IAP has been shown to reduce abdominal wall blood flow by the direct, compressive effects leading to local ischemia and edema.[110] This can decrease abdominal wall compliance and exacerbate IAH.[69] Abdominal wall muscle and fascial ischemia may contribute to infectious and noninfectious wound complications (eg, dehiscence, herniation, necrotizing fasciitis) often seen in this patient population.

IMPORTANCE OF INTRA-ABDOMINAL PRESSURE IN OTHER CLINICAL CONDITIONS
Abdominal Compartment Syndrome in Pediatric Patients

Omphalocele and gastroschisis are the original clinical conditions that are closely associated with the phenomenon of increased IAP.[111,112] We owe a debt of gratitude to the pediatric surgeons who were the first to deal with defects of the abdominal wall and the consequences of their closure.[113] Several series from the past decade document the manifestations of elevated IAP in children undergoing such repairs, the beneficial effects of monitoring IAP, and the role of elevated IAP in the increased incidence of necrotizing enterocolitis. Please pay attention to IAP in children!

Abdominal Compartment Syndrome in Burn Patients

Patients with large burns (50% or greater or with associated inhalation injury) are at risk of developing IAH.[114] Patients with burns on greater than 70% of total body surface area are at risk of developing ACS, particularly if they have a concurrent inhalation injury. The development of IAH and ACS is related to the volume of crystalloid fluid infused during the burn resuscitation and does not require abdominal injury or operation or even the presence of abdominal wall burn eschar.[114–120]

However, these patients have very large burns, often severe inhalation injuries, and frequently die later in their hospitalization from complications of their burns that are unrelated to their ACS.

- Burn patients are at great risk to develop large-volume resuscitation-related secondary ACS.
- Burn patients who develop IAH mostly have more then 50% total body surface area (TBSA) burns.
- A variety of management options exist for IAH and ACS in burn patients, all of which may be of some benefit.[117,120]
  - sedation
  - pharmacologic paralysis
  - abdominal wall escharotomy
  - percutaneous catheter decompression of the peritoneal cavity
  - surgical decompression

Abdominal Compartment Syndrome in Hematological Patients

Recent studies have alluded to the increased incidence and consequences of IAH in hematological patients,[121] the causes of which are multifactorial:

- Growth factor–induced capillary leak syndrome with concomitant large-volume fluid resuscitation and third-space sequestration
- Chemotherapy-induced ileus, colonic pseudo-obstruction (Ogilvie's syndrome), mucositis, or gastroenteritis
- Sepsis and infectious complications aggravating intestinal and capillary permeability
- Extramedullary hematopoiesis as seen with chronic myeloid leukemia resulting in hepatosplenomegaly, chronic IAH, and chronic (irreversible) pulmonary hypertension
- The mechanisms of veno-occlusive disease seen after stem cell transplantation may be triggered by or related to increased IAP.

Abdominal Compartment Syndrome in Morbidly Obese Patients

Recent studies show that obese patients have higher baseline IAP values.[122] As with IAH in the critically ill, elevated IAP in the morbidly obese patient can have far-reaching effects on end-organ function. Disease processes common in morbidly obese patients such as obesity hypoventilation syndrome, pseudotumor cerebri, gastroesophageal reflux, and stress urinary incontinence are now being recognized as being caused by the increased IAP occurring with an elevated body mass index.[13,42,123] Furthermore, the increased incidence of poor fascial healing and incisional hernia rates have been related to the IAH-induced reductions in rectus sheath and abdominal wall blood flow.

- IAH-related complications of morbid obesity generally respond to weight loss.[44]

- The morbidly obese are at a greater risk of developing ACS because of preexisting baseline IAH and organ dysfunction.
- Clinicians should have a low threshold for monitoring IAP in obese patients because of the so-called "silent IAH."

Intra-Abdominal Pressure During Pregnancy

In the second and the third trimesters of pregnancy, the uterus occupies a major part of the abdominal cavity, and in the supine position breathlessness and blood pressure drop ("supine hypotension syndrome") are seen.[124] These symptoms are the result of restriction of the diaphragm and compression of the inferior vena cava. However, overall IAP is usually not elevated.[125] Furthermore, the symptoms are alleviated in the lateral, sitting, or standing positions. Because of hormonal influences during pregnancy, the abdominal wall is slowly stretched, increasing its compliance, which reduces the potential for increase in IAP caused by the expanding uterus. However, if IAP increases as a result of other reasons, eg, pneumoperitoneum at laparoscopy, perfusion of the uterus and the fetus might be severely compromised.[126]

INTRODUCING A NEW CONCEPT: THE POLYCOMPARTMENT SYNDROME

Within a specific compartment, the CS can be localized like a pelvic compartment syndrome or global like ACS; thus, we suggest the terms localized CS (LCS) and global CS (GCS). Scalea and colleagues[127] alluded to the term multiple compartment syndrome (MCS) in a study of 102 patients with increased intra-abdominal (IAP), intrathoracic, and intracranial pressure (ICP) after severe brain injury. Seventy-eight patients had an ICS and underwent a decompressive craniectomy (DC). The DC in these 78 patients resulted in a significant decrease in ICP from 24 to 14 mm Hg. The other 24 patients had a multiple CS and underwent both a decompressive craniectomy and a decompressive laparotomy (DL). The combination of DC and DL in these 24 patients led to a decrease in ICP from around 32 to 14 mm Hg after DC and from 28 to 19 mm Hg after DL (the effect being different depending on whether DC or DL was performed first). After DL, the IAP decreased from 28 to around 18 mm Hg and so did mean airway pressure from 37 to 27 cmH2O. The authors concluded that increased ICP can result from primary traumatic brain injury as well as from increased IAP, which has been documented before.[32,33,128] Patients with multiple CS showed a trend toward higher mortality (42% versus 31%), although it did not reach statistical significance. Multiple CS should therefore be considered in multiple injured patients with increased ICP that does not respond to therapy.[127]

Since the term multi or multiple CS is mostly used in the literature referring to multiple limb trauma with CS needing decompressive fasciotomy and to avoid confusion, the term polycompartment syndrome was finally coined.[129] Because of the central position of the abdomen and the effects of IAP on nearly all other compartments, IAH and ACS play a central role in the development of poly CS (**Fig. 3**). The increased IAP hence will affect ICP, ITP, CVP, and PAOP.

FLUID RESUSCITATION, MULTIPLE ORGAN FAILURE, AND POLYCOMPARTMENT SYNDROME

Clearly the relationship between fluid resuscitation and IAH is very complex since fluid overload is a leading cause of IAH, but fluid loading may

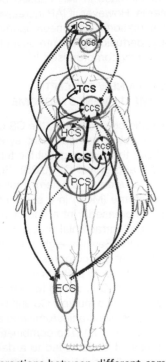

Fig. 3. Interactions between different compartments. The arrows indicate possible interactions between different compartments. Solid lines show direct effects by mechanical pressure forces. Dotted lines show indirect distant effects between compartments. ACS, abdominal compartment syndrome; CCS, cardiac compartment syndrome; ECS, extremity compartment syndrome; HCS, hepatic compartment syndrome; ICS, intracranial compartment syndrome; OCS, orbital compartment syndrome; PCS, pelvic compartment syndrome; RCS, renal compartment syndrome; TCS, thoracic compartment syndrome.

also protect against some of the detrimental effects of IAH on organ function. Therefore, we dedicate a section of this article to this complex issue.

Why Do We Like Fluids?

The importance of increasing circulating blood volume in hypovolemic shock has been apparent for decades and the implementation of guidelines and protocols for fluid management in trauma has saved countless lives. After the success obtained in hypovolemic shock, aggressive fluid resuscitation has been studied in distributive shock as well. Burn resuscitation is a well-known example, where mortality was significantly decreased using aggressive crystalloid resuscitation. In septic shock as well, fluid resuscitation is the first and foremost therapeutic action recommended in the Surviving Sepsis Campaign Guidelines.[51] Traditionally, fluid resuscitation protocols are aimed at correction of "basic" physiologic parameters such as blood pressure, central venous pressure (CVP), and urine output. The advantages of this approach are multiple and easy to understand: these parameters are readily available at the bedside and do not require expensive and operator-dependent equipment, leading to broader applicability worldwide. Over time, the only significant evolution regarding the use of fluid resuscitation as such has been the gradual increase in emphasis on the importance of time. Both in trauma and burns, delayed fluid resuscitation has been associated with increased mortality. ATLS guidelines as well as burn resuscitation guidelines have stressed the importance of prompt administration of fluids for a long time.[130] The importance of time in sepsis was highlighted more recently in the landmark paper by Rivers and colleagues[52] and current sepsis guidelines have embraced this concept completely.[51]

Which Fluids Do We Like?

The goal of fluid resuscitation is to restore circulating blood volume, which may mean substitution of external losses, supplying volume to a dilated vascular system, or supplementing internal losses due to third spacing or capillary leak. This has traditionally been accomplished using isotonic crystalloid solutions, which contain mainly NaCl. Since the Na+ ion is an extracellular ion, crystalloid solutions will be evenly distributed throughout the extracellular body water compartment after intravenous (IV) administration. In the search for fluids that would selectively expand the intravascular compartment, colloids, both synthetic and natural, were evaluated. According to Starling's equation, they should tip the balance in favor of fluid movement from the interstitial to the intravascular compartment and thus plasma volume expansion (**Fig. 4**). However, several studies could not show a survival benefit in favor of colloid resuscitation using either albumin or synthetic colloid solutions in several clinical situations. Furthermore, colloids are more expensive; albumin and gelatins were manufactured as derivatives from human and animal tissue and therefore carried a small risk for disease transmission; and synthetic colloids were associated with adverse effects such as anaphylaxis, renal failure, and coagulation defects. These findings resulted in the incorporation of crystalloid solutions in guidelines as the gold standard for fluid resuscitation, especially in North American literature and guidelines. This has led to administration of enormous amounts of crystalloid solution in the first 24 hours after major trauma, burns, or septic shock. In several studies, mean administration of more than 30 L of crystalloids over 24 hours has been reported! In situations associated with capillary leak, this approach leads to development of massive tissue edema and the iatrogenic complications that ensue may lead to the polycompartment syndrome and multiple organ failure and death. Reports of mortality secondary to massive fluid resuscitation after trauma or shock are appearing increasingly over the past 10 years.

Do We Like Fluids Too Much?

The dangers of underresuscitation in terms of amount or timing of fluid administration are clear, but the adverse effects of overresuscitation, especially using crystalloids, are only recently being recognized. There is increasing evidence that increased compartment pressures and especially IAH may be the missing link between overresuscitation, multiple organ failure, and death.[131] As early as 1999, IAH and ACS were described in patients who received massive fluid resuscitation after extra-abdominal injury.[132] The mechanism through which massive fluid resuscitation causes IAH is probably related to capillary leak and edema, both of the abdominal wall (leading to decreased abdominal wall compliance) and of the bowel wall (leading to increased abdominal volume). In a retrospective series by Maxwell and colleagues,[132] the incidence of abdominal decompression among non–abdominal trauma victims was found to be 0.5%. The mean amount of fluids administered was 19 ± 5 L of crystalloid and 29 ± 10 units of packed red blood cells, the mortality was 67%, and nonsurvivors were decompressed approximately 20 hours later than survivors. The authors suggested that the incidence of secondary

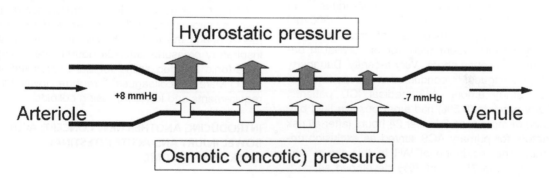

Force	Pressure	Arteriole	Venule
INTO interstitium	P_c	30 mmHg	15 mmHg
	π_i	6 mmHg	6 mmHg
INTO capillaries	π_c	- 28 mmHg	- 28 mmHg
	P_i	- 0 mmHg	- 0 mmHg
	Net pressure	**+ 8 mmHg**	**-7 mmHg**
		INTO interstitium	INTO capillaries

$$J_v = K_f([P_c - P_i] - \sigma[\pi_c - \pi_i])$$

Fig. 4. The Starling equation. Capillaries act rather like a leaky hosepipe: although the bulk of the fluid continues along the pipe, the pressure forces come out of the walls. Hydrostatic (blood) pressure is not the only force acting to cause fluid movement in and out of the capillaries. The plasma proteins that cannot cross the capillary walls exert an osmotic pressure to draw water back into the capillaries, which outweighs the hydrostatic pressure at the venous end of the capillaries. The net pressure at the arteriolar site is +8 mm Hg and forces fluids into the interstitium; the net pressure at the venular site is −7 mm Hg and drives fluids back into the capillaries. Each day about 20 L is lost while 16 L is regained. J_v is the net fluid movement between compartments The other factors are: Capillary hydrostatic pressure (P_c) Interstitial hydrostatic pressure (P_i) Capillary oncotic pressure (π_c) Interstitial oncotic pressure (π_i) Filtration coefficient (K_f) Reflection coefficient (σ)

ACS may be higher than previously thought in non–abdominal trauma victims and that early decompression may improve outcome since some improvement in organ function after decompression was seen. They recommended IAP monitoring in patients receiving high amounts of fluid resuscitation. A landmark paper by Balogh and colleagues[133] confirmed these findings. In their series, 11 (9%) of 128 standardized shock resuscitation patients developed secondary ACS. All cases were recognized and decompressed within 24 hours of hospital admission. After decompression, the bladder pressure and the systemic vascular resistance decreased, while the mean arterial pressure, cardiac index, and static lung compliance increased. The mortality rate was 54%. Those who died failed to respond to decompression with increased cardiac index and a sustained decrease in IAP. In analogy to trauma, secondary ACS has since been described also in burns and sepsis. The multiple-center studies on the prevalence and incidence of IAH in mixed ICU patients also showed that a positive net fluid balance as well as a positive cumulative fluid balance were predictors for poor outcome: nonsurvivors had a positive cumulative fluid balance of about 6 L versus 1 L in survivors.[25,26] Similar results have also been found by Alsous and colleagues:[134] at least 1 day of negative fluid balance ($\leq$ −500 mL) achieved by the third day of treatment was a good independent predictor of survival in patients with septic shock. Very recently, Daugherty and colleagues[135] conducted a prospective cohort study among 468 medical ICU patients. Forty patients (8.5%) had a net positive fluid balance of more than 5 L after 24 hours (after all risk factors for primary ACS served as exclusion criteria). The incidence of IAH in this group was a staggering 85% and 25% developed secondary ACS. The study was not powered to detect differences in mortality and outcome parameters were not statistically different between patients with or without IAH and ACS. Nevertheless, there was a trend toward higher mortality in the IAH groups and mortality figures reached 80% in the ACS group. Although epidemiologic research regarding this subject is virtually nonexistent, the increase in reported series seems to indicate increasing incidence of this highly lethal complication. In light of this increasing body of evidence regarding the association between massive fluid resuscitation, intra-abdominal hypertension, organ dysfunction, and mortality, it seems wise to at least incorporate IAP as a parameter in all future studies regarding fluid management, and to put into question current clinical practice guidelines, not in terms of whether to administer fluids at all, but in terms of the parameters we use to guide our treatment.

So How Should We Use Our Fluids?

As a result of the increasing problems with massive fluid resuscitation, many researchers have gone back to the concept of small volume resuscitation. This concept, to achieve the same physiologic goals as in "classical" crystalloid resuscitation using smaller volumes, implies the use of hypertonic or hyperosmotic solutions. In the American literature there is growing interest in the use of hypertonic saline for several indications.[136,137] The European literature and clinical practice, having never abandoned colloid administration completely, has focused mainly on new synthetic colloids such as 130-kD hydroxyethyl starch (HES – Voluven). Attempts to combine both strategies have led to several studies using mixed hypertonic saline and colloid infusions, eg, hyperHES, a solution consisting of NaCl 7.2% in HES with mixed results. Although good results have been obtained with small-volume resuscitation in most of these studies, many of them unfortunately make no mention of IAP or incidence of IAH and ACS at all. In the area of burn resuscitation there are some exceptions: Oda and colleagues[138] did report a reduced risk for abdominal compartment syndrome (as well as lower fluid requirements during the first 24 hours and lower peak inspiratory pressures after 24 hours) when using hypertonic lactated saline for burn resuscitation and O'Mara and colleagues[139] reported lower fluid requirements and lower IAP using colloids.

INTRODUCING ANOTHER NEW CONCEPT: ACUTE BOWEL INJURY AND ACUTE INTESTINAL DISTRESS SYNDROME

Although few epidemiologic data are available to confirm this observation, it is our impression that the incidence of primary IAH/ACS is decreasing owing to increased awareness of the problem among surgeons, who are more likely to leave the abdomen open in high-risk surgery cases.[140–142] This observation was also mentioned by Kimball and colleagues[143] in a series of ruptured aortic aneurysm cases and in a recent survey.[144]

The focus of attention is shifting to secondary ACS and rightfully so. This syndrome is highly prevalent in critically ill patients and leads to even higher mortality than primary IAH. As described by Kimball and colleagues[143] and Kirkpatrick and colleagues,[145] a variety of noxious stimuli (such as infection, trauma, burns, and sepsis) can lead to activation of the innate immune system and neutrophil activation. This systemic immune response causes release of cytokines into the circulation leading to systemic inflammatory response syndrome (SIRS) and capillary leak. Apart from direct negative impact on cellular organ function, this syndrome also exerts its deleterious effect through accumulation of extravascular fluids in the tissues and local ischemia. This mechanism of injury is widely recognized and accepted in the lung, where it is classified as acute lung injury (ALI) or acute respiratory distress syndrome (ARDS). However, the same pathologic process occurs in the gut, but this concept is much slower to seep into general ICU practice.

Why is this the case? It is undoubtedly true that bowel function is much harder to quantify than, for example, lung function. PaO2/FiO2 ratios are very easy to calculate at the bedside and monitoring parameters such as extravascular lung water index (EVLWI) have been demonstrated to be accurate prognostic predictors. However, the role of the gut as the motor of organ dysfunction syndrome cannot be denied and difficulties in assessing gut function should not deter us from recognizing that concept. In fact, in analogy to ALI and AKI, we propose the introduction of a concept named acute bowel injury (ABI), which is manifested through bowel edema and the ensuing IAH. Even more than other organ dysfunction syndromes, ABI goes hand in hand with the polycompartment syndrome and has a negative impact on distant organ systems through the development of IAH, and can contribute to the development of AKI and ALI.

HOW DO WE DEFINE ACUTE BOWEL INJURY AND ACUTE INTESTINAL DISTRESS SYNDROME?

No specific markers of bowel function have been identified, apart from the very crude on/off parameter of enteral feeding tolerance. However, since capillary leak and bowel edema are cornerstones of this syndrome, ABI can probably best been defined in terms of IAP levels. Another plus for IAP is that it has already been linked to prognosis in several epidemiologic studies. One might argue than that the ABI concept is just another word for IAH. However, ABI reflects a more basic concept of complex bowel injury caused by a first hit (either directly, such as in abdominal sepsis or trauma, or indirectly such as in ischemia due to hypovolemic or distributive shock), followed by a second hit in the form of capillary leak, bowel edema, and local ischemia, of which (secondary) IAH is the result (**Fig. 5**). If the vicious cycle is not stopped this will eventually lead to acute intestinal distress syndrome (AIDS) and ACS. In the light of the increased permeability as the motor of the first and second

hit some suggested the term acute intestinal permeability syndrome (AIPS). This can evolve to a more intuitive understanding of the complexity of the pathologic process instead of a purely mechanical viewpoint of increased pressure in a confined anatomic space.

CLINICAL MANAGEMENT

The management of patients with IAH is based on the following four principles:[27,146,147]

- specific procedures to reduce IAP and the consequences of ACS
- general support (intensive care) of the critically ill patient
- surgical decompression
- optimization after surgical decompression to perhaps counteract some of the specific adverse effects associated with decompression

Medical Treatment

Before surgical decompression is considered, less invasive medical treatment options should be optimized. The relation between abdominal contents and IAP is not linear but exponential (**Fig. 6**) and this curve is shifted to the left and upward when abdominal wall compliance is decreased. Therefore IAH can be treated by improving abdominal wall compliance and by decreasing intra-abdominal volume or both. Different medical treatments have been suggested to decrease IAP.[64] These are based on five different mechanisms:

- Improvement of abdominal wall compliance
- Evacuation of intraluminal contents
- Evacuation of abdominal fluid collections
- Correction of capillary leak and positive fluid balance
- Specific treatments

An algorithm for the clinical management of IAH and ACS is proposed in **Fig. 7**. **Box 2** gives an overview of the different medical treatment options.

Improvement of abdominal wall compliance
Sedation can help to control IAH by increasing abdominal wall compliance. Neuromuscular blockade has also been shown to decrease IAP, a phenomenon known for a long time in the operating theater.[33,75,148–150] Fentanyl, on the contrary, may acutely increase IAP by stimulation of active phasic expiratory activity.[151] Body positioning and the use of skin pressure decreasing interfaces will also affect IAP.[73,74,80] A percutaneous procedure to increase abdominal capacity/compliance

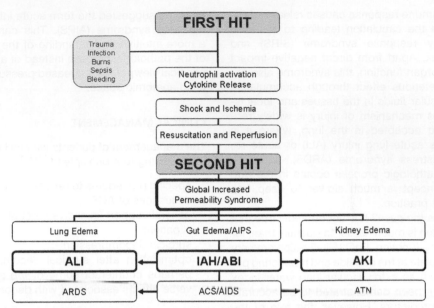

Fig. 5. The two-hit model causing the polycompartment syndrome. ABI, acute bowel injury; ACS, abdominal compartment syndrome; AIDS, acute intestinal distress syndrome; AIPS, acute intestinal permeability syndrome; AKI, acute kidney injury; ALI, acute lung injury; ARDS, acute respiratory distress syndrome; ATN, acute tubular necrosis; IAH, intra-abdominal hypertension.

and to decrease IAP, based on the principles of abdominal wall components separation was recently validated in a porcine ACS model.[152] In burn patients, a similar procedure had the same beneficial effects.[120]

Evacuation of intra-luminal contents
Ileus is common in most critically ill patients. Non-invasive evacuation of abdominal contents should

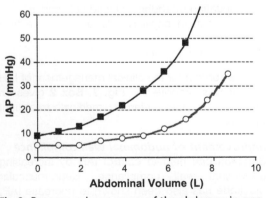

Fig. 6. Pressure volume curves of the abdomen in a patient with poor abdominal wall compliance (*closed squares*) compared with a patient with normal (*open circles*) abdominal wall compliance. (*Adapted from* Malbrain ML. Different techniques to measure intra-abdominal pressure (IAP): time for a critical reappraisal. Intensive Care Med 2004;30:357–71; with permission.)

be tried by means of gastric tube placement and suctioning, rectal tube, and enemas and possibly endoscopic decompression.[153–156] This can be done in conjunction with gastro- and or colonoprokinetics such as erythromycin (200 mg IV every 6 hours), metoclopramide (10 mg IV every 8 hours), neostygmine or prostygmine (2 mg diluted in up to 50 mL iv given slowly by infusion).[157–162]

Evacuation of abdominal fluid collections
Drainage of tense ascites may result in a decrease in IAP.[90,163–166] In patients with liver cirrhosis and esophageal varices, paracentesis helps to decrease variceal wall tension and the risk for rupture and bleeding.[167] Paracentesis is also the treatment of choice in burn patients with secondary ACS.[120,168,169] In the case of hematomas, blood collections, or a local abscess, CT-guided fine-needle aspiration has recently been described in the setting of IAH and ACS.

Correction of capillary leak and positive fluid balance
In the initial phase of ACS, fluid loss should be compensated to prevent splanchnic hypoperfusion.[58,170,171] Low-dose infusion of dobutamine, but not dopamine, also corrects the intestinal mucosal perfusion impairment induced by moderate increases in intra-abdominal pressure.[172] Because of the nature of the illness and injury associated

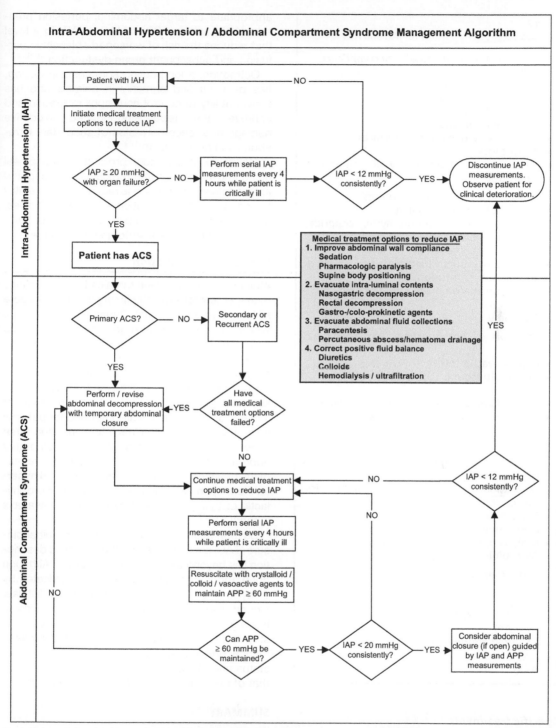

Fig. 7. Intra-abdominal hypertension/abdominal compartment syndrome management.

with ACS, these patients retain large volumes of sodium and water. Because of the capillary leak this will exacerbate tissue edema and third spacing, creating a vicious cycle of ongoing IAH. In the early stages, diuretic therapy in combination with albumin can be considered to mobilize the edema, but only if the patient is hemodynamically stable. Many patients, however, will develop anuria as renal blood flow is reduced. In these cases, the institution of renal replacement therapy should not be delayed, with fluid removal by intermittent dialysis or CVVH.[173–175]

> **Box 2**
> **Medical treatment options for IAH and ACS**
>
> *Improvement of abdominal wall compliance*
> - Sedation
> - Pain relief (not fentanyl!)
> - Neuromuscular blockade
> - Body positioning
> - Negative fluid balance
> - Skin pressure decreasing interfaces
> - Weight loss
> - Percutaneous abdominal wall component separation
>
> *Evacuation of intraluminal contents*
> - Gastric tube and suctioning
> - Gastroprokinetics (erythromycin, cisapride, metoclopramide)
> - Rectal tube and enemas
> - Colonoprokinetics (neostygmine, prostygmine bolus, or infusion)
> - Endoscopic decompression of large bowel
> - Colostomy
> - Ileostomy
>
> *Evacuation of peri-intestinal and abdominal fluids*
> - Ascites evacuation
> - CT- or ultrasound (US)-guided aspiration of abscess
> - CT- or US-guided aspiration of hematoma
> - Percutaneous drainage of (blood) collections
>
> *Correction of capillary leak and positive fluid balance*
> - Albumin in combination with diuretics (furosemide)
> - Correction of capillary leak (eg, antibiotics, source control)
> - Colloids instead of crystalloids
> - Dobutamine (not dopamine!)
> - Dialysis or CVVH with ultrafiltration
> - Ascorbinic acid in burn patients
>
> *Specific therapeutic interventions*
> - Continuous negative abdominal pressure (CNAP)
> - Negative external abdominal pressure (NEXAP)
> - Targeted abdominal perfusion pressure (APP)
> - (experimental: Octreotide and melatonin in ACS)

Specific treatments

Recently the application of continuous negative abdominal pressure by means of a cuirass has been studied in animals and humans showing a decrease in IAP and increase in end-expiratory lung volumes.[34,38,176–178]

In a similar manner to targeting cerebral perfusion pressure (CPP = MAP − ICP) or coronary perfusion pressure (CoPP = DBP − PAOP), it may be appropriate to target abdominal perfusion pressure (APP), where APP = MAP − IAP, to a level that reduces the risk of worsened splanchnic perfusion and subsequent organ dysfunction.[48,63,64]

Octreotide, a long-acting somatostatin analog, has been studied primarily in animals and has shown ability to control neutrophil infiltration and improve the reperfusion-induced oxidative damage after decompression of secondary intra-abdominal hypertension.[179]

Melatonin, a secretory product of the pineal gland known to have free radical scavenging and antioxidative properties, has recently shown ability to reduce lipid peroxidation in cell membranes, a process that promotes cell death, as the functional integrity of these structures is damage.[180]

Surgical Decompression

Although decompression remains the only definite management for ACS, the timing of this procedure still remains controversial. During the intervention, specific anesthetic challenges need to be solved and after decompression the patient is at risk for ischemia reperfusion injury, venous stasis, and fatal pulmonary embolism.[181] Maintaining adequate preload and abdominal perfusion pressure are the keys to success.[49,58,63] Open abdomen treatment (or laparostomy) was initially intended for patients with diffuse intra-abdominal infections, and often used in combination with a planned relaparotomy approach. Because of the increased awareness of the deleterious effects of intra-abdominal hypertension, open abdomen treatment, either prophylactic or therapeutic, is more common nowadays in the ICU.[102,182]

Several methods for temporary abdominal closure (TAC) are available, but their detailed description lies beyond the scope of this text.[183] Although open abdomen treatment can be complicated by delayed fascial closure, enterocutaneous fistulae, wound infections, and intractable fluid losses, leading to frequent reoperations and longer ICU stay, a large study has shown that the decreased mental, physical, emotional, and behavioral health status after decompressive laparotomy returns to that of the general population after 1 year.[184]

SUMMARY

First suggested in 1863 by Marey, ACS is the end stage of the physiologic sequellae of increased IAP, termed IAH. Recent observations suggest an increasing frequency of this complication in all types of patients. Even chronic elevations of IAP seem to affect the various organ systems in the body. The presence of IAH and ACS are significant causes of organ failure, increased resource use, decreased economic productivity, and increased mortality among a wide variety of patient populations.[25,29] Despite its obvious clinical implications, too little attention is paid to IAP, IAH, and ACS. Although there is much research interest in the subject, there are still too many unanswered questions that cloud our understanding of the pathophysiology of this syndrome.

In analogy to AKI and ALI, there is certainly a need for basic research into the underlying mechanisms of the new concepts of acute bowel injury and the polycompartment syndrome. Ischemia/reperfusion injury research in particular seems to show a lot of promise into this pathogenesis. At the same time, clinical research is also necessary.

Currently no good multicentric randomized interventional controlled clinical trial has tackled the question of whether an increase of IAP is a phenomenon or an epiphenomenon and whether any intervention to normalize IAP or APP will eventually affect patient outcome. Until that study exists, there will always be believers and nonbelievers.[185] The development of a management algorithm for IAH/ACS compares with the multifaceted approach emerging for early goal-directed therapy in sepsis.[52] The world society of the abdominal compartment syndrome (WSACS) invites interested researchers to join the society, to adhere to the consensus definitions posted at the Web site, and to submit some prospective data for the next world congress (www.wcacs.org), to be held in Dublin, Ireland, June 24 to 27, 2009. For those who carry the mandate to future IAH/ACS research, the path ahead is clear: using available evidence, we must develop an IAH/ACS therapeutic bundle and apply it in a multiple center, prospective, outcome trial. In a separate effort, attempts should be made to better understand the causes and evolution of ABI, AIDS/AIPS, and the polycompartment syndrome. In our opinion, it is one of the great scientific adventures of the future to link all the data that we have today on organ dysfunction, be it ALI, AKI, or ABI, and bring them together in a single broad-based concept that can explain the different aspects of the systemic inflammatory response syndrome and provide clues for treatment, not only aimed at the organs involved, but at the core of what kills our patients.

REFERENCES

1. Malbrain ML, Cheatham ML, Kirkpatrick A, et al. Results from the International Conference of experts on intra-abdominal hypertension and abdominal compartment syndrome. I. Definitions. Intensive Care Med 2006;32:1722–32.

2. Fietsam R Jr, Villalba M, Glover JL, et al. Intra-abdominal compartment syndrome as a complication of ruptured abdominal aortic aneurysm repair. Am Surg 1989;55:396–402.

3. Malbrain ML, De laet I, Cheatham M. Consensus conference definitions and recommendations on intra-abdominal hypertension (IAH) and the abdominal compartment syndrome (ACS)—the long road to the final publications, how did we get there? Acta Clin Belg Suppl 2007;62:44–59.

4. Malbrain ML, Cheatham ML, Kirkpatrick A, et al. Abdominal compartment syndrome: it's time to pay attention! Intensive Care Med 2006;32:1912–4.

5. Malbrain ML. You don't have any excuse, just start measuring abdominal pressure and act upon it! Minerva Anestesiol 2008;74:1–2.

6. Ivatury RR. Abdominal compartment syndrome: a century later, isn't it time to accept and promulgate? Crit Care Med 2006;34:2494–5.

7. Kirkpatrick AW, Brenneman FD, McLean RF, et al. Is clinical examination an accurate indicator of raised intra-abdominal pressure in critically injured patients? Can J Surg 2000;43:207–11.

8. Sugrue M, Bauman A, Jones F, et al. Clinical examination is an inaccurate predictor of intraabdominal pressure. World J Surg 2002;26:1428–31.

9. Malbrain ML. Different techniques to measure intra-abdominal pressure (IAP): time for a critical reappraisal. Intensive Care Med 2004;30:357–71.

10. Malbrain M, Jones F. Intra-abdominal pressure measurement techniques. In: Ivatury R, Cheatham M, Malbrain M, Sugrue M, editors. Abdominal compartment syndrome. Georgetown (TX): Landes Bioscience; 2006. p. 19–68.

11. Sanchez NC, Tenofsky PL, Dort JM, et al. What is normal intra-abdominal pressure? Am Surg 2001;67:243–8.

12. Sugerman H, Windsor A, Bessos M, et al. Intra-abdominal pressure, sagittal abdominal diameter and obesity comorbidity. J Intern Med 1997;241:71–9.

13. Sugerman HJ. Effects of increased intra-abdominal pressure in severe obesity. Surg Clin North Am 2001;81:1063–75, vi.

14. Davis PJ, Koottayi S, Taylor A, et al. Comparison of indirect methods of measuring intra-abdominal pressure in children. Intensive Care Med 2005;31:471–5.

15. Saggi B, Ivatury R, Sugerman HJ. Surgical critical care issues: abdominal compartment syndrome. In: Holzheimer RG, Mannick JA, editors. Surgical treatment evidence-based and problem-oriented. München: W. Zuckschwerdt Verlag München; 2001.

16. De Potter TJ, Dits H, Malbrain ML. Intra- and interobserver variability during in vitro validation of two novel methods for intra-abdominal pressure monitoring. Intensive Care Med 2005;31:747–51.

17. De Waele J, Pletinckx P, Blot S, et al. Saline volume in transvesical intra-abdominal pressure measurement: enough is enough. Intensive Care Med 2006;32:455–9.

18. Malbrain ML, Deeren DH. Effect of bladder volume on measured intravesical pressure: a prospective cohort study. Crit Care 2006;10:R98.

19. Ball CG, Kirkpatrick AW. 'Progression towards the minimum': the importance of standardizing the priming volume during the indirect measurement of intra-abdominal pressures. Crit Care 2006; 10:153.

20. De Iaet I, Hoste E, De Waele JJ. Transvesical intra-abdominal pressure measurement using minimal instillation volumes: how low can we go? Intensive Care Med 2008;34:746–50.

21. Malbrain ML. The assumed problem of air bubbles in the tubing during intra-abdominal pressure measurement—author reply. Intensive Care Med 2004; 30:1693.

22. Schachtrupp A, Henzler D, Orfao S, et al. Evaluation of a modified piezoresistive technique and a water-capsule technique for direct and continuous measurement of intra-abdominal pressure in a porcine model. Crit Care Med 2006;34: 745–50.

23. Schachtrupp A, Tons C, Fackeldey V, et al. Evaluation of two novel methods for the direct and continuous measurement of the intra-abdominal pressure in a porcine model. Intensive Care Med 2003;29: 1605–8.

24. Balogh Z, Jones F, D'Amours S, et al. Continuous intra-abdominal pressure measurement technique. Am J Surg 2004;188:679–84.

25. Malbrain ML, Chiumello D, Pelosi P, et al. Incidence and prognosis of intraabdominal hypertension in a mixed population of critically ill patients: a multiple-center epidemiological study. Crit Care Med 2005;33:315–22.

26. Malbrain ML, Chiumello D, Pelosi P, et al. Prevalence of intra-abdominal hypertension in critically ill patients: a multicentre epidemiological study. Intensive Care Med 2004;30:822–9.

27. Cheatham ML, Malbrain ML, Kirkpatrick A, et al. Results from the International Conference of experts on intra-abdominal hypertension and abdominal compartment syndrome. II. Recommendations. Intensive Care Med 2007;33:951–62.

28. Suominen PK, Pakarinen MP, Rautiainen P, et al. Comparison of direct and intravesical measurement of intraabdominal pressure in children. J Pediatr Surg 2006;41:1381–5.

29. Malbrain ML. Is it wise not to think about intraabdominal hypertension in the ICU? Curr Opin Crit Care 2004;10:132–45.

30. Malbrain ML, Deeren D, De Potter TJ. Intra-abdominal hypertension in the critically ill: it is time to pay attention. Curr Opin Crit Care 2005;11:156–71.

31. Citerio G, Berra L. Central nervous system. In: Ivatury R, Cheatham M, Malbrain M, Sugrue M, editors. Abdominal compartment syndrome. Georgetown (TX): Landes Bioscience; 2006. p. 144–56.

32. Citerio G, Vascotto E, Villa F, et al. Induced abdominal compartment syndrome increases intracranial pressure in neurotrauma patients: a prospective study. Crit Care Med 2001;29:1466–71.

33. Deeren D, Dits H, Malbrain MLNG. Correlation between intra-abdominal and intracranial pressure in nontraumatic brain injury. Intensive Care Med 2005;31:1577–81.

34. Bloomfield G, Saggi B, Blocher C, et al. Physiologic effects of externally applied continuous negative abdominal pressure for intra-abdominal hypertension. J Trauma 1999;46:1009–14 [discussion: 14–6].

35. Bloomfield GL, Dalton JM, Sugerman HJ, et al. Treatment of increasing intracranial pressure secondary to the acute abdominal compartment syndrome in a patient with combined abdominal and head trauma. J Trauma 1995;39:1168–70.

36. Bloomfield GL, Ridings PC, Blocher CR, et al. Effects of increased intra-abdominal pressure upon intracranial and cerebral perfusion pressure before and after volume expansion. J Trauma 1996;40: 936–41 [discussion: 41–3].

37. Bloomfield GL, Ridings PC, Blocher CR, et al. A proposed relationship between increased intra-abdominal, intrathoracic, and intracranial pressure. Crit Care Med 1997;25:496–503.

38. Saggi BH, Bloomfield GL, Sugerman HJ, et al. Treatment of intracranial hypertension using non-surgical abdominal decompression. J Trauma 1999;46:646–51.

39. Irgau I, Koyfman Y, Tikellis JI. Elective intraoperative intracranial pressure monitoring during laparoscopic cholecystectomy. Arch Surg 1995;130: 1011–3.

40. Joseph DK, Dutton RP, Aarabi B, et al. Decompressive laparotomy to treat intractable intracranial hypertension after traumatic brain injury. J Trauma 2004;57:687–93 [discussion: 93–5].

41. Josephs LG, Este-McDonald JR, Birkett DH, et al. Diagnostic laparoscopy increases intracranial pressure. J Trauma 1994;36:815–8 [discussion: 8–9].

42. Sugerman HJ, DeMaria EJ, Felton WL III, et al. Increased intra-abdominal pressure and cardiac filling pressures in obesity-associated pseudotumor cerebri. Neurology 1997;49:507–11.

43. Sugerman HJ, Felton IW III, Sismanis A, et al. Continuous negative abdominal pressure device to

treat pseudotumor cerebri. Int J Obes Relat Metab Disord 2001;25:486–90.

44. Sugerman H, Windsor A, Bessos M, et al. Effects of surgically induced weight loss on urinary bladder pressure, sagittal abdominal diameter and obesity co-morbidity. Int J Obes Relat Metab Disord 1998;22:230–5.

45. Kashtan J, Green JF, Parsons EQ, et al. Hemodynamic effect of increased abdominal pressure. J Surg Res 1981;30:249–55.

46. Ridings PC, Bloomfield GL, Blocher CR, et al. Cardiopulmonary effects of raised intra-abdominal pressure before and after intravascular volume expansion. J Trauma 1995;39:1071–5.

47. Richardson JD, Trinkle JK. Hemodynamic and respiratory alterations with increased intra-abdominal pressure. J Surg Res 1976;20:401–4.

48. Malbrain ML, Cheatham ML. Cardiovascular effects and optimal preload markers in intra-abdominal hypertension. In: Vincent J-L, editor. Yearbook of intensive care and emergency medicine. Berlin: Springer-Verlag; 2004. p. 519–43.

49. Cheatham M, Malbrain M. Abdominal perfusion pressure. In: Ivatury R, Cheatham M, Malbrain M, Sugrue M, editors. Abdominal compartment syndrome. Georgetown (TX): Landes Bioscience; 2006. p. 69–81.

50. Cheatham M, Malbrain M. Cardiovascular implications of elevated intra-abdominal pressure. In: Ivatury R, Cheatham M, Malbrain M, Sugrue M, editors. Abdominal compartment syndrome. Georgetown (TX): Landes Bioscience; 2006. p. 89–104.

51. Dellinger RP, Carlet JM, Masur H, et al. Surviving Sepsis Campaign guidelines for management of severe sepsis and septic shock. Intensive Care Med 2004;30:536–55.

52. Rivers E, Nguyen B, Havstad S, et al. Early goal-directed therapy in the treatment of severe sepsis and septic shock. N Engl J Med 2001;345: 1368–77.

53. Cheatham ML, Block EF, Nelson LD, et al. Superior predictor of the hemodynamic response to fluid challenge in critically ill patients. Chest 1998;114: 1226–7.

54. Cheatham ML, Nelson LD, Chang MC, et al. Right ventricular end-diastolic volume index as a predictor of preload status in patients on positive end-expiratory pressure. Crit Care Med 1998;26: 1801–6.

55. Schachtrupp A, Graf J, Tons C, et al. Intravascular volume depletion in a 24-hour porcine model of intra-abdominal hypertension. J Trauma 2003;55: 734–40.

56. Michard F, Alaya S, Zarka V, et al. Global end-diastolic volume as an indicator of cardiac preload in patients with septic shock. Chest 2003;124: 1900–8.

57. Michard F, Teboul JL. Predicting fluid responsiveness in ICU patients: a critical analysis of the evidence. Chest 2002;121:2000–8.

58. Simon RJ, Friedlander MH, Ivatury RR, et al. Hemorrhage lowers the threshold for intra-abdominal hypertension-induced pulmonary dysfunction. J Trauma 1997;42:398–403 [discussion: 4–5].

59. Burchard KW, Ciombor DM, McLeod MK, et al. Positive end expiratory pressure with increased intra-abdominal pressure. Surg Gynecol Obstet 1985;161:313–8.

60. Pelosi P, Ravagnan I, Giurati G, et al. Positive end-expiratory pressure improves respiratory function in obese but not in normal subjects during anesthesia and paralysis. Anesthesiology 1999;91: 1221–31.

61. Sugrue M, D'Amours S. The problems with positive end expiratory pressure (PEEP) in association with abdominal compartment syndrome (ACS). J Trauma 2001;51:419–20.

62. Sussman AM, Boyd CR, Williams JS, et al. Effect of positive end-expiratory pressure on intra-abdominal pressure. South Med J 1991;84:697–700.

63. Cheatham ML, White MW, Sagraves SG, et al. Abdominal perfusion pressure: a superior parameter in the assessment of intra-abdominal hypertension. J Trauma 2000;49:621–6 [discussion: 6–7].

64. Malbrain ML. Abdominal perfusion pressure as a prognostic marker in intra-abdominal hypertension. In: Vincent JL, editor. Yearbook of intensive care and emergency medicine. Berlin: Springer-Verlag; 2002. p. 792–814.

65. Mertens zur Borg IR, Verbrugge SJ, Olvera C. Pathophysiology: respiratory. In: Ivatury R, Cheatham M, Malbrain M, Sugrue M, editors. Abdominal compartment syndrome. Georgetown (TX): Landes Bioscience; 2006. p. 105–18.

66. Ranieri VM, Brienza N, Santostasi S, et al. Impairment of lung and chest wall mechanics in patients with acute respiratory distress syndrome: role of abdominal distension. Am J Respir Crit Care Med 1997;156:1082–91.

67. Gattinoni L, Pelosi P, Suter PM, et al. Acute respiratory distress syndrome caused by pulmonary and extrapulmonary disease. Different syndromes? Am J Respir Crit Care Med 1998;158:3–11.

68. Mutoh T, Lamm WJ, Embree LJ, et al. Abdominal distension alters regional pleural pressures and chest wall mechanics in pigs in vivo. J Appl Physiol 1991;70:2611–8.

69. Mutoh T, Lamm WJ, Embree LJ, et al. Volume infusion produces abdominal distension, lung

compression, and chest wall stiffening in pigs. J Appl Physiol 1992;72:575–82.

70. Pelosi P, Quintel M, Malbrain ML. Effect of intra-abdominal pressure on respiratory mechanics. Acta Clin Belg Suppl 2007;62:78–88.

71. Quintel M, Pelosi P, Caironi P, et al. An increase of abdominal pressure increases pulmonary edema in oleic acid-induced lung injury. Am J Respir Crit Care Med 2004;169:534–41.

72. De Keulenaer BL, De Backer A, Schepens DR, et al. Abdominal compartment syndrome related to noninvasive ventilation. Intensive Care Med 2003;29:1177–81.

73. Hering R, Vorwerk R, Wrigge H, et al. Prone positioning, systemic hemodynamics, hepatic indocyanine green kinetics, and gastric intramucosal energy balance in patients with acute lung injury. Intensive Care Med 2002;28:53–8.

74. Hering R, Wrigge H, Vorwerk R, et al. The effects of prone positioning on intraabdominal pressure and cardiovascular and renal function in patients with acute lung injury. Anesth Analg 2001;92:1226–31.

75. De Waele JJ, Benoit D, Hoste E, et al. A role for muscle relaxation in patients with abdominal compartment syndrome? Intensive Care Med 2003;29:332.

76. Diebel LN, Wilson RF, Dulchavsky SA, et al. Effect of increased intra-abdominal pressure on hepatic arterial, portal venous, and hepatic microcirculatory blood flow. J Trauma 1992;33:279–82 [discussion: 82–3].

77. Wendon J, Biancofiore G, Auzinger G. Intraabdominal hypertension and the liver. In: Ivatury R, Cheatham M, Malbrain M, Sugrue M, editors. Abdominal compartment syndrome. Georgetown (TX): Landes Bioscience; 2006. p. 138–43.

78. Biancofiore G, Bindi ML, Boldrini A, et al. Intraabdominal pressure in liver transplant recipients: incidence and clinical significance. Transplant Proc 2004;36:547–9.

79. Biancofiore G, Bindi ML, Romanelli AM, et al. Intraabdominal pressure monitoring in liver transplant recipients: a prospective study. Intensive Care Med 2003;29:30–6.

80. Michelet P, Roch A, Gainnier M, et al. Influence of support on intra-abdominal pressure, hepatic kinetics of indocyanine green and extravascular lung water during prone positioning in patients with ARDS: a randomized crossover study. Crit Care 2005;9:R251–7.

81. Schein M. Abdominal compartment syndrome: historical background. In: Ivatury R, Cheatham M, Malbrain M, Sugrue M, editors. Abdominal compartment syndrome. Georgetown (TX): Landes Bioscience; 2006. p. 1–7.

82. Biancofiore G, Bindi ML, Romanelli AM, et al. Postoperative intra-abdominal pressure and renal function after liver transplantation. Arch Surg 2003;138:703–6.

83. Sugrue M, Hallal A, D'Amours S. Intra-abdominal pressure hypertension and the kidney. In: Ivatury R, Cheatham M, Malbrain M, Sugrue M, editors. Abdominal compartment syndrome. Georgetown (TX): Landes Bioscience; 2006. p. 119–28.

84. Sugrue M, Buist MD, Hourihan F, et al. Prospective study of intra-abdominal hypertension and renal function after laparotomy. Br J Surg 1995;82: 235–8.

85. Sugrue M, Jones F, Deane SA, et al. Intra-abdominal hypertension is an independent cause of postoperative renal impairment. Arch Surg 1999;134: 1082–5.

86. Kirkpatrick AW, Colistro R, Laupland KB, et al. Renal arterial resistive index response to intraabdominal hypertension in a porcine model. Crit Care Med. 2006;35(1):207–13.

87. Bradley SE, Mudge GH, Blake WD, et al. The effect of increased intra-abdominal pressure on the renal excretion of water and electrolytes in normal human subjects and in patients with diabetes insipidus. Acta Clin Belg 1955;10:209–23.

88. Harman PK, Kron IL, McLachlan HD, et al. Elevated intra-abdominal pressure and renal function. Ann Surg 1982;196:594–7.

89. Kron IL, Harman PK, Nolan SP. The measurement of intra-abdominal pressure as a criterion for abdominal re-exploration. Ann Surg 1984;199: 28–30.

90. Luca A, Feu F, Garcia-Pagan JC, et al. Favorable effects of total paracentesis on splanchnic hemodynamics in cirrhotic patients with tense ascites. Hepatology 1994;20:30–3.

91. Jacques T, Lee R. Improvement of renal function after relief of raised intra-abdominal pressure due to traumatic retroperitoneal haematoma. Anaesth Intensive Care 1988;16:478–82.

92. Morris JA Jr, Eddy VA, Blinman TA, et al. The staged celiotomy for trauma. Issues in unpacking and reconstruction. Ann Surg 1993;217:576–84.

93. Shelly MP, Robinson AA, Hesford JW, et al. Haemodynamic effects following surgical release of increased intra-abdominal pressure. Br J Anaesth 1987;59:800–5.

94. Cullen DJ, Coyle JP, Teplick R, et al. Cardiovascular, pulmonary, and renal effects of massively increased intra-abdominal pressure in critically ill patients. Crit Care Med 1989;17:118–21.

95. Smith JH, Merrell RC, Raffin TA. Reversal of postoperative anuria by decompressive celiotomy. Arch Intern Med 1985;145:553–4.

96. Richards WO, Scovill W, Shin B, et al. Acute renal failure associated with increased intra-abdominal pressure. Ann Surg 1983;197:183–7.

97. Stothert JC. Evaluation of decapsulation of the canine kidney on renal function following acute ischemia. J Surg Res 1979;26:560–4.

98. Gewertz BL, Krupski W, Wheeler HT, et al. Effect of renal decapsulation on cortical hemodynamics in the postischemic kidney. J Surg Res 1980;28:252–9.

99. Ivatury R, Diebel L. Intra-abdominal hypertension and the splanchnic bed. In: Ivatury R, Cheatham M, Malbrain M, Sugrue M, editors. Abdominal compartment syndrome. Georgetown (TX): Landes Bioscience; 2006. p. 129–37.

100. Diebel LN, Dulchavsky SA, Brown WJ. Splanchnic ischemia and bacterial translocation in the abdominal compartment syndrome. J Trauma 1997;43:852–5.

101. Diebel LN, Dulchavsky SA, Wilson RF. Effect of increased intra-abdominal pressure on mesenteric arterial and intestinal mucosal blood flow. J Trauma 1992;33:45–8 [discussion: 8–9].

102. Balogh Z, Moore FA. Postinjury secondary abdominal compartment syndrome. In: Ivatury R, Cheatham M, Malbrain M, Sugrue M, editors. Abdominal compartment syndrome. Georgetown (TX): Landes Bioscience; 2006. p. 170–7.

103. Raeburn CD, Moore EE. Abdominal compartment syndrome provokes multiple organ failure: animal and human supporting evidence. In: Ivatury R, Cheatham M, Malbrain M, Sugrue M, editors. Abdominal compartment syndrome. Georgetown (TX): Landes Bioscience; 2006. p. 157–69.

104. Sugrue M, Jones F, Lee A, et al. Intraabdominal pressure and gastric intramucosal pH: is there an association? World J Surg 1996;20:988–91.

105. Ivatury RR, Porter JM, Simon RJ, et al. Intra-abdominal hypertension after life-threatening penetrating abdominal trauma: prophylaxis, incidence, and clinical relevance to gastric mucosal pH and abdominal compartment syndrome. J Trauma 1998;44:1016–21 [discussion: 21–3].

106. Balogh Z, McKinley BA, Cocanour CS, et al. Supranormal trauma resuscitation causes more cases of abdominal compartment syndrome. Arch Surg 2003;138:637–42 [discussion: 42–3].

107. Balogh Z, McKinley BA, Cox CS Jr, et al. Abdominal compartment syndrome: the cause or effect of postinjury multiple organ failure. Shock 2003;20: 483–92.

108. Moore FA. The role of the gastrointestinal tract in postinjury multiple organ failure. Am J Surg 1999; 178:449–53.

109. Eleftheriadis E, Kotzampassi K, Papanotas K, et al. Gut ischemia, oxidative stress, and bacterial translocation in elevated abdominal pressure in rats. World J Surg 1996;20:11–6.

110. Diebel L, Saxe J, Dulchavsky S. Effect of intra-abdominal pressure on abdominal wall blood flow. Am Surg 1992;58:573–5.

111. Wesley JR, Drongowski R, Coran AG. Intragastric pressure measurement: a guide for reduction and closure of the silastic chimney in omphalocele and gastroschisis. J Pediatr Surg 1981;16:264–70.

112. Rizzo A, Davis PC, Hamm CR, et al. Intraoperative vesical pressure measurements as a guide in the closure of abdominal wall defects. Am Surg 1996; 62:192–6.

113. Kuhn MA, Tuggle DW. Abdominal compartment syndrome in the pediatric patient. In: Ivatury R, Cheatham M, Malbrain M, Sugrue M, editors. Abdominal compartment syndrome. Georgetown (TX): Landes Bioscience; 2006. p. 217–22.

114. Ivy ME. Secondary abdominal compartment syndrome in burns. In: Ivatury R, Cheatham M, Malbrain M, Sugrue M, editors. Abdominal compartment syndrome. Georgetown (TX): Landes Bioscience; 2006. p. 178–86.

115. Demling RH, Crawford G, Lind L, et al. Restrictive pulmonary dysfunction caused by the grafted chest and abdominal burn. Crit Care Med 1988; 16:743–7.

116. Greenhalgh DG, Warden GD. The importance of intra-abdominal pressure measurements in burned children. J Trauma 1994;36:685–90.

117. Hobson KG, Young KM, Ciraulo A, et al. Release of abdominal compartment syndrome improves survival in patients with burn injury. J Trauma 2002; 53:1129–33.

118. Ivy ME, Atweh NA, Palmer J, et al. Intra-abdominal hypertension and abdominal compartment syndrome in burn patients. J Trauma 2000;49: 387–91.

119. Ivy ME, Possenti PP, Kepros J, et al. Abdominal compartment syndrome in patients with burns. J Burn Care Rehabil 1999;20:351–3.

120. Latenser BA, Kowal-Vern A, Kimball D, et al. A pilot study comparing percutaneous decompression with decompressive laparotomy for acute abdominal compartment syndrome in thermal injury. J Burn Care Rehabil 2002;23:190–5.

121. Ziakas PD, Voulgarelis M, Felekouras E, et al. Myelofibrosis-associated massive splenomegaly: a cause of increased intra-abdominal pressure, pulmonary hypertension, and positional dyspnea. Am J Hematol 2005;80:128–32.

122. Hamad GG, Peitzman AB. Morbid obesity and chronic intra-abdominal hypertension. In: Ivatury R, Cheatham M, Malbrain M, Sugrue M, editors. Abdominal compartment syndrome. Georgetown (TX): Landes Bioscience; 2006. p. 187–94.

123. Sugerman HJ. Increased intra-abdominal pressure in obesity. Int J Obes Relat Metab Disord 1998;22:1138.

124. Ueland K, Novy MJ, Peterson EN, et al. Maternal cardiovascular dynamics. IV. The influence of gestational age on the maternal cardiovascular

response to posture and exercise. Am J Obstet Gynecol 1969;104:856–64.

125. Lemaire BM, van Erp WF. Laparoscopic surgery during pregnancy. Surg Endosc 1997;11:15–8.

126. O'Rourke N, Kodali BS. Laparoscopic surgery during pregnancy. Curr Opin Anaesthesiol 2006;19:254–9.

127. Scalea TM, Bochicchio GV, Habashi N, et al. Increased intra-abdominal, intrathoracic, and intracranial pressure after severe brain injury: multiple compartment syndrome. J Trauma 2007;62:647–56.

128. De laet I, Citerio G, Malbrain ML. The influence of intraabdominal hypertension on the central nervous system: current insights and clinical recommendations, is it all in the head? Acta Clin Belg Suppl 2007;62:89–97.

129. Malbrain ML, Wilmer A. The polycompartment syndrome: towards an understanding of the interactions between different compartments! Intensive Care Med 2007;33:1869–72.

130. De laet IE, De Waele JJ, Malbrain MLNG. Fluid resuscitation and intra-abdominal hypertension. In: Vincent J-L, editor. Yearbook of intensive care and emergency medicine. Berlin: Springer-Verlag; 2008. p. 536–48.

131. Kirkpatrick AW, De Waele JJ, Ball CG, et al. The secondary and recurrent abdominal compartment syndrome. Acta Clin Belg Suppl 2007;62:60–5.

132. Maxwell RA, Fabian TC, Croce MA, et al. Secondary abdominal compartment syndrome: an underappreciated manifestation of severe hemorrhagic shock. J Trauma 1999;47:995–9.

133. Balogh Z, McKinley BA, Cocanour CS, et al. Secondary abdominal compartment syndrome is an elusive early complication of traumatic shock resuscitation. Am J Surg 2002;184:538–43 [discussion: 43–4].

134. Alsous F, Khamiees M, DeGirolamo A, et al. Negative fluid balance predicts survival in patients with septic shock: a retrospective pilot study. Chest 2000;117:1749–54.

135. Daugherty EL, Hongyan L, Taichman D, et al. Abdominal compartment syndrome is common in medical intensive care unit patients receiving large-volume resuscitation. J Intensive Care Med 2007;22:294–9.

136. Morishita Y, Harada T, Moriyama Y, et al. Simultaneous retrieval of the heart and liver from a single donor: an evaluation through preservation and transplantation. J Heart Transplant 1988;7:269–73.

137. Tyagi S, Kaul UA, Nair M, et al. Balloon angioplasty of the aorta in Takayasu's arteritis: initial and long-term results. Am Heart J 1992;124:876–82.

138. Oda J, Ueyama M, Yamashita K, et al. Hypertonic lactated saline resuscitation reduces the risk of abdominal compartment syndrome in severely burned patients. J Trauma 2006;60:64–71.

139. O'Mara MS, Slater H, Goldfarb IW, et al. A prospective, randomized evaluation of intra-abdominal pressures with crystalloid and colloid resuscitation in burn patients. J Trauma 2005;58:1011–8.

140. Reintam A, Parm P, Kitus R, et al. Primary and secondary intra-abdominal hypertension—different impact on ICU outcome Intensive Care Med 2008;34(9):1624–31.

141. Vidal M, Ruiz Weisser J, Gonzalez F, et al. Incidence and clinical effects of intraabdominal hypertension in critically ill patients. Crit Care Med 2008;36(6):1823–31.

142. Malbrain ML, De Laet I. AIDS is coming to your ICU: be prepared for acute bowel injury and acute intestinal distress syndrome. Intensive Care Med 2008;34(9):1565–9.

143. Kimball EJ. Intra-abdominal hypertension and the abdominal compartment syndrome: 'ARDS' of the gut. Int J Intensive Care 2006;1–7, Spring.

144. De Laet IE, Hoste FA, De Waele JJ. Survey on the perception and management of the abdominal compartment syndrome among Belgian surgeons. Acta Chir Belg 2007;107:648–52.

145. Kirkpatrick AW, Balogh Z, Ball CG, et al. The secondary abdominal compartment syndrome: iatrogenic or unavoidable? J Am Coll Surg 2006;202:668–79.

146. Mayberry JC. Prevention of abdominal compartment syndrome. In: Ivatury R, Cheatham M, Malbrain M, Sugrue M, editors. Abdominal compartment syndrome. Georgetown (TX): Landes Bioscience; 2006. p. 221–9.

147. Parr M, Olvera C. Medical management of abdominal compartment syndrome. In: Ivatury R, Cheatham M, Malbrain M, Sugrue M, editors. Abdominal compartment syndrome. Georgetown (TX): Landes Bioscience; 2006. p. 230–7.

148. Macalino JU, Goldman RK, Mayberry JC. Medical management of abdominal compartment syndrome: case report and a caution. Asian J Surg 2002;25:244–6.

149. Kimball EJ, Mone M. Influence of neuromuscular blockade on intra-abdominal pressure. Crit Care Med 2005;33:A38.

150. Kimball WR, Loring SH, Basta SJ, et al. Effects of paralysis with pancuronium on chest wall statics in awake humans. J Appl Physiol 1985;58:1638–45.

151. Drummond GB, Duncan MK. Abdominal pressure during laparoscopy: effects of fentanyl. Br J Anaesth 2002;88:384–8.

152. Voss M, Pinheiro J, Reynolds J, et al. Endoscopic components separation for abdominal compartment syndrome. Am J Surg 2003;186:158–63.

153. Bauer JJ, Gelernt IM, Salky BA, et al. Is routine postoperative nasogastric decompression really necessary? Ann Surg 1985;201:233–6.

154. Cheatham ML, Chapman WC, Key SP, et al. A meta-analysis of selective versus routine

nasogastric decompression after elective laparotomy. Ann Surg 1995;221:469–76.

155. Moss G, Friedman RC. Abdominal decompression: increased efficency by esophageal aspiration utilizing a new nasogastric tube. Am J Surg 1977; 133:225–8.

156. Savassi-Rocha PR, Conceicao SA, Ferreira JT, et al. Evaluation of the routine use of the nasogastric tube in digestive operation by a prospective controlled study. Surg Gynecol Obstet 1992;174: 317–20.

157. Ponec RJ, Saunders MD, Kimmey MB. Neostigmine for the treatment of acute colonic pseudo-obstruction. N Engl J Med 1999;341:137–41.

158. Wilmer A, Dits H, Malbrain ML, et al. Gastric emptying in the critically ill—the way forward. Intensive Care Med 1997;23:928–9.

159. Madl C, Druml W. Gastrointestinal disorders of the critically ill. Systemic consequences of ileus. Best Pract Res Clin Gastroenterol 2003;17: 445–56.

160. Malbrain ML. Abdominal pressure in the critically ill. Curr Opin Crit Care 2000;6:17–29.

161. Gorecki PJ, Kessler E, Schein M. Abdominal compartment syndrome from intractable constipation. J Am Coll Surg 2000;190:371.

162. van der Spoel JI, Oudemans-van Straaten HM, Stoutenbeek CP, et al. Neostigmine resolves critical illness-related colonic ileus in intensive care patients with multiple organ failure—a prospective, double-blind, placebo-controlled trial. Intensive Care Med 2001;27:822–7.

163. Sugrue M. Abdominal compartment syndrome. Curr Opin Crit Care 2005;11:333–8.

164. Corcos AC, Sherman HF. Percutaneous treatment of secondary abdominal compartment syndrome. J Trauma 2001;51:1062–4.

165. Cabrera J, Falcon L, Gorriz E, et al. Abdominal decompression plays a major role in early postparacentesis haemodynamic changes in cirrhotic patients with tense ascites. Gut 2001;48: 384–9.

166. Reckard JM, Chung MH, Varma MK, et al. Management of intraabdominal hypertension by percutaneous catheter drainage. J Vasc Interv Radiol 2005;16:1019–21.

167. Escorsell A, Gines A, Llach J, et al. Increasing intra-abdominal pressure increases pressure, volume, and wall tension in esophageal varices. Hepatology 2002;36:936–40.

168. Gotlieb WH, Feldman B, Feldman-Moran O, et al. Intraperitoneal pressures and clinical parameters of total paracentesis for palliation of symptomatic ascites in ovarian cancer. Gynecol Oncol 1998; 71:381–5.

169. Navarro-Rodriguez T, Hashimoto CL, Carrilho FJ, et al. Reduction of abdominal pressure in patients with ascites reduces gastroesophageal reflux. Dis Esophagus 2003;16:77–82.

170. Friedlander MH, Simon RJ, Ivatury R, et al. Effect of hemorrhage on superior mesenteric artery flow during increased intra-abdominal pressures. J Trauma 1998;45:433–89.

171. Gargiulo NJ 3rd, Simon RJ, Leon W, et al. Hemorrhage exacerbates bacterial translocation at low levels of intra-abdominal pressure. Arch Surg 1998;133:1351–5.

172. Agusti M, Elizalde JI, Adalia R, et al. Dobutamine restores intestinal mucosal blood flow in a porcine model of intra-abdominal hyperpressure. Crit Care Med 2000;28:467–72.

173. Oda S, Hirasawa H, Shiga H, et al. Management of intra-abdominal hypertension in patients with severe acute pancreatitis with continuous hemodiafiltration using a polymethyl methacrylate membrane hemofilter. Ther Apher Dial 2005;9:355–61.

174. Kula R, Szturz P, Sklienka P, et al. A role for negative fluid balance in septic patients with abdominal compartment syndrome? Intensive Care Med 2004;30:2138–9.

175. Vachharajani V, Scott LK, Grier L, et al. Medical management of severe intra-abdominal hypertension with aggressive diuresis and continuous ultrafiltration. Internet J Emerg Intensive Care Med 2003;6. Available at: http://www.ispub.com/ostia/index.phpxmlFilePath=journals/ijeicm/vol6n2/ultr.

176. Valenza F, Irace M, Guglielmi M, et al. Effects of continuous negative extra-abdominal pressure on cardiorespiratory function during abdominal hypertension: an experimental study. Intensive Care Med 2005;31:105–11.

177. Valenza F, Bottino N, Canavesi K, et al. Intra-abdominal pressure may be decreased non-invasively by continuous negative extra-abdominal pressure (NEXAP). Intensive Care Med 2003;29:2063–7.

178. Valenza F, Gattinoni L. Continuous negative abdominal pressure. In: Ivatury R, Cheatham M, Malbrain M, Sugrue M, editors. Abdominal compartment syndrome. Georgetown (TX): Landes Bioscience; 2006. p. 238–51.

179. Kacmaz A, Polat A, User Y, et al. Octreotide improves reperfusion-induced oxidative injury in acute abdominal hypertension in rats. J Gastrointest Surg 2004;8:113–9.

180. Sener G, Kacmaz A, User Y, et al. Melatonin ameliorates oxidative organ damage induced by acute intra-abdominal compartment syndrome in rats. J Pineal Res 2003;35:163–8.

181. Mertens zur Borg IR, Verbrugge SJ, Kolkman KA. Anesthetic considerations in abdominal compartment syndrome. In: Ivatury R, Cheatham M, Malbrain M, Sugrue M, editors. Abdominal compartment syndrome. Georgetown (TX): Landes Bioscience; 2006. p. 252–63.

182. Balogh Z, Moore FA, Goettler CE, et al. Management of abdominal compartment syndrome. In: Ivatury R, Cheatham M, Malbrain M, Sugrue M, editors. Abdominal compartment syndrome. Georgetown (TX): Landes Bioscience; 2006. p. 264–94.

183. De Laet IE, Ravyts M, Vidts W, et al. Current insights in intra-abdominal hypertension and abdominal compartment syndrome: open the abdomen and keep it open! Langenbecks Arch Surg 2008;393(6):833–47.

184. Cheatham ML, Safcsak K, Llerena LE, et al. Long-term physical, mental, and functional consequences of abdominal decompression. J Trauma 2004;56:237–41 [discussion: 41–2].

185. Kimball EJ, Kim W, Cheatham ML, et al. Clinical awareness of intra-abdominal hypertension and abdominal compartment syndrome in 2007. Acta Clin Belg 2007;62(Suppl):66–73.

186. Burch JM, Moore EE, Moore FA, et al. The abdominal compartment syndrome. Surg Clin North Am 1996;76:833–42.

187. Ivatury RR, Sugerman HJ, Peitzman AB. Abdominal compartment syndrome: recognition and management. Adv Surg 2001;35:251–69.

ICU Management of Acute Liver Failure

Michael L. Schilsky, MD[a,b,c,*], Shyoko Honiden, MD[a,d],
Lindsay Arnott, RN, MHA, CCTC[b,e], Sukru Emre, MD[b,e]

KEYWORDS

• Acute liver failure • Liver transplant • Cerebral edema
• Coagulopathy • Liver assist devices • Hypothermia

Acute liver failure (ALF) is defined as the development of impaired hepatic synthetic function with coagulopathy and the development of hepatic encephalopathy in the absence of underlying liver disease in less than 2 to 3 months time.[1] In the setting of ALF, hepatic encephalopathy may be associated with life-threatening cerebral edema, whereas by contrast this association is absent in patients who have chronic liver failure with encephalopathy. The recovery from the loss of functional liver mass in acute liver injury occurs more readily than in the chronic setting because of the lack of long-standing fibrosis and portal hypertension, and the host's overall better nutritional status. Therefore, if the individual can be supported properly throughout the acute event, and the inciting injury is removed or ameliorated, recovery will follow the rapid regeneration of liver cells. For those in whom spontaneous recovery is not possible, liver transplant may be life-saving.

PATHOGENESIS OF ACUTE LIVER FAILURE

The specific pathogenesis of the liver injury is dependent to a large degree on the etiology. There are features of injury common to most etiologies of ALF, however. Injury to hepatocytes causes cell damage or cell death by necrosis or apoptosis; however, these processes may coexist.[2] Triggering of the mitochondrial permeability transition by injury typically is associated with apoptosis if ATP stores are preserved, and necrosis if there is ATP depletion.[2] Examples of mitochondrial injury associated with apoptosis include acute Wilson disease[3] and Reye's syndrome.[4] In the early phase of injury from warm and cold ischemia, hepatocytes and endothelial cells activate the mitochondrial permeability transition, and mitochondrial injury results in ATP depletion and ensuing necrosis.

Necrotic injury of liver cells leads to a loss of cell membrane integrity and eventual rupture and cell death with the release of cytosolic proteins including lactate dehydrogenase (LDH), alanine aminotransferase (ALT), aspartate aminotransferase (AST), and ferritin. Cellular glutathione is diminished, especially following ALF with acetaminophen.[5] This increases cellular susceptibility to oxidative injury and impairs the ability to conjugate and detoxify some toxic substances. Other detoxification mechanisms are impaired, including the transport systems for bilirubin, leading cholestasis and conjugated hyperbilirubinemia.

An important feature of acute and chronic liver injury is the general loss of Kuppfer cell function that results in reduced clearance of endotoxin and other substrates regularly presented to

[a] Department of Medicine, Yale New Haven Transplantation Center, 333 Cedar Street, New Haven, CT 06520, USA
[b] Department of Surgery, Yale New Haven Transplantation Center, 333 Cedar Street, New Haven, CT 06520, USA
[c] Section of Transplant and Immunology, Division of Digestive Diseases, Yale New Haven Transplantation Center, 333 Cedar Street, New Haven, CT 06520, USA
[d] Division of Pulmonology and Critical Care, Yale New Haven Transplantation Center, 333 Cedar Street, New Haven, CT 06520, USA
[e] Section of Transplant and Immunology, Yale New Haven Transplantation Center, 333 Cedar Street, New Haven, CT 06520, USA
* Corresponding author. Yale University Medical Center, 333 Cedar Street, LMP 1080, New Haven, CT 06520.
E-mail address: michael.schilsky@yale.edu (M.L. Schilsky).

Clin Chest Med 30 (2009) 71–87
doi:10.1016/j.ccm.2008.10.001

hepatocytes by means of the portal system, increasing the risk of infection.[6]

The site of injury within the liver plays an important role in determining the ability of the liver to regenerate. Arterial blood and portal blood rich in oxygen and nutrients are supplied in the portal tract where the liver progenitor cells, ductal hepatocytes, or oval cells are present.[7] Injury to the portal zone inhibits the regenerative response, while injury to the central zone with sparing of the portal zone permits more frequent spontaneous recovery. The central zone is more susceptible to ischemic injury. Other toxic injuries may differ in their site of action because of differences in the metabolism of central hepatocytes compared with portal hepatocytes.

ETIOLOGIES OF ACUTE LIVER FAILURE AND SPECIFIC THERAPIES

The specific etiology of ALF is the most important determinant of outcome.[8] The frequency of specific types of liver injury varies in different geographic locations.[8,9] The following section focuses on specific etiologies and therapies for ALF.

Toxins

Acetaminophen remains by far the most common cause of toxic liver injury.[8] Liver failure caused by acetaminophen typically is associated with ingestion of at least 4 mg and more frequently greater than 10 g of the drug. Lesser amounts of acetaminophen may cause liver failure in the setting of alcohol use or underlying liver disease, presumably because of activation of the microsomal enzymes that metabolize acetaminophen, although the degree of increased susceptibility has been questioned by some.[10] In theory, this increased susceptibility should be worse in women who have a reduced threshold for alcohol-related liver injury because of reduced alcohol dehydrogenase activity relative to males.[11] Interestingly, in patients who have muscular dystrophy, there appears to be an increased susceptibility to severe liver injury with therapeutic dosages of acetaminophen for as yet uncertain reasons.[12] Acetaminophen is metabolized in hepatocytes by cytochrome enzymes to the toxic metabolite N-acetyl P-benzoquinoneimine (NAPQI) that normally is detoxified by conjugation with glutathione. Depletion of glutathione leads to accelerated liver injury by virtue of reduced detoxification of NAPQI. N-acetylcysteine (NAC) is administered to patients with toxic acetaminophen ingestion to replenish glutathione stores.[13] Acetaminophen-induced injury is concentrated in the central zones of the liver, and portal tracts are mostly spared excepting in extreme injury, permitting spontaneous recovery in as many as 80% with timely NAC therapy.[8] Serum levels of acetaminophen in the blood are typically proportional to the amount of acetaminophen ingested and permit stratification of the risk for liver failure if the time of ingestion is known. Recently, acetaminophen adducts were measured in some patients in whom acetaminophen ingestion was uncertain.[14] Whether the acetaminophen alone was causative in these individuals and whether these levels can be used to prognosticate injury in a similar fashion to acetaminophen alone remain to be determined. NAC previously had been administered to patients as an oral solution that was as efficacious as the intravenous preparation.[15] Intravenous preparations, however, are now available and are preferable in the setting of ALF, because they eliminate problems related to absorption, especially in patients who have been given charcoal or other adsorbents.[16] Reactions to the medication, allergic or cardiac dysrhythmia that can be related to the rate of infusion, are rare and typically reversible with the use of antihistamines and discontinuation of the NAC.

Amanita poisoning from the heat-stable toxin contained in the mushroom *Amanita phalloides* and *Amanita virosa* may lead to acute liver injury. Initially, these patients suffer gastrointestinal symptoms of vomiting and diarrhea.[17] This is followed by liver injury and then development of secondary injury to other organ systems. Mortality approaches 10% to 30%. Treatment with silibinin or with penicillin G early on in high dosages may ameliorate the hepatic injury.[18]

Other drugs and herbal compounds may cause severe acute liver injury, and the site within the liver that is affected, central versus portal, in part may determine the ability to spontaneously recovery from the injury. Many of these injuries are idiosyncratic. There may be some predisposition to developing severe drug- induced liver injury due to individual differences in drug metabolism, however.[19] Examples for which this is suspected include isoniazid, ketoconazole, disulfuram, valproate, and amiodarone, among others. Other toxic injuries, one excellent example being halothane, may trigger severe immune-mediated liver injury upon re-exposure.[20]

Viral Hepatitis

Viral infection with hepatotrophic viruses such as hepatitis A, B, and E is associated more often with acute liver injury with recovery; however, a small percent of patients who have each of these infections will develop acute liver failure.[8,9] There are no specific therapies for hepatitis A or E, but there are antiviral agents that inhibit the replication of hepatitis B. Although use of antiviral agents in patients who have acute hepatitis B virus (HBV) seems logical, studies from India and the United States experience from the Acute Liver Failure Study Group (ALFSG) fail to demonstrate that treatment reduces the risk for ALF.[21,22] For patients who have acute HBV with liver failure, however, use of antiviral agents may be warranted if for no other reason than to suppress the virus in a patient destined for liver transplant to reduce the risk of recurrence in the graft. Acute HBV may be even more severe if there is coinfection or superinfection with hepatitis D virus (HDV). Acute outbreaks of HBV and HDV infection have been reported in association with injection drug use.[23] Hepatitis E is rarely fatal; however, in pregnant patients in India who had acute hepatitis E virus (HEV) infection, liver failure and death without transplantation were reported to be as high as 20% of affected individuals.[24] Another recent report suggests that this high mortality with HEV during pregnancy is not seen in other geographic regions, and the reason for these differences are as yet unknown.[25]

Other viral infections that are associated with ALF include herpes simplex virus, varicella zoster virus, and cytomegalovirus.[8] Rarely, ALF may be caused by Epstein-Barr virus (EBV) infection.[26]

Metabolic

ALF may result from underlying metabolic liver disease. Liver failure caused by copper toxicosis in Wilson disease is unusual in that underlying liver disease is present, often previously unrecognized, and ALF occurs on the background of advanced fibrosis or cirrhosis of the liver.[27] This accounts for the almost uniform mortality of these patients without transplantation, because there is little hepatic reserve.[28] ALF caused by Wilson disease typically is accompanied by a nonimmune hemolytic anemia, and may be recognized by a low alkaline phosphatase to bilirubin ratio (less than four) and ALT to AST ratio of less than 2, markedly elevated serum copper greater than 200 μg/dL, and 24-hour urine copper often greater than 200 μg.[27,29] Although Kayser-Fleischer rings are pathognomonic, they are present only in approximately 30% to 50% of patients diagnosed with Wilson disease in the setting of ALF;[27] thus, the absence of rings does not exclude the diagnosis. Ceruloplasmin levels, useful for the diagnosis of most other patients who have Wilson disease, are poorly predictive in the setting of ALF.[29] Renal insufficiency is often present because of tubular damage caused by acute copper exposure. Treatments that acutely lower circulating copper levels of the patient by some form of plasma exchange or other treatment such as albumin dialysis may help in acutely stabilizing the patient by breaking the cycle of liver and renal tubular injury and hemolysis. These therapies delay but do not stay the need for transplant in these patients, however. Treatment with copper chelation and zinc, mainstays of medical treatment for Wilson disease, may be best used for those who have chronic liver failure and has little influence on the outcome of patients who have this acute presentation.[27]

Acute fatty liver of pregnancy (AFLP) is an unusual disorder where the metabolic disruption in the fetus causes maternal–fetal distress.[30] This disorder typically presents in the third trimester with marked elevation of liver tests and may progress rapidly to jaundice and liver failure. Fifty percent of the patients have preeclampsia. Fatty liver may be suspected on noninvasive imaging, but the type and percent of the fat content cannot be estimated. Liver biopsy is the standard for diagnosis, with fatty change concentrated in the centrilobular hepatocytes. Delivery of the fetus is necessary for maternal and fetal survival. Underlying defects in fetal fatty acid metabolism have been demonstrated.[31] More recently, use of plasma exchange was studied in six patients who had AFLP 2 to 8 days after delivery, and may have improved outcomes with reduced hospital stays and prevention of multiorgan failure syndrome.[32] Although this needs further study, the relatively low risk of performing this procedure suggests it could be tried as adjunctive therapy for these individuals.

Preeclampsia during pregnancy can be associated with HELLP syndrome (hemolysis, elevated liver enzymes, and low platelets).[33] This disorder also occurs most commonly in patents in the last stage of pregnancy, but may develop after delivery. Delivery of the fetus is the only known treatment that may arrest the progression of the disease.

Vascular

Acute obstruction of hepatic venous outflow or Budd Chiari syndrome may result in ALF. This often is recognized by the presence of hepatomegaly, new and rapid onset of ascites, and imaging studies showing hepatic venous thrombosis. Acute decompression of the obstruction with transhepatic intrahepatic portosystemic shunt (TIPS)[34] or surgical portosystemic shunt procedure[35] may prevent further hepatic injury. If there is underlying cirrhosis or continued decompensation, transplantation may become necessary.[34–36] This disorder frequently is associated with hypercoagulable states or disorders causing hypercoaguability.[36,37] If the patient survives the acute injury, remodeling of the liver and efforts for vascular decompression and anticoagulation may improve or stabilize hepatic function with time.

Ischemic hepatitis or shock liver is associated with acute liver injury mainly in the central zone. Typically there is a history of significant hypotension that precedes the development of the injury. Treatment of the underlying condition that led to the hepatic injury is critical for recovery.[38]

Other vascular causes of acute liver injury includes sinusoidal obstruction syndrome that occurs with smaller vessel veno-occlusive disease[39] and infiltrative disease associated with malignancy, more commonly with lymphoma but also from other tumors.[40]

Autoimmune

Autoimmune hepatitis rarely may present with ALF. Some patients may have acute or chronic disease if the earlier injury was unrecognized. Up to 30% of patients who have acute presentation of autoimmune hepatitis will not have the typical serum markers for autoimmune hepatitis.[41] Some patients may respond to high-dose steroid treatment following the exclusion of viral hepatitis. Liver biopsy may help to identify these individuals, and transjugular liver biopsy may be warranted in selected patients despite coagulopathy.

EVALUATION OF THE PATIENT WITH ACUTE LIVER FAILURE

The most critical element to patient survival with ALF is its early recognition. This permits rapid identification of the etiology of the liver failure, initiation of etiology-specific treatments when appropriate, and importantly the proper mobilization of personnel involved in various aspects of patient care.

The first phase of the evaluation includes obtaining a detailed history from the patient if possible or from others who may know the patient's medical history. Physical examination should assess the patient's mental status and evaluate liver and spleen size and presence or absence of ascites. Lack of stigmata of chronic liver disease such as spider angiomata, splenomegaly, or gynecomastia is typical in ALF. Neurologic evaluation should note pupil size and reactivity and reflexes, presence or absence of clonus, and the presence or absence of hepatic encephalopathy.

Encephalopathy should be graded using a standard scale such as the Glasgow coma scale or West Haven Criteria. It is important to recognize that patients with the earliest phase of encephalopathy may demonstrate only very subtle signs, and the use of standard testing such as the trails test[42] can help establish the presence of early impairment even in the absence of lethargy or demonstrated tremor or asterixis. The neurologic evaluation needs to be monitored frequently in patients who have rapidly accelerating disease, as changes may occur in hours.

Initial laboratory testing and imaging that should be performed on patients who have ALF are outlined in **Box 1**. Many of the tests will help assess the degree of impairment of the liver and other organs such as the kidney. Other tests should be obtained to determine the etiology of the injury, identify any other toxic ingestion, exclude active infection, and provide a basis for comparison with future or historical laboratory determinations. Blood typing is necessary for any factor replacement by the blood bank, and for matching of organs for potential transplant candidates. Two separate blood types are needed for patient listing for liver transplant with the United Network for Organ Sharing (UNOS). The frequency of the full panel for blood testing (complete blood cell count [CBC], international normalized ratio [INR], electrolytes, liver tests) is typically twice daily in more stable patients, but specific testing such as blood glucose levels should be obtained more frequently.

Imaging of the liver should focus on liver size, spleen size, and demonstration of a patent portal and hepatic veins and hepatic artery. Presence of a smaller size liver with splenomegaly suggests the presence of underlying chronic liver disease, while hepatomegaly may accompany the acute vascular obstruction of venous outflow associated with Budd Chiari. The absence of detectable liver lesions is also important, especially in patients who have a suspected history of malignancy. If renal dysfunction is present, imaging should include the kidneys and exclude any obstruction and look for changes in size or texture that could suggest chronic kidney disease.

Very detailed social work and psychiatric evaluations are important in patients where there is suspected history of substance use or underlying psychiatric disorder. Information from these consultants may be helpful for managing the patient with respect to the use of careful sedation and cognizance of substance use and risk for withdrawal. If the patient has a history of suicidal drug ingestion, a careful evaluation may help determine eligibility for liver transplant.

Box 1
Initial laboratory testing for patients with acute liver failure
Blood testing
Complete blood cell count with platelets
Electrolytes and renal function – Na, K, Cl, CO_2, BUN, Cr
International normalized ratio
Factors 5, 7
Liver panel
Alanine aminotransferase
Aspartate aminotransferase
Alkaline phosphatase
Total bilirubin
Direct bilirubin
Albumin
Gamma glutamyl transpeptidase
Blood lactate
Ammonia
Blood gas with pH
HIV testing (rapid)
Viral markers
Hepatitis A virus IgM
HBcAb IgM
HBsAg
HBsAb
HBcAb total
Hepatitis C virus Ab
Hepatitis B virus DNA
Hepatitis C virus RNA
Hepatitis E virus Ab
Hepatitis E virus polymerase chain reaction (PCR) (in appropriate patients with travel history)
Cytomegalovirus (CMV) PCR
CMV Ab
Herpes simplex virus (HSV) PCR
HSV Ab
Epstein-Barr virus Ab
Autoimmune markers
Antinuclear antibody
Antismooth muscle antibody
Anti-liver kidney microsomal
Metabolic markers
Uric acid
Serum copper and urine copper
Hypercoagulable markers
Lupus anticoagulant
Factor 5 Leiden
Toxicology screen and drug panel
Acetaminophen
Opiates
Barbiturates
Cocaine
Alcohol
Pregnancy testing (females)
beta human chorionic gonadotropin
Urinalysis and microscopic analysis
Urine electrolytes and osmolarity
Blood cultures
Urine cultures
Imaging and other testing
Chest radiograph
Abdominal ultrasound with Doppler study of the liver
ECG
Echocardiogram with estimation of pulmonary artery pressures

Logistical considerations should permit daily multidisciplinary team meetings with transplant surgeons, hepatologists, and intensivists, and may include consultants from other disciplines (**Table 1**). This last group may include nephrologists, infectious disease specialists, cardiologists, radiologists, anesthesiologists, neurologists, hematologists, and others. The purpose of these meetings is to discuss changes in patient management and help determine whether any new interventions or consultations are needed. Daily communication between the care team and the patient's family is very important given the rapidly changing clinical picture.

ASSESSING THE PATIENT FOR LIVER TRANSPLANTATION

Although liver transplantation is not required for many patients who have ALF, in appropriate

Table 1
Consultations for patients with acute liver failure

Consultant	Role	Testing
Intensivist	Evaluate patient status and need for ventilatory, hemodynamic, or renal support Establish vascular access Coordinate contact with consultants	Physical examination Laboratory testing Oxygen saturation monitoring Chest radiograph ECG
Hepatology	Help assess etiology of the liver disease and the use of specific therapies, begin evaluation and education for liver transplant	Physical examination Laboratory testing Liver imaging
Transplant surgery	Assess patient as a surgical candidate, educate patient and family about options for transplantation and their outcomes	Physical examination Laboratory testing Liver imaging
Social work	Assess patients social supports, identify any pattern of substance use or underlying psychiatric disturbance, help identify resources to assist patient and family	Interview of patient Interview of family or other patient support
Psychiatry	Assess status of patient's mental health, determine if there is untreated psychiatric illness, assess ability of the patient and family to cooperate with medical treatments	Interview of patient Interview of family or other patient support Contact mental health providers for the patient
Neurology	Assess neurologic changes, help with monitoring of any intervention for cerebral edema	Physical examination Laboratory testing Brain imaging
Neurosurgery	Placement of cerebral pressure monitor and helping assess neurologic status of treated patient	Physical examination Laboratory testing Brain imaging Cerebral pressure tracings
Cardiology	Evaluate for evidence of any underlying cardiac illness and make recommendations for hemodynamic management	Physical examination Laboratory testing ECG Echocardiogram
Nephrology	Assess renal function and provide assistance with renal replacement therapy and electrolyte management	Laboratory testing Monitoring of hemodynamics and urine excretion Renal imaging
Nutrition	Assess ability to eat and nutritional support needs	Examination and interview of the patient and caregivers
Transplant coordinator	Assess eligibility for transplant Review information needed for listing for liver transplant Educate patient and family about transplantation	Interview with patient and family Coordinate information about patient transplant listing status with transplant surgery and hepatology

candidates, liver transplant will be lifesaving. The decision as to whether a patient will recover with conservative management or require transplantation has been the subject of many different reports and case series; however, the Kings College Criteria remain the current standard for clinicians.[43] These criteria are used to predict death in patients presenting with ALF in the setting of acetaminophen and other causes of ALF (**Box 2**). Patients who had a high probability of death were considered to be candidates for liver transplantation. Other studies have attempted to look at etiology-specific indices (ie, Dhawan and colleagues[44] and Korman and colleagues for Wilson disease)[29] or have tried to use other additional serum-based tests to help predict survival (Schiodt

Box 2
Kings Criteria for increased mortality in acute liver failure

Acetaminophen- induced acute liver failure (ALF)

> Hepatic encephalopathy coma grades 3 to 4
>
> Arterial pH <7.3
>
> Prothrombin time (PT) greater than 100 seconds
>
> Serum creatinine greater than 300 μg/mL (3.4 mg/dL)

Nonacetaminophen-induced ALF

> PT of greater than 100 seconds or three of the following five criteria:
>
> 1. Age less than 10 years or greater than 40 years
> 2. ALF caused by non-A, non-B, non-C hepatitis, halothane hepatitis, or idiosyncratic drug reactions
> 3. Jaundice present more than 1 week before onset of encephalopathy
> 4. PT greater than 50 seconds
> 5. Serum bilirubin greater than 300 mmol/L (17.5 mg/dL)

and colleagues;[45] Gc protein, phosphate for acetaminophen),[46] and these may be used adjunctively along with the Kings Criteria to help with the clinical decision as to whether to move toward transplant. Decision making with respect to the timing of transplantation is difficult for transplant surgeons and hepatologists. Although established criteria such as Kings College Criteria have been used to predict poor outcomes without transplantation, the right decision can be made only by the transplant team after following the patient's clinical course and disease progression.

Once transplantation is considered, the patient must undergo a rapid multidisciplinary evaluation to determine candidacy. Unlike standard transplant evaluations, where there is time to obtain very detailed medical records from other treating physicians or to evaluate difficult social or psychiatric issues that could be barriers to candidacy for transplantation, in the setting of ALF, a rapid judgment must be made. The first step in this process is a conscious decision to engage the transplant team in the care of the patient. In units that are run by liver teams or where the liver team initiates the admission or transfer of the patient to the ICU, this is automatic. In other ICUs, however, the liver transplant team must be consulted. Either way,

a cooperative effort to rapidly complete the evaluation and meetings to discuss important care decisions should take place. It is useful to have very clear protocols for the evaluation, along with predetermined lines of communication in place, so that time is not lost following the decision to move forward with the evaluation.

The job of the transplant hepatologist working in concert with the transplant surgeon is to critically assess the patient with respect to appropriate indications for transplantation, and assure that no contraindications to transplantation exist. Along with the transplant coordinator, he or she also must be able to educate the patient and family about the timing for transplantation and potential outcomes. To be actively listed for liver transplantation, patients must meet the minimal listing criteria for transplant at the center where they are being evaluated, and to be considered for the highest status for transplant, must have ALF with encephalopathy, coagulopathy with INR greater than 2, and be in an intensive care setting.[47] Whether the patient is intubated and requires other system support such as renal replacement therapy also is taken into consideration. A rapid social work and possible psychiatric evaluation may require the participation of family members or other patient supports if the patient cannot conduct an interview. This is especially important if there is a prior history of substance use or a history of suicide or serious mental health issue. Active substance use or multiple suicide attempts are contraindications for candidacy for liver transplantation. Other issues where family and friends and the patient's prior treating physicians play an important role is in obtaining a history of any recent malignancies or infectious disease that may preclude or delay listing for transplantation.

Other medical evaluation for transplantation includes imaging of the liver to exclude liver masses and establish the patency of the hepatic vasculature, cardiac evaluation, neurologic evaluation, interventions if there is advancing encephalopathy, and help from other consultants such as nephrologists if there is concurrent renal insufficiency or renal failure. Cardiac evaluation is especially important for patients older than 45 years or those who have a prior cardiac history or history of multiple risk factors for cardiac disease. For critically ill patients, the ECG, bedside echocardiography, and chest radiograph typically are obtained. If necessary, central lines can be converted to pulmonary artery catheters for direct monitoring while the patient is in the ICU.

The transplant coordinator, financial counselors, and social worker are important team members who should be engaged immediately in the transplant process. Often they must rapidly educate and work with a family that was not prepared for the acute illness and incapacitation of the patient. It is important that these family members receive information regarding the transplant process, have the resources to care for the patient, obtain the necessary post-transplant medications, and obtain emergent assistance for care of any dependents of the patient.

Once the initial evaluation is complete, the transplant team often will hold an emergent meeting to discuss patient candidacy that will include representatives from all members of the care team for the patient. If a patient is found to meet listing criteria and has no contraindications to transplant, emergent listing as status 1A will be made with UNOS, the federally contracted agency that controls organ distribution. If a patient has contraindications to listing that are correctable, then listing can be delayed until the appropriate issues are resolved. If, however, the decision is made not to list the patient for transplantation, this information must be shared with the patient and family members and with the care team in a timely fashion to help with care decisions.

ICU-BASED INTERVENTIONS

Advances in critical care medicine and in management strategies have reduced mortality for ALF to approximately 33% according to the USALF Study Group Registry.[8] This mortality is attributed to three complications in particular: cerebral edema, multiorgan dysfunction syndrome (MODS), and sepsis. The following section will review ICU-based management strategies and interventions that have evolved to address the various organ dysfunctions associated with ALF.

NEUROLOGIC FAILURE: CEREBRAL EDEMA AND INTRACRANIAL HYPERTENSION

Management of intracranial hypertension (ICH) remains challenging. Left untreated, mortality can exceed 90%, and some estimate that up to a third of patients succumb to brainstem herniation while awaiting an organ. Clinically recognizable risk factors associated with cerebral edema include: high-grade encephalopathy (grades 3 to 4), elevated serum ammonia (greater than 150 to 200 μm),[48,49] rapid/hyperacute progression of liver injury to hepatic encephalopathy, infection or systemic inflammatory syndrome (SIRS), and requirement for vasopressor support or renal replacement therapy.[50] Neuroimaging is not reliable in diagnosing early ICH[51] but may help exclude other problems such as intracranial

bleeding or stroke. Invasive intracranial pressure (ICP) monitoring remains the only objective gold standard for measuring and monitoring ICH.

INTRACRANIAL PRESSURE MONITORING: GENERAL CONSIDERATIONS

In clinical practice, ICP monitoring for patients who have ALF remains controversial, in part because randomized controlled trials are lacking to guide clinicians through nuanced scenarios in which invasive monitoring may or may not be helpful. The lack of an accepted consensus protocol for managing cerebral edema hampers attempts at rigorous multicenter research studies. To fuel the controversy further, in nonrandomized studies, such devices have not been shown to improve survival.[52] Despite lack of consensus, many centers place ICP monitors to actively manage cerebral edema In patients who have advanced (stage 3 or 4) encephalopathy. Such devices have the additional benefit of providing important prognostic information regarding neurologic recovery after orthotopic liver transplant (OLT), and may serve as one additional data point used in the complex decision making that occurs in identifying the ideal transplantation candidate. For example, severe sustained ICP greater than 40 mm Hg (or cerebral perfusion pressure less than 40 mm Hg) for over 2 hours is associated with brainstem herniation or poor neurologic recovery post-OLT.

Furthermore, because early edema can be clinically silent, placement of a device may allow for early detection and intervention. Some have argued that ICP monitoring also may be helpful in patients who have a good prognosis (ie, unlikely to require liver transplant), but with severe encephalopathy. Aggressive treatment in this subset may reduce mortality and morbidity by stabilizing neurologic function and allowing a longer time for hepatic recovery. On the other hand, because of the uniformly high mortality of ALF in patients who have extremely poor prognosis without the option for liver transplant, this subset of patients is unlikely to benefit from invasive monitoring.

Intracranial bleeding, an often-cited complication of ICP monitoring, is encountered in 10% to 20% of patients. Most intracranial bleeding is mild and of little clinical significance.[52] Among patients who have severe coagulopathy, reduction of INR has been managed successfully with the use of recombinant factor 7a, although whether this translates into a reduced risk for bleeding complications is uncertain.[53] Correction of coagulopathy should be continued for approximately 48 hours after the insertion of probes/catheters to prevent bleeding. Undoubtedly, the experience of the team in placing ICP monitors is important in keeping this complication rate low.

INTRACRANIAL PRESSURE MONITORING: PRACTICAL CONSIDERATIONS

Even after a decision is made to proceed with invasive ICP monitoring, the ideal location of placement remains unclear. In general, intraventricular placement carries the highest risk of bleeding (although with the added therapeutic potential), and epidural placement the lowest risk. The latter approach however, suffers from less accuracy in ICP measurement. The subdural position is the most commonly used location in the United States, according to a recent survey.[52] Ultimately, until definitive evidence accumulates, local expertise and comfort level will define where and how the monitors are placed.

INTRACRANIAL HYPERTENSION: GENERAL MANAGEMENT PRINCIPLES

In general, patients should be kept in a quiet room with minimal stimulus, including infrequent endotracheal suctioning. The head of the bed should be elevated to 30° (to improve CSF drainage), and neck rotation or flexion should be limited (to avoid compromise of jugular venous drainage). Fevers should be controlled by cooling, because acetaminophen and nonsteroidal anti-inflammatory drugs (NSAIDS) should be avoided, and rigoring or shivering also avoided, as these may exacerbate ICP.[54] When invasive monitoring is available, the ICP should be maintained below 25 mm Hg. The mean arterial pressure (MAP) should be adequate to maintain cerebral perfusion pressure (CPP) between 50–80 mm Hg. Care should be taken to avoid an overly robust CPP (some have argued a range between 50 and 65 mm Hg as ideal in this fragile population), as this may exacerbate cerebral hyperemia.

Meticulous attention needs to be paid to metabolic and acid–base abnormalities including hyper- and hypoglycemia, hyponatremia, hyperlactatemia, and hypercapnia, as these have been shown to contribute to higher ICP. Mannitol can be used as first-line therapy and given as repeated boluses, provided serial serum osmolality remains below 320 mOsm/L. Its use is limited once patients develop significant renal injury. In patients requiring renal support, continuous venovenous hemofiltration is preferred over traditional hemodialysis to prevent rapid fluid shifts and swings in blood pressure.[55] In contrast to mannitol, hypertonic saline can be used as a prophylactic measure with few adverse effects, with a goal of achieving sodium

of 145 to 155 mEq/L.[56] Evidence, however, is limited to a single randomized controlled trial, and hypertonic saline never has been tested formally as a treatment of established ICH in patients who have ALF.

If osmotic therapies fail to adequately control ICP, other adjunctive measures to reduce ICP include:

Barbiturate coma (to reduce brain metabolism, although incremental benefit is unclear if the patient is already in stage 4 encephalopathy with coma)
Indomethacin
Paralytic agents
Phenytoin (may reduce cerebral edema regardless of seizure activity)

There are no good data that show lactulose or other nonabsorbable oral antibiotics, such as rifaxamin, improve ICP; however, these may help lower ammonia and are of theoretic benefit. There is no role for corticosteroids given cerebral edema is of cytotoxic, as opposed to vasogenic origin in the patient who has ALF. In the midst of relative therapeutic disappointments, one modality that is garnering increasing attention is therapeutic hypothermia.

KEEPING IT COOL: THERAPEUTIC HYPOTHERMIA

Moderate hypothermia (32°C to 33°C) so far appears to be a formidable tool for managing refractory ICP elevations.[57,58] Therapeutic hypothermia simultaneously alters multiple pathways important in the pathogenesis of cerebral edema and ICH and leads to:

Reductions in brain energy metabolism (both metabolic and electrophysiologic components)
Possible suppression of subclinical seizure activity
Normalization of cerebral blood flow and autoregulation
Reduced delivery of ammonia to the brain
Amelioration in anaerobic glycolysis and oxidative stress in astrocytes
Decrement in brain extracellular glutamate and normalization of brain osmolarity
Reversal of SIRS
Nitric oxide metabolism[59]

In some patients, cooling also may restore vascular responsiveness and has the added benefit of less vasopressor requirement.[57]

On a practical level, the markedly vasodilated state typical of patients who have ALF allows for efficient heat exchange from external cooling devices. Although endovascular devices have been used in cardiac arrest and traumatic brain injury (TBI), such invasive devices are probably not necessary to achieve modest hypothermia, and are not ideal given bleeding and infection risks in this patient population. For example, in preliminary studies, goal temperatures have been reached within 1 hour of initiating cooling blankets.[57,59] Therapeutic hypothermia consistently reduces ICP and cerebral blood flow (CBF). It additionally improves CPP and has been used for the treatment of refractory ICH and as a bridge for OLT. Intraoperative surges in ICP (during the reperfusion and dissection phases of the procedure in particular) also may be averted with maintenance of moderate hypothermia in the operating room.[59] Finally, its role as a prophylactic measure also has been explored in a small pilot study (see Box 2).[60]

Potential adverse effects of cooling include arrhythmia, infection (which increases with degree and duration of hypothermia), bleeding, electrolyte imbalance, hyperglycemia, and alteration in drug metabolism. Many of these abnormalities are difficult to distinguish from physiologic changes that commonly accompany ALF itself, making recognition difficult. Theoretic concerns exist regarding the negative effect of hypothermia upon liver regeneration, but there may be beneficial effects in limiting progression of liver injury.

Regardless, there remain many unanswered questions regarding therapeutic hypothermia, including optimal target population, timing, degree and duration of treatment, hypothermia, and rewarming techniques. Although one patient in Jalan's series was cooled for up to 5 days, duration of safety is unknown, and the markers that can be used to indicate adequate hepatic recovery (and therefore safe discontinuation of therapy) are unclear. Rapid rewarming can exacerbate electrolyte abnormalities and lead to hemodynamic instability and worsening CPP. In the TBI literature, safe rewarming has been documented at a range of rates from 1°C/h to 1°C/d. Given the special hemodynamic issues inherent in this population, some have suggested a conservative rate, perhaps at 1°C per 12 hours.[49]

NEUROLOGIC MANIFESTATIONS: SEIZURES

Seizures can aggravate cerebral edema and ICH, but they also can be a manifestation of ICP surges. There is at least one study that has shown a benefit of phenytoin infusion in preventing subclinical seizure activity,[61] although a recent clinical trial noted no benefit.[62] Hypothermia reduces seizure activity in experimental models of epilepsy, and may be an additional important mechanism of action of hypothermia in ALF.[63,64] Presently the authors do not recommend prophylaxis for seizures, but continuous EEG monitoring has become available and may be useful for patients at high risk for seizures.

RESPIRATORY FAILURE: MECHANICAL VENTILATION

The ideal timing for endotracheal intubation is not always clear. When considering interhospital patient transfer to a liver transplant center, one of the discussions commonly includes whether the patient should be intubated before transfer, as neurologic deterioration can be very rapid. Intubation should be considered strongly once advanced encephalopathy becomes evident at grade 3 or more. In addition to preventing gross aspiration events, mechanical ventilation and judicious sedation may help manage extreme agitation, which can contribute to dangerous surges in ICP.

Development of acute lung injury/acute respiratory distress syndrome (ARDS) is not uncommon among patients who have ALF and cerebral edema. Attention should be paid to pCO2 once a low tidal volume ARDS protocol is instituted, to counter the detrimental effects of severe hypercarbia on ICP. Prophylactic hyperventilation, on the other hand, has not been shown to modify the ultimate development of cerebral edema.[65] For patients suspected of having brainstem herniation, acute hyperventilation can be used emergently.

Higher positive-end expiratory pressure (PEEP) theoretically also can increase ICP, but the level in which this becomes clinically significant in a particular patient is unclear. In general, using the lowest level of PEEP that can maintain adequate oxygenation is recommended.

SEDATION AND ANALGESIA

Because agitation (including excessive coughing and straining) and pain can exacerbate ICP elevations, adequate analgesia and judicious sedation are required, particularly before and after placement of invasive devices such as endotracheal tubes and ICP monitors.

In reality, there are not enough data to suggest a standard agent or dosing regimen in this scenario. In general, short-acting agents are preferred, although it is important to note that all sedative drugs are subject to delayed metabolism. Recovery time from propofol tends to be shorter than from benzodiazepines and may allow for more reliable serial neurologic testing when this agent is withdrawn. Despite adverse effects on hemodynamics, prohibitive cost, and infusion syndromes that can be seen with prolonged use, propofol has the added benefit of decreasing CBF and lowering ICP.[66] Both propofol and benzodiazepines can increase γ-aminobutyric acid (GABA) neurotransmission and theoretically exacerbate hepatic encephalopathy. For treatment of pain, bolus doses of fentanyl are preferred as the first-line agent. Morphine and meperidine are not recommended because of active metabolites. In the case of meperidine, seizure thresholds may be lowered.

HEMODYNAMIC FAILURE: SHOCK MANAGEMENT

Hypotension is common in patients who have ALF and is marked by a state of high cardiac output and reduced systemic vascular resistance. This hemodynamic picture closely mimics septic shock, and differentiating between the two can be challenging. Concurrent infectious workup is mandatory. Relative adrenal insufficiency occurs frequently, but treatment with moderate-dose corticosteroids is reserved for those unresponsive to pressors. In one series, 62% of patients who had ALF were found to have an abnormal response to high-dose corticotrophin stimulation.[67,68] As in other states of shock, assessment of volume status and adequate resuscitation, if appropriate, is a crucial first step. Vasopressors can be used adjunctively to maintain a MAP above 50 mm Hg, with a goal CPP of 50 to 80. Surges in MAPs also should be avoided as this may lead to cerebral hyperemia.

The risks and benefits of individual vasopressor agents have not been evaluated carefully, but extrapolation of data from TBI suggests that norepinephrine should be preferred, as it is associated with consistent and predictable increases in CPP. There are conflicting data on the use of newer agents, such as vasopressin or terlipressin. In one study, terlipressin caused cerebral vasodilation and increased ICP at low doses that did not alter systemic hemodynamics.[67] In a rat model, vasopressin appears to accelerate development of cerebral edema.[69] More recently however, in another small study, terlipressin appeared to increase CPP and CBP in patients who had ALF without detrimental effects on ICP or increase in cerebral metabolic rate.[70]

VENOUS ACCESS DEVICES

Catheter-related infections are a major source of avoidable complications in patients who have ALF.[71,72] As such, when placing venous access devices, meticulous attention to catheter care is paramount. Routine placement of multiple catheters is unnecessary, and placement of venous access devices probably should occur only as the need arises.

IMPORTANCE OF CARDIAC DYSFUNCTION

Recent data suggest myocardial injury may occur in ALF. Although classically felt to spare the heart, nearly 75% of patients in the US Acute Liver Failure Study Group cohort demonstrated an elevation of troponin 1 of 0.1 ng/mL or more. Importantly, patients who had elevated troponins experienced arrhythmias and higher coma grades (stage 3 or 4) at a rate two and four times respectively compared with those patients who had normal troponins.[73] Mortality rates (before and after transplant) were significantly higher in patients who had elevated troponins in a level-dependent manner, such that patients in the highest quintile (troponin 1 greater than 3.0 ng/mL) ultimately died at a rate of 33.3%. Advanced coma occurred in 71.4% of these patients. The corresponding rate for patients who had normal troponin was 10.2% and 22.4%. Troponin levels may be an important biomarker with prognostic implications in ALF.

HEMATOLOGIC FAILURE: DEALING WITH COAGULOPATHY

Despite severe derangements in coagulation profile, clinically significant spontaneous bleeding remains relatively uncommon. Because subclinical vitamin K deficiency contributes to coagulopathy in up to 25% of patients, empiric administration of vitamin K 10 mg intravenously given as a single dose is recommended.[74] Prophylactic transfusions to normalize coagulation profile in all patients who have ALF is unnecessary, as it has not been shown to alter the risk of significant bleeding or future transfusion requirement. Additionally, it carries a risk of volume overload and pulmonary edema (particularly in patients facing deteriorating renal function), and it obscures the trend of prothrombin time, which is useful as a prognostic marker.

For patients who have clinically significant bleeding or before placement of invasive devices, an attempt at improving coagulopathy should be made. Although strict guidelines do not exist, a rough target would be to correct the INR to approximately 1.5 and platelet count to approximately 50,000/mm^3 before procedures with the use of fresh frozen plasma (FFP) and platelets. Concomitant administration of cryoprecipitate is recommended for patients who have significant hypofibrinogenemia (less than 100 mg/dL). When FFP fails to adequately normalize PT/INR, the use of recombinant factor 7a (rF7) can be considered and has been used successfully to facilitate placement of ICP monitors.[53] FFP or cryoprecipitate should be administered before rF7 (40 μg/kg) if fibrinogen levels are less than 100 mg/dL to replete factors involved in the clotting cascade. The procedure generally should be performed within 30 to 60 minutes of infusion of rF7. Repeat prophylactic doses of rF7 are probably not necessary after successful device placement, unless there is clinical evidence of oozing or bleeding (duration of action greater than 2 hours).

RENAL FAILURE MANAGEMENT

Renal insufficiency that progresses to renal failure may accompany liver failure. The causes may be multifactorial, including ischemia from hypotension that may cause acute tubular necrosis, hepatorenal syndrome, and other direct toxic injuries such as copper induced tubular injury in Wilson disease,[27] and contrast-induced nephropathy if contrast studies were recently performed. Urine sodium may be low in hypovolemic states, hepatorenal syndrome, and with contrast nephropathy. It is important to establish as best as possible whether the patient is euvolemic to avoid excess fluid administration that can exacerbate cerebral edema and cause pulmonary congestion and accelerate ascites formation. This may necessitate central pressure monitoring or indirect estimates of volume by measurement of end diastolic volume in the heart by echocardiography. In patients who have worsening renal function or acidemia, renal replacement therapy should be started early to avoid volume overload and to help with control of acid–base status and electrolyte balance. Continuous veno-venous hemofiltration with dialysis as opposed to standard hemodialysis is the preferred method for achieving renal replacement therapy because of the reduced shifts in blood pressure associated with its use. If the patient moves forward to transplantation, the continuous veno-venous hemofiltration may be continued intra- and perioperatively as necessary.

INFECTIOUS DISEASE CONSIDERATIONS

Infections are the most common cause of death and morbidity in patients who have ALF. With severe injury to the liver, Kuppfer cell function is impaired, and clearance of normal gut bacteria that translocate is less efficient. This increases the risk of patients who have ALF to infection. The most common site of bacterial infection is the lung, then urinary tract and blood.[71,72,75–77] The most frequently identified organisms are *Staphylococcus, Streptococcus* and enteric gram- negative bacilli. Fungal infections, in particular *Candida*, may be present in up to one third of patients who have ALF. Catheter-related sepsis is a serious concern,

and avoidance of unnecessary intravenous lines and careful attention to proper hygiene and changing of access are important.

Although it is not universally accepted that all patients who have ALF should be treated with prophylactic antibiotics, there is justification for careful surveillance for infection in all of these patients and a low threshold for treatment. Survival has not been shown to be altered by the use of prophylactic antibiotics; however, the numbers of patients studied may not have been large enough to definitively preclude benefits of prophylactic treatment.[71,72,75–77]

On admission, a chest radiograph is performed, and urinalysis and urine and blood cultures should be obtained routinely. For any patient on a ventilator, sputum smear and cultures also should be obtained. These cultures and radiograph surveillance should continue every 48 to 72 hours or if the clinical status worsens.

Empiric use of antibiotics is recommended when surveillance cultures are positive, when encephalopathy is rapidly progressive, when there is hemodynamic instability with refractory hypotension or systemic signs of infection such as elevated temperature, tachycardia, and leukocytosis. Leukocytosis, however, may occur merely as a result of the liver injury, and the differential of the CBC should be watched for changes from baseline values. Antifungal therapy may be particularly warranted in patients who have had prior antibiotic treatment and for those who have renal failure.

The choice of an antimicrobial agent must take into account the need to cover a broad spectrum of gram-positive and -negative organisms. In general, third-generation cephalosporin drugs are recommended. Once speciation from any culture is possible, antimicrobial therapy may be narrowed accordingly. When line infection is suspected, vancomycin should be started pending results of cultures. All dosages must be adjusted based on renal function, and levels obtained when appropriate to help guide therapy further. Aminoglycosides are to be avoided if possible, owing to their potential for nephrotoxicity. Antifungal therapy should be given empirically and in the setting of prolonged use of antibacterial agents or the lack of a prompt response to institution of antibacterial therapy.

NUTRITION FOR THE PATIENT WITH ACUTE LIVER FAILURE

Patients are prone to hypoglycemia in acute liver injury because of loss of glycogen stores, impairment of gluconeogenesis, and increased circulating insulin. Intravenous supplementation with glucose solutions is recommended if the patient is not being fed. Marked hyperglycemia should be avoided, because this may impair control of intracranial pressure;[78] however the benefits of attempting tight control must be weighed against the risk of hypoglycemia.

There is a need for nutritional supplementation in ALF, because these patients are catabolic.[79] The means of supplementation will vary with the ability of the patient to eat. In patients who have minimal hepatic encephalopathy, oral feeding is possible, but with advancing encephalopathy, oral feeding may need to be discontinued if there is a risk of aspiration. This clearly holds for patients transitioning from grade 2 to grade 3 hepatic coma. If oral feeding is discontinued, then enteral supplementation by means of feeding tube is recommended, at a minimum to provide the gut with some trophic feeds to reduce the risk of bacterial translocation.

Caloric goals for patients who have ALF should be approximately 25 to 30 kcal/kg/d. Parenteral or enteral nutrition may be used if oral feeding is not possible. The fear of parenteral nutrition-induced liver failure does not appear to be founded in the setting of ALF;[80] however careful attention to prevent line sepsis must be taken. Protein intake of approximately 1 g/kg/d does not appear to worsen hyperammonemia. Excess glutamine supplementation should be avoided given glutamine's role in the production of ammonia and development of cerebral edema in ALF.

LIVER SUPPORT DEVICES

Liver support devices may benefit patients who have liver failure by being used as a bridge to liver transplantation or liver recovery; however their utility only has been tested in nonrandomized studies to date.[81] The results of ongoing multicenter trials are awaited. There are two main types of liver support devices that have been developed:

- Artificial (cell-free systems) such as those based on plasma filtration and removal of substances by use of dialysis or charcoal or other ion exchange columns
- Bioartificial systems that rely upon the use of liver cells (human or nonhuman) to perform detoxification and secretion of hepatocytes derived factors[82]

Both of these aim to remove known and unknown toxins that are released or are not cleared in the setting of liver failure. Some treatments such as hemofiltration and hemodialysis have difficulty with removal of toxins bound to larger molecules such as albumin, and newer techniques have evolved that also can deal with these substances. Specific units for which clinical data are emerging include the molecular adsorbents recirculating system, and fractionated plasma separation and adsorption (SEPAD- Prometheus).[83] Although neither of these units has been shown to change survival in the setting of ALF, other endpoints such as changes in degree of hepatic encephalopathy and lowering of serum bilirubin have been achieved. Interestingly, there are reports of the use of molecular absorption recirculation system for acute Wilson disease where copper was lowered and patients stabilized before transplantation.[84] This also has been achieved using hemofiltration and plasma exchange.[85]

Fewer data are available for bioartificial support devices that use human hepatocytes, such as the extracorporeal liver assist device, and some limited data are available regarding the HepatAssist device (Arbios Systems, inc., HepaLife Technologies, Boston, Massachusetts), which uses porcine hepatocytes. The difficulty with these systems is the need to have viable cells available on demand for use for patients who have liver failure. Another concern is the development of antibodies to foreign proteins that can occur with nonhuman devices.

At present, the use of these devices remains experimental; however, results of new studies that are ongoing and technological advances suggests that one should remain optimistic about the development of a useful device for liver support in the near future. For those in whom the devices are being tried, one must pay careful attention to blood coagulation, glucose levels, and levels of antibiotics and antifungals that can be altered by these potential treatments.

LIVER TRANSPLANTATION

Patients who have ALF not recovering despite medical/supportive treatment are candidates for liver transplantation. It is the authors' policy to list patients who have ALF meeting the minimal listing criteria as UNOS status 1A immediately after completing medical and UNOS-required evaluations. When a suitable liver offer becomes available, transplantation will be performed. The availability of deceased donor liver allograft is unpredictable, however, because of a shortage of organ donors and the current organ allocation system. As a result, patients who have ALF may die because of brain herniation while waiting for transplant or become nontransplantable secondary to sepsis and multiorgan system failure.

Types of transplants offered for patient who have ALF are deceased donor liver transplantation, living donor liver transplantation (LDLT) and auxiliary orthotopic liver transplantation (APOLT). Although there have been case reports, LDLT in the adult ALF setting has not been accepted uniformly as a result of the short time period for living donor evaluation, leading to possible mishaps that can cause adverse living donor outcomes. APOLT is an appealing concept, in which usually the right lobe of the native liver is removed, and right lobe of the donor liver is transplanted in an orthotopic fashion. The native liver part left in place will regenerate within 6 to 8 months following the operation, at which point immunosuppressive therapy is tapered gradually, letting the allograft be rejected. Thus the patient can live with his/her own liver without lifelong immunosuppressive medication use. This operation is technically more challenging, however, and issues related to maintaining the blood supply to the graft and recipient native liver are more complex.

OUTCOMES OF PATIENTS WITH ACUTE LIVER FAILURE

Survival of patients who have ALF depends on the etiology of ALF, with spontaneous or nontransplant recovery being the best in patients with acetaminophen-induced injury who receive timely treatment with NAC. For those patients who undergo emergent liver transplantation, the outcomes are good for long-term survival but below those for patients who have chronic liver diseases or liver cancer. The 1-, 3-, and 5-year graft survivals following transplant in a published series from a single center with a large experience in transplantation for acute liver failure were 63.2%, 58.0%, and 56.6%, respectively.[85] This is approximately 10% to 20% lower than transplantation for chronic liver diseases where 5-year survivals are typically 70% to 80%. Causes of graft loss in the patients who had ALF were patient death from sepsis, neurologic complications, and primary graft nonfunction, the last occurring at a much higher frequency (13.2%) than for nonemergent transplantation. The cause for this is likely because of donor and host factors: the use of more marginal grafts due to the urgency of transplantation and the placement of grafts into patients with multiorgan failure. The risk of transplantation must be weighed against the risk of death without transplantation and presence of any contraindications to transplantation. This risk–benefit analysis must be thought through carefully for each individual patient before deciding to move toward transplant or to continue with conservative management alone.

The early identification of ALF and the etiology of the liver failure along with the judicious use of transplant and the advances in ICU management of these patients have contributed greatly to the improved overall survival of patients who have ALF. Survival now approaches 66%, compared with a once dismal 20% survival. Further advances in ICU management including the future use of liver support devices, advances in techniques and organ distribution for liver transplant, and the early recognition of liver failure by medical personnel will contribute to even better future outcomes.

REFERENCES

1. Trey, Davidson. The management of fulminant hepatic failure. Prog Liver Dis 1970;3:282–98.
2. Rutherford A, Chung RT. Acute liver failure: mechanisms of hepatocytes injury and regeneration. Semin Liver Dis 2008;28:167–74.
3. Strand S, Hofmann WJ, Grambihler A, et al. Hepatic failure and liver cell damage in acute Wilson's disease involve CD95 (APO-1/Fas)-mediated apoptosis. Nat Med 1998;4:588–93.
4. Trost LC, Lemasters JJ. Role of the mitochondrial permeability transition in salicylate toxicity to cultured rat hepatocytes: implications for the pathogenesis of Reye's syndrome. Toxicol Appl Pharmacol 1997;147:431–41.
5. Smilkstein MJ, Knapp GL, Kulig KW, et al. Efficacy of oral N-acetylcysteine in the treatment of acetaminophen overdose. Analysis of the national multicenter study (1976 to 1985). N Engl J Med 1988;319:1557–62.
6. Hawker F. Liver dysfunction in critical illness. Anaesth Intensive Care 1991;19:165–81.
7. Lindros K. Ozonation of cytochrome P450 expression, drug metabolism, and toxicity in liver. Gen Pharmacol 1997;28:191–6.
8. Ostapowicz G, Fontana RJ, Schiødt FV, et al. Results of a prospective study of acute liver failure at 17 tertiary care centers in the United States. Ann Intern Med 2002;137:947–54.
9. Polson J, Lee WM. Etiologies of acute liver failure: location, location, location. Liver Transpl 2007;13: 1362–3.
10. Prescott LF. Paracetamol, alcohol and the liver. Br J Clin Pharmacol 2000;49:291–301.
11. Lieber CS. Susceptibility to alcohol-related liver injury. Alcohol Alcohol Suppl 1994;2:315–26.
12. Pearce B, Grant IS. Acute liver failure following therapeutic paracetamol administration in patients with muscular dystrophies. Anaesthesia 2008;63:89–91.
13. Miners JO, Drew R, Birkett DJ. Mechanism of action of paracetamol protective agents in mice in vivo. Biochem Pharmacol 1984;33:2995–3000.
14. Davern TJ, James LP, Hinson J, et al. Measurement of serum acetaminophen–protein adducts in

patients with acute liver failure. Gastroenterology 2006;130:687–94.

15. Perry HE, Shannon MW. Efficacy of oral versus intravenous N-acetylcysteine in acetaminophen overdose: results of an open-label, clinical trial. J Pediatr 1998;132(1):149–52.

16. Ekins BR, Ford DC, Thompson MI, et al. The effect of activated charcoal on N-acetylcysteine absorption in normal subjects. Am J Emerg Med 1987;5:483–7.

17. Broussard CN, Aggarwal A, Lacey SR, et al. Mushroom poisoning—from diarrhea to liver transplantation. Am J Gastroenterol 2001;96:3195–8.

18. Floersheim GL, Eberhard M, Tschumi P, et al. Effects of penicillin and silymarin on liver enzymes and blood clotting factors in dogs given a boiled preparation of amanita phalloides. Toxicol Appl Pharmacol 1978;46:455–62.

19. Abboud G, Kaplowitz N. Drug-induced liver injury. Drug Saf 2007;30:277–94.

20. Trey C, Lipworth L, Chalmers TC, et al. Fulminant hepatic failure. Presumable contribution to halothane. N Engl J Med 1968;279:798–801.

21. Kumar M, Satapathy S, Monga R, et al. A randomized controlled trial of lamivudine to treat acute hepatitis B. Hepatology 2007;45:97–101.

22. HBV acute ALFSG experience. In press.

23. Lettau LA, McCarthy JG, Smith MH, et al. Outbreak of severe hepatitis due to delta and hepatitis B viruses in parenteral drug abusers and their contacts. N Engl J Med 1987;317(20):1256–62.

24. Patra S, Kumar A, Trivedi SS, et al. Maternal and fetal outcomes in pregnant women with acute hepatitis E virus infection. Ann Intern Med 2007;147:28–33.

25. Navaneethan U, Al Mohajer M, Shata MT. Hepatitis E and pregnancy: understanding the pathogenesis. Liver Int 2008;9:1190–9.

26. Feranchak AP, Tyson RW, Narkewicz MR, et al. Fulminant Epstein-Barr viral hepatitis: orthotopic liver transplantation and review of the literature. Liver Transpl Surg 1998;4:469–76.

27. Roberts E, Schilsky ML. A practice guideline on Wilson disease. Hepatology 2008;47:2089–111.

28. Sokol RJ, Francis PD, Gold SH, et al. Orthotopic liver transplantation for acute fulminant Wilson disease. J Pediatr 1985;107:549–52.

29. Korman JD, Volenberg I, Balko J, et al. Screening for Wilson disease in acute liver failure by serum testing: a comparison of currently used tests. Hepatology 4:1030–2.

30. Castro MA, Fassett MJ, Reynolds TB, et al. Reversible peripartum liver failure: a new perspective on the diagnosis, treatment, and cause of acute fatty liver of pregnancy, based on 28 consecutive cases. Am J Obstet Gynecol 1999;181:389–95.

31. Ibdah JA, Bennett MJ, Rinaldo P, et al. A fetal fatty-acid oxidation disorder as a cause of liver disease in pregnant women. N Engl J Med 1999;340:1723–31.

32. Martin JN Jr, Briery CM, Rose CH, et al. Postpartum plasma exchange as adjunctive therapy for severe acute fatty liver of pregnancy. J Clin Apher 2008;23(4):138–43.

33. Barton JR, Sibai BM. Care of the pregnancy complicated by HELLP syndrome. Gastroenterol Clin North Am 1992;21:937–50.

34. Ochs A, Sellinger M, Haag K, et al. Transjugular intrahepatic portosystemic stent–shunt (TIPS) in the treatment of Budd-Chiari syndrome. J Hepatol 1993;18:217–25.

35. Orloff MJ, Daily PO, Orloff SL, et al. A 27-year experience with surgical treatment of Budd-Chiari syndrome. Ann Surg 2000;232(3):340–52.

36. Menon KV, Shah V, Kamath PS. The Budd-Chiari syndrome. N Engl J Med 2004;350:578–85.

37. Patel RK, Lea NC, Heneghan MA, et al. Prevalence of the activating JAK2 tyrosine kinase mutation V617F in the Budd-Chiari syndrome. Gastroenterology 2006;130:2031–8.

38. Ebert EC. Hypoxic liver injury. Mayo Clin Proc 2006;81:1232–6.

39. Reiss U, Cowan M, McMillan A, et al. Hepatic veno-occlusive disease in blood and bone marrow transplantation in children and young adults: incidence, risk factors, and outcome in a cohort of 241 patients. J Pediatr Hematol Oncol 2002;24:746–50.

40. Alexopoulou A, Koskinas J, Deutsch M, et al. Acute liver failure as the initial manifestation of hepatic infiltration by a solid tumor: report of 5 cases and review of the literature. Tumori 2006;92:354–7.

41. Krawitt EL. Autoimmune hepatitis. N Engl J Med 2006;354:54–66.

42. Nilson L, Barregård L, Bäckman L. Trail making test in chronic toxic encephalopathy: performance and discriminative potential. Clin Neuropsychol 1999;13(3):314–27.

43. O'Grady JG, Alexander GJ, Hayllar KM, et al. Early indicators of prognosis in fulminant hepatic failure. Gastroenterology 1989;97:439–45.

44. Dhawan A, Taylor RM, Cheeseman P, et al. Wilson's disease in children: 37-year experience and revised King's score for liver transplantation. Liver Transpl 2005;11:441–8.

45. Schiødt FV, Bangert K, Shakil AO, et al. Predictive value of actin-free Gc-globulin in acute liver failure. Liver Transpl 2007;13:1324–9.

46. Gow PJ, Sood S, Angus PW. Serum phosphate as a predictor of outcome in acetaminophen-induced fulminant hepatic failure. Hepatology 2003;37:711–2.

47. Allocation of livers. Available at: www.unos.org/PoliciesandBylaws2/policies/pdfs/policy_8.pdf. Accessed November 26, 2008.

48. Clemmesen JO, Larsen FS, Kondrup J, et al. Cerebral herniation in patients with acute liver failure is

correlated with arterial ammonia concentration. Hepatology 1999;29:648–53.

49. Tofteng F, Hauerberg J, Hansen BA, et al. Persistent arterial hyperammonemia increases the concentration of glutamine and alanine in the brain and correlates with intracranial pressure in patients with fulminant hepatic failure. J Cereb Blood Flow Metab 2006;26:21–7.

50. Stravitz RG, Lee WM, Kramer AH, et al. Therapeutic hypothermia for acute liver failure: toward a randomized, controlled trial in patients with advanced hepatic encephalopathy. Neurocrit Care 2008;9:90–6.

51. Munoz SJ, Robinson M, Northrup B, et al. Elevated intracranial pressure and computed tomography of the brain in fulminant hepatocellular failure. Hepatology 1991;13:209–12.

52. Vaquero J, Fontana RJ, Larson AM, et al. Complications and use of intracranial pressure monitering in patients with acute liver failure and severe encephalopathy. Liver Transpl 2005;11:1581–9.

53. Shami VM, Caldwell SH, Hespenheide EE, et al. Recombinant activated factor VII for coagulopathy in fulminant hepatic failure compared to conventional therapy. Liver Transpl 2003;9:138–43.

54. Vaquero J, Rose C, Butterworth RF. Keeping cool in acute liver failure: rationale for the use of mild hypothermia. J Hepatol 2005;43:1067–77.

55. Winney RJ, Kean DM, Best JJ, et al. Changes in brain water with haemodialysis. Lancet 1986;9:1107–8.

56. Murphy N, Auzinger G, Bernel W, et al. The effect of hypertonic sodium chloride on intracranial pressure in patients with acute liver failure. Hepatology 2004; 39:464–70.

57. Jalan R, Damink SW, Deutz NE, et al. Moderate hypothermia for uncontrolled intracranial hypertension in acute liver failure. Lancet 1999;354:1164–8.

58. Jalan R, Damink SW, Deutz NE, et al. Moderate hypothermia in patients with acute liver failure and uncontrolled intracranial hypertension. Gastroenterology 2004;127:1338–46.

59. Vaquero J, Blei AT. Mild hypothermia for acute liver failure: a review of mechanisms of action. J Clin Gastroenterol 2005;39(Suppl 2):S147–57.

60. Jalan R. Intracranial hypertension in acute liver failure: pathophysiological basis of rational management. Semin Liver Dis 2003;23:271–82.

61. Ellis AJ, Wendon JA, Williams R. Subclinical seizure activity and prophylactic phenytoin infusion in acute liver failure: a controlled clinical trial. Hepatology 2000;32:536–41.

62. Bhatia V, Batra Y, Acharya SK. Prophylactic phenytoin does not improve cerebral edema or survival in acute liver failure—a controlled clinical trial. J Hepatol 2004;41:89–96.

63. Baldwin M, Frost LL. Effect of hypothermia on epileptiform activity in the primate temporal lobe. Science 1956;124:931–2.

64. Liu Z, Gatt A, Mikati M, et al. Effect of temperature on kainic acid-induced seizures. Brain Res 1993;631:51–8.

65. Ede RJ, Gimson AE, Bihari D, et al. Controlled hyperventilation in the prevention of cerebral oedema in fulminant hepatic failure. J Hepatol 1986;2:43–51.

66. Wijdicks EFM, Nyberg SL. Propofol to control intracranial pressure in fulminant hepatic failure. Transplant Proc 2002;34:1220–2.

67. Harry R, Auzinger G, Wendon J. The effects of supraphysiological doses of corticosteroids in hypotensive liver failure. Liver Int 2003;23:71–7.

68. Harry R, Auzinger G, Wendon J. The clinical importance of adrenal insufficiency in acute hepatic dysfunction. Hepatology 2002;36:395–402.

69. Chung C, Gottstein J, Vaquero J, et al. Vasopressin infusion accelerates the development of brain edema in rats after portacaval anastomosis. Hepatology 2002;36:380A.

70. Eefsen M, Dethloff T, Frederisen JH, et al. Comparison of terlipressin and noradrenalin on cerebral perfusion, intracranial pressure, and cerebral extracellular concentrations of lactate and pyruvate in patients with acute liver failure in need of inotropic support. J Hepatol 2007;47:381–6.

71. Rolando N, Harvey F, Brahm J, et al. Prospective study of bacterial infection in acute liver failure. Hepatology 1990;11:49–53.

72. Vaquero J, Polson J, Chung C, et al. Infection and the progression of hepatic encephalopathy in acute liver failure. Gastroenterology 2003;125:755–64.

73. Parekh NK, Hynan LS, De Lemos J, et al. Elevated troponin I levels in acute liver failure: is myocardial injury an integral part of acute liver failure? Hepatology 2007;45:1489–95.

74. Pereira SP, Rowbotham D, Fitt S, et al. Pharmacokinetics and efficacy of oral versus intravenous mixed-micellar phylloquinone (vitamin K_1) in severe acute liver disease. J Hepatol 2005;42:365–70.

75. Rolando N, Philpott-Howard J, Williams R. Bacterial and fungal infection in acute liver failure. Semin Liver Dis 1996;16:389–402.

76. Rolando N, Harvey F, Brahm J, et al. Fungal infection: a common, unrecognised complication of acute liver failure. J Hepatol 1991;12:1–9.

77. Rolando N, Gimson A, Wade J, et al. Prospective controlled trial of selective parenteral and enteral antimicrobial regimen in fulminant liver failure. Hepatology 1993;17:196–201.

78. Kodakat S, Gopal P, Wendon J. Hyperglycemia is associated with intracranial hypertension in patients with acute liver failure. Liver Transpl 2001;7:C21.

79. Walsh TS, Wigmore SJ, Hopton P, et al. Energy expenditure in acetaminophen-induced fulminant hepatic failure. Crit Care Med 2000;28:649–54.

80. Salvino R, Ghanta R, Seidner DL, et al. Liver failure is uncommon in adults receiving long-term parenteral nutrition. JPEN J Parenter Enteral Nutr 2006;30:202–8.

81. Stadlbauer V, Jalan R. Acute liver failure: liver support therapies. Curr Opin Crit Care 2007;13:215–21.

82. Curr Opinion.

83. Skwarek A, Grodzicki M, Nyckowski P, et al. The use Prometheus FPSA system in the treatment of acute liver failure: preliminary results. Transplant Proc 2006;38:209–11.

84. Sen S, Felldin M, Steiner C, et al. Albumin dialysis and molecular adsorbents recirculating system (MARS) for acute Wilson's disease. Liver Transpl 2002;8:962–7.

85. Farmer DG, Anselmo DM, Ghobrial RM, et al. Liver transplantation for fulminant hepatic failure: experience with more than 200 patients over a 17-year period. Annals of Surgery 2003;237:666–76.

Obstetric Disorders in the ICU

Ghada Bourjeily, MD[a],*, Margaret Miller, MD[b]

KEYWORDS

- Pre-eclampsia • Eclampsia • Pulmonary edema
- Amniotic fluid embolism • Venous thromboembolism
- Ovarian hyperstimulation syndrome • HELLP
- Acute fatty liver of pregnancy

Maternal mortality in the developed world, even in patients admitted to intensive care units (ICUs), is rare. Unfortunately, mortality rates in the developing world are much higher. Recent statistics have shown that the lifetime risk of dying in pregnancy is 1 in 65 in Asia and parts of Africa, whereas that same risk is 1 in 8700 in Switzerland. Risks for mortality during pregnancy and childbirth include lack of education, single marital status, multiparity, lack of prenatal care, and non-Hispanic black race. The lowest rate of mortality is seen in non-Hispanic whites in the developed world. Traditional customs, social bias, and cultural factors also may affect mortality rates. Most maternal deaths (up to 70%) occur antepartum, whereas 27% of mothers who die do so in the first 6 weeks postpartum.

Obstetric disorders account for 55% to 80% of admissions to the ICUs in the obstetric population.[1,2] Despite this, medical conditions are emerging as the leading cause of maternal mortality, partly because of marked improvement in surgical and obstetric care in the developed world. The rise in maternal mortality related to medical conditions can be explained by multiple factors: (1) medical care is improved and women with chronic illnesses are reaching childbearing years, (2) many women in the western world are older at the time of their first pregnancy, (3) reproductive technologies have improved significantly in the past 20 years (consequently, older women and women with chronic illnesses are more likely to successfully conceive), and (4) severe medical conditions may be exacerbated by the physiologic changes of pregnancy,[3] leading to a sicker pregnant population.

The lower mortality associated with obstetric disorders may be explained by the fact that in many cases, delivery or surgical intervention is associated with quick reversal of the underlying pathology and clinical improvement. Risk factors for critical illness and consequent ICU admissions were suggested in a 14-year study of 1023 admissions to the ICU.[4] Risk factors include age older than 35 years (OR = 1.4, CI 1.05–1.81; P = .02), black race (OR = 1.8, CI = 1.38–2.30; P < .001), race other than black or white (OR = 5.9, CI = 2.60–12.77; P < .001), treatment in a minor teaching hospital (OR = 2.0, CI = 1.48–2.60; P < .001), and transfer to a higher level hospital (OR = 2.5, CI = 1.23–5.14; P = .01). Overall, the proportion of pregnant women admitted to nonobstetric ICUs is small, which makes the exposure of the average intensivist to pregnancy-related issues limited. The focus of this article is to review the most frequent disorders leading to ICU admissions in the obstetric population.

PRE-ECLAMPSIA

Pre-eclampsia (PEC) is an idiopathic multisystemic disorder that is specific to human pregnancy and the puerperium. It is essentially a placental disorder because complete molar pregnancies

[a] Department of Medicine, Pulmonary and Critical Care, Women & Infants Hospital, Warren Alpert Medical School of Brown University, 100 Dudley Street, Providence, RI 02905, USA
[b] Department of Medicine, Obstetric and Consultative Medicine, Women & Infants Hospital, Warren Alpert Medical School of Brown University, 100 Dudley Street, Providence, RI 02905, USA
* Corresponding author.
E-mail address: gbourjeily@wihri.org (G. Bourjeily).

Clin Chest Med 30 (2009) 89–102
doi:10.1016/j.ccm.2008.10.004
0272-5231/08/$ – see front matter © 2009 Elsevier Inc. All rights reserved.

chestmed.theclinics.com

that contain no fetal tissue have been associated with PEC. PEC and eclampsia were the second most likely cause of maternal mortality in a study published in 1988[5] and accounted for 15% of maternal deaths. More recent statistics from the confidential enquiry into maternal mortality in the United Kingdom found hypertensive disorders to directly cause 14 deaths per 1 million maternities (**Tables 1** and **2**).[6] Fortunately, maternal mortality rates related to PEC have declined significantly over the past two decades,[6,7] but PEC-associated infant mortality remains elevated and was reported to be 47.2 per 1000 births.[7]

The development of PEC has been thought to be secondary to abnormal placentation, which suggests that PEC is determined at an early stage in gestation. Failure of the second phase of trophoblast invasion results in the lack of destruction of the muscularis layer of the spiral arterioles. Persistence of this layer hinders the ability of those arterioles to vasodilate and accommodate the increase in blood flow.[8] Subsequently, placental hypoperfusion and hypoxia lead to the release of factors in the maternal circulation that are thought to be responsible for endothelial dysfunction, hypertension, and other manifestations of PEC. Endothelial dysfunction is thought to occur in part as a result of a functional defect in vascular endothelial growth factor, related to elevated levels of vascular endothelial growth factor antagonists such as s-Flt1 and endoglin. However, other factors are involved in the pathogenesis.

Clinically, the most conservative definition of PEC is blood pressure of 140/90 mm Hg or more in a previously normotensive woman and proteinuria more than 300 mg/dL or 2+ or more on a urine dipstick with or without peripheral edema. This definition has been used in most clinical studies. The Canadian Society of Obstetrics and However,

gynecology recently issued a report that accepted the diagnosis of PEC in the absence of proteinuria (http://www.sogc.org/guidelines/documents/gui206CPG0803_001.pdf9) (**Table 3**).[9] PEC occurs in 8% to 10% of pregnancies, but in most cases it is mild to moderate and does not necessitate critical care services. It is increased in frequency in patients with a prior history of PEC, a family history in a first-degree relative, underlying renal disease, thrombophilia, secondary hypertension, or systemic lupus erythematosis. A few life-threatening complications of PEC may require an ICU admission.

Eclampsia

Eclampsia is defined as seizures or coma in the setting of PEC without any evidence of other neurologic disorders. The cause of the convulsions is thought to be related to cerebral vasospasm with local ischemia, hypertensive encephalopathy, vasogenic edema, or endothelial damage. Approximately half the cases of eclampsia occur before term (< 37 weeks' gestation), with more than 20% occurring before 31 weeks' gestation. Most seizures are self-limited and last 3 to 4 minutes at most, and most usually occur before the patient even has intravenous access, which makes it difficult to properly compare the therapeutic effects of drugs. It is thought that seizure prophylaxis and control are best achieved with magnesium sulfate ($MgSO_4$) infusions, however. Benzodiazepines also may be used, and they control the seizures in most cases within 5 minutes; however, use of benzodiazepines close to delivery may be associated with severe respiratory depression in the newborn, so if they are required for seizure control it is recommended that a neonatologist be present for delivery. When comparing $MgSO_4$ to phenytoin and benzodiazepines, the eclampsia trial collaborative group showed that $MgSO_4$ is superior to

Table 1
Numbers of direct deaths attributed to eclampsia and pre-eclampsia and mortality rates per 100,000 maternities, United Kingdom: 1985–2005

Triennium	Number	Rate	95% CI	
1985–1987	27	1.19	0.82	1.73
1988–1990	27	1.14	0.79	1.66
1991–1993	20	0.86	0.56	1.33
1994–1996	20	0.91	0.59	1.41
1997–1999	16	0.75	0.46	1.22
2000–2002	14	0.70	0.42	1.16
2003–2005	18	0.85	0.54	1.35

Data from Lewis G, editor. The Confidential Enquiry into Maternal and Child Health (CEMACH). Saving mothers' lives: reviewing maternal deaths to make motherhood safer. 2003–2005. The seventh report on confidential enquiries into maternal deaths in the United Kingdom. London: CEMACH; 2007.

Table 2
Number of deaths from pre-eclampsia or eclampsia, United Kingdom: 2003–2005

Triennium	Cerebral					Pulmonary				Hepatic		Other	All	Total
	Intracranial Hemorrhage	Subarachnoid	Infarct	Edema	All	ARDS	Edema	Other	All	Rupture	Failure/Necrosis			
1985–1987	11	0	0	0	11	9	1	2	12	0	1	3	4	27
1988–1990	10	2	2	0	14	9	1	0	10	0	1	2	3	27
1991–1993	5	0	0	0	5	8	3	0	11	0	0	4	4	20
1994–1996	3	1	0	3	7	6	2	0	8	2	1	2	5	20
1997–1999	7	0	0	0	7	2	0	0	2	2	0	5	7	16
2000–2002	9	0	0	0	9	1	0	0	1	0	0	4	4	14
2003–2005	10	0	2	0	12	0	0	0	0	0	2	4	6	18

Abbreviation: ARDS, adult respiratory distress syndrome.
Data from Lewis G, editor. The Confidential Enquiry into Maternal and Child Health (CEMACH). Saving mothers' lives: reviewing maternal deaths to make motherhood safer. 2003–2005. The seventh report on confidential enquiries into maternal deaths in the United Kingdom. London: CEMACH; 2007.

both drugs in the prevention of recurrent eclamptic seizures.[10] MgSO$_4$ was also shown to be associated with 8% lower likelihood of ICU admission and need for ventilatory support when compared with phenytoin.[10] Patients treated with magnesium infusion should have patellar reflex monitoring and monitoring of respiratory rate and urine output. Respiratory arrest caused by magnesium toxicity can be reversed with calcium. Blood pressure control is also essential in the setting of eclampsia.

Pulmonary Edema

Pulmonary edema complicates 0.05% of low-risk pregnancies and 2.9% of all cases of PEC (**Fig. 1**).[11] Starling forces dictate the capillary–interstitial fluid exchange that occurs in the lungs, and the development of pulmonary edema is governed largely by the plasma colloid oncotic pressure-pulmonary capillary wedge pressure gradient.[12] Pulmonary edema in patients with PEC can be either cardiogenic or noncardiogenic and may be caused by various mechanisms. First, plasma colloid oncotic pressure falls during normal pregnancy from 23.2 mm Hg in the first trimester to 21.1 mm Hg at term[13] to 16 mm after delivery. The fall is even more pronounced in cases of PEC.[14] This significant drop in colloid oncotic pressure in PEC can be explained by renal albumin losses and impaired liver synthesis. The precipitous drop in the postpartum period can be explained further by blood loss, fluid shifts from the extravascular to the intravascular space, and excessive crystalloid infusions. Second, increased capillary wedge pressure may be related to left ventricular dysfunction, intravenous fluids, or the phenomenon of autotransfusion observed with uterine contractions in labor. In fact, 300 to 500 mL of blood are pumped from the uterine circulation into the systemic circulation with every contraction. Third, capillary endothelial damage can occur because pulmonary edema has been observed in the setting of normal colloid oncotic pressure–wedge gradient and normal wedge pressure. Finally, left ventricular dysfunction, which may be either systolic or diastolic, can be present. Pulmonary edema secondary to systolic dysfunction may occur in patients with severe hypertension, leading to a sudden increase in afterload or underlying heart disease, such as peripartum cardiomyopathy or cardiomyopathy predating the pregnancy related to various causes.[15] The development of pulmonary edema in these cases is facilitated by the drop in the oncotic-hydrostatic pressure gradient. Diastolic dysfunction has been described in obese, chronically hypertensive women with superimposed PEC.

Table 3
Classification of the hypertensive disorders of pregnancy

Primary Diagnosis	Definition of Pre-Eclampsia[a]
Pre-existing hypertension	
With comorbid conditions[b]	
With pre-eclampsia → (after 20 weeks' gestation)	Resistant hypertension or new or worsening proteinuria or one or more adverse conditions
Gestational hypertension	
With comorbid conditions[b]	
With pre-eclampsia → (after 20 weeks' gestation)	New proteinuria or one/more adverse conditions[c]

Women may be classified into more than one subgroup.

Abbreviations: ALT, alanine aminotransferase; AST, aspartate aminotransferase; LDH, lactate dehydrogenase.

[a] Severe pre-eclampsia corresponds to pre-eclampsia with onset before 34 weeks' gestation, with heavy proteinura (3–5 g/d according to other international guidelines) or with one or more adverse conditions.

[b] Comorbid conditions, such as type I or II diabetes mellitus, renal disease, or an indication for antihypertensive therapy outside pregnancy.

[c] Other adverse conditions consist of maternal symptoms (persistent or new/unusual headache, visual disturbances, persistent abdominal right upper quadrant pain, severe nausea or vomiting, chest pain, or dyspnea), maternal signs of end-organ dysfunction (eclampsia, severe hypertension, pulmonary edema, or suspected abruptio placentae), abnormal maternal laboratory testing (elevated serum creatinine [according to local laboratory criteria]; elevated AST, ALT or LDH [according to local laboratory criteria] with symptoms; platelet count <100 × 109/L; or serum albumin <20 g/L); or fetal morbidity (oligohydramnios, intrauterine growth restriction, absent or reversed end-diastolic flow in the umbilical artery by Doppler velocimetry, or intrauterine fetal death [www.sogc.org/guidelines]).

From von Dadelszen P, Magee L. What matters in preeclampsia are the associated adverse outcomes: the view from Canada. Current Opin Obstet Gynecol 2008;20:111; with permission.

A confounding factor suggested in the literature as a possible cause for the development of pulmonary edema is intravenous administration of $MgSO_4$ for seizure prevention in pre-eclampsia.

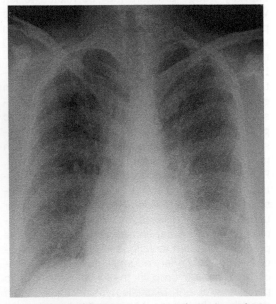

Fig. 1. 44-year-old G1P0 with pre-eclampsia and cardiogenic pulmonary edema.

In a study of 294 patients who received $MgSO_4$ for the prevention of pre-eclamptic seizures, however, only 4 patients developed pulmonary edema,[16] which makes this causative relationship less likely.

Pulmonary edema develops most commonly (70%–80% of cases) in the postpartum period.[11,14] It can be explained by the postpartum changes that include a significant drop in colloid oncotic pressure and the increase in preload that occurs with uterine contractions, the relief of vena caval obstruction after delivery of the conception products, and the mobilization of extravascular fluid that occurs in the initial 24 to 72 hours postpartum. Diseased kidneys are also commonly incapable of handling this rapid increase in intravascular volume. On the other hand, the small proportion of patients who experiences pre-eclampsia and develop pulmonary edema in the antenatal period is usually multiparous and older and has chronic hypertension.[11]

Hemodynamic profiles of patients with severe PEC/eclampsia vary in the literature from an elevated cardiac output and a normal systemic vascular resistance in the preclinical stage to an elevated cardiac output and elevated systemic vascular resistance or an elevated systemic vascular resistance with a depressed cardiac output or even normal systemic vascular resistance.[17–21] Variations in the data may depend partly on the methods used to measure hemodynamics[20] but also may suggest the presence of different hemodynamic profiles in PEC. It is not entirely clear whether patients may progress from one profile to the other. In a study that followed serial hemodynamic measurements in an obstetric population using a finger arterial pressure waveform registration device, patients with PEC without fetal growth restriction were found to have a higher cardiac output at different stages in pregnancy than patients with PEC with fetal growth restriction.[22] For those reasons, hemodynamic monitoring may be necessary in patients with severe, complicated PEC who do not respond to initial therapy to help clarify the hemodynamic profile and tailor therapy accordingly.

Treatment of pulmonary edema is basically unchanged compared with the general population and should be modified depending on whether pulmonary edema is thought to be cardiogenic or noncardiogenic in nature. Pregnant women generally respond to lower doses of diuretics than nonpregnant women, and most patients respond to 10 mg of furosemide administered intravenously. Afterload reduction and blood pressure control may be achieved with administration of intravenous hydralazine or labetolol.

Hypertensive Emergency

PEC may present with severe hypertension with a potential for end-organ damage, including retinal hemorrhage, papilledema, pulmonary edema, severe headache, and renal failure. Acute cerebral complications (eg, intracranial hemorrhage, massive cerebral edema) are particularly worrisome because they account for more than 75% of maternal deaths secondary to PEC. The goal of treatment is to prevent end-organ damage while still maintaining adequate uteroplacental perfusion.

Optimal blood pressure goals in the management of severe PEC are controversial. There is a general consensus that blood pressure of more than 180 mm Hg (systolic) or 110 mm Hg (diastolic) should be treated urgently in all cases and that patients who present with evidence of end-organ damage benefit from treatment of blood pressure more than 160 mm Hg (systolic) or 100 mm Hg (diastolic). In patients with no evidence of end-organ damage, no data suggest a clear benefit from treating blood pressure less than 180 mm Hg systolic or 110 mm Hg diastolic. Because PEC is a disorder characterized by diffuse vasospasm, many experts believe that allowing blood pressure to run in the moderate to severe range is the safest

approach for avoiding worsening of ischemia and maintaining an adequate uteroplacental flow.

If urgent lowering of blood pressure is required, intravenous labetalol or intravenous hydralazine may be used. Some evidence suggests that labetalol may be the better choice,[23] but studies comparing one antihypertensive to another are limited.[24] Short-acting nifedipine is also a reasonable alternative and begins to work within 30 minutes when given orally. Previous reports of nifedipine drug interactions with magnesium seem to be ill founded, and calcium channel blockers and magnesium may be used concurrently.[25] Nitroglycerin has been used for many indications in pregnancy, such as acute blood pressure control, acute coronary syndrome, and uterine relaxation. It seems to be safe in pregnancy, but data are limited. Nitroprusside has been associated with a risk of cyanide accumulation in the fetus.

Oliguric Renal Failure

Renal failure in the setting of PEC is usually rapidly reversible. For patients with oliguria and rising creatinine, treatment with small fluid boluses (250 mL) may improve urine output. Fluids should be given with caution because pregnant women with PEC are at risk for pulmonary edema, which is more likely to be associated with poor obstetric outcomes than mild renal failure. Less commonly, acute tubular necrosis or cortical necrosis may occur, especially if significant hypotension has occurred, which may be the case with placental abruption or disseminated intravascular coagulation–related hemorrhage. Prolonged oliguria is unusual in cases of PEC. If renal function deteriorates rapidly, other diagnoses, such as hemolytic uremic syndrome and thrombotic thrombocytopenic purpura, should be considered.

HEMOLYSIS, ELEVATED LIVER ENZYMES, AND LOW PLATELETS

Hemolysis, elevated liver enzymes, and low platelets (HELLP) is a constellation of findings that includes hemolysis with a microangiopathic blood smear, elevated liver function tests, and thrombocytopenia. HELLP complicates 1 in 1000 pregnancies but is much more common in patients with severe PEC, occurring in up to 20% of patients.[26] In the same series, HELLP was diagnosed antenatally in up to 70% of patients,[26] and most patients were diagnosed before 37 weeks' gestation. It is not clear whether HELLP is a manifestation of PEC or an independent entity altogether. Although maternal mortality is in the range of 1% in patients with HELLP, perinatal mortality associated with this syndrome ranges between 7% and 20%.[27] It is important to differentiate HELLP from thrombotic thrombocytopenic purpura/hemolytic uremic syndrome because the distinction has an impact on prognostic and therapeutic factors. Complications should be sought if liver enzymes are significantly elevated, which suggests hepatic infarction or congestion (**Fig. 2**), or if severe abdominal pain is present, which may suggest a subcapsular hematoma.

Delivery is the ultimate treatment for HELLP syndrome; however, the timing and urgency of delivery depend on fetal maturity, fetal well-being, and the severity of maternal disease. The decision to deliver should be made in conjunction with maternal fetal medicine specialists. The use of corticosteroids has been controversial. A Cochrane review of randomized and quasi-randomized clinical trials concluded that there were insufficient data to determine whether corticosteroid use in HELLP had any significant effect on maternal and fetal morbidity and mortality.[28] A subsequent large study by Fonseca and colleagues[29] that randomized patients to receive therapy with either dexamethasone or placebo found no difference in recovery of platelet number, lactate dehydrogenase, or aspartate aminotransferase. There was no difference in the duration of hospitalization, need for transfusion, or maternal complications.

ACUTE FATTY LIVER OF PREGNANCY

Acute fatty liver of pregnancy is a complication unique to human pregnancy that occurs in the second half of pregnancy, usually in the third trimester. This condition affects 1 in 13,000 pregnancies but is usually associated with a high mortality. Acute fatty liver of pregnancy is characterized by the deposition of microvesicular fat in the hepatocytes; the clinical presentation may

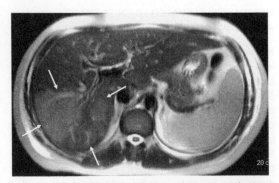

Fig. 2. 34-year-old G1P0 with pre-eclampsia and HELLP and transaminases >1000. Axial T2-weighted MRI of the liver demonstrates geographic increased signal intensity in the posterior right hepatic lobe (*arrows*) due to hepatic congestion.

include fulminant hepatic failure with coagulopathy, coma, and renal failure. In 50% of cases, acute fatty liver of pregnancy was associated with PEC at one point in the course of the disease.[30] Diagnosis is made definitively by a liver biopsy; however, because of the invasive nature of this test, it is not always performed. Delivery should be contemplated as soon as the diagnosis of acute fatty liver of pregnancy is made. The condition tends to improve with early recognition and delivery. Transfer to a liver unit may be necessary in severe cases, and some patients may require liver transplantation. It is important to counsel patients regarding the potential for recurrence in subsequent pregnancies.

TOCOLYTIC-INDUCED PULMONARY EDEMA

Preterm birth is defined as birth before 37 weeks' gestation. Preterm birth—with its many consequences—is by far the leading cause of infant mortality in the United States. Preterm labor occurred in 12.5% of births in 2005, but in general, 30% of cases of preterm labor remit spontaneously.[31] A significant number of patients require medical intervention to delay labor with the intention of either having enough time to administer glucocorticoids to help with fetal organ/lung maturity or to prolong the pregnancy in the case of a treatable risk factor for preterm labor.

The main agents used in the treatment of preterm labor include beta-adrenergics, $MgSO_4$ or calcium channel blockers. Tocolytic-induced pulmonary edema is a potential complication of these agents; however, recent data suggest that the incidence of pulmonary edema associated with beta-adrenergic agents is 0.3%.[32] Among beta-agonists, ritodrine is the only drug that is approved by the US Food and Drug Administration for the treatment of PTL; however, this drug is not manufactured in the United States any longer. Terbutaline is the most commonly used beta-adrenergic. The development of pulmonary edema with betasympathomimetics may be multifactorial. Increased plasma volume encountered in pregnancy is a predisposing factor.[33] Fluid overload related to the release of antidiuretic hormone, renin, angiotensin, and aldosterone by beta-agonists leading to increased salt and water retention likely plays a role.[34] The administration of additional fluid may worsen the fluid balance. Decreased diastolic filling time related to tachycardia is another important factor, especially in women with underlying heart disease. The administration of multiple tocolytics was found to be present in all identified cases of tocolytic-induced pulmonary edema in one large series.[35]

Pulmonary edema is occasionally related to increased vascular permeability, especially in the setting of an infectious process leading to preterm labor or superimposed PEC. Pulmonary edema also has been described with the use of nifedipine for tocolysis. The data are not convincing, however, either because the pulmonary complication may not be pulmonary edema based on the case description[36] or because the co-administration of other tocolytics, glucocorticoids, or intravenous fluids makes the association less potent.[37]

$MgSO_4$ has been associated with the development of pulmonary edema, with an incidence of 6.3% in one study.[38] Risk factors for the development of pulmonary edema include higher magnesium and intravenous infusion rates. Other causes, such as the concomitant use of other tocolytics, less concentrated infusions, and large net positive fluid balances, were also described as risk factors in that study.[38] These conditions likely represent risk factors for the development of pulmonary edema of any cause rather than being specific to magnesium-induced pulmonary edema. The use of $MgSO_4$ in PEC for seizure prevention also was not shown to be associated with a higher rate of pulmonary edema than that in the general population with pre-eclampsia.[16]

Indomethacin is another drug used for the treatment of preterm labor. This drug carries a black box warning against the increased incidence of cardiovascular events because of a risk of premature narrowing or closure of the patent ductus arteriosus with prolonged use. Atosiban is a tocolytic that is used commonly in Europe but is not available in the United States. Atosiban is a potential alternative because it has not been associated with any cardiovascular complications.

Treatment of tocolytic-induced pulmonary edema involves the withdrawal of the offending agent and treatment with supplemental oxygen as needed, fluid restriction, and diuresis. Minimizing the risk of tocolytic-induced pulmonary edema can be achieved by administering the lowest possible infusion rates and minimizing the duration of the infusion while monitoring heart rate.

AMNIOTIC FLUID EMBOLISM

Amniotic fluid embolism (AFE) is a rare but potentially catastrophic obstetric complication. The incidence of AFE varies significantly in the literature from 1 in 8000 to 1 in 80,000 live births.[39–41] Despite a low incidence, morbidity and mortality remain significant, with mortality reports ranging from 26% to 86%.[42,43] Survivors of the initial event and the cardiopulmonary collapse are likely to develop serious complications, such as disseminated intravascular coagulation and adult respiratory distress syndrome, and neurologic complications related to a hypoxic injury. In an analysis of a national registry, Clark and colleagues[40] found that neurologic sequelae in survivors of AFE occur in more than 80% of cases.

The pathogenesis of AFE is poorly understood. Risk factors such as the use of oxytocin, uterine tetany, male fetus, multiparity, and advanced maternal age have been debated in the literature.[40,43] The inciting event to the development of acute cardiopulmonary collapse was thought to be the presence of fetal debris and fetal squamous cells in the pulmonary vasculature, leading to a mechanical obstruction or stimulating an immunohumoral cascade that leads to the cardiovascular collapse. Later studies showed fetal squamous cells to be present in the pulmonary vasculature of patients who died of anesthetic complications and not AFE.[44] Hemodynamic changes associated with AFE support a humoral cause rather than an obstructive one in the pathogenesis of AFE.[45]

Hypoxia, one of the hallmarks of the disease, occurs early in the presentation. It is thought to be related to either an acute ventilation perfusion mismatch that results from the embolic event or the development of cardiogenic pulmonary edema secondary to left ventricular dysfunction. Hypoxia persists in the course of the disease and is thought to be secondary to a profound alveolar capillary membrane damage and noncardiogenic pulmonary edema. Hypotension is another manifestation of AFE. Human data are scarce on hemodynamic changes in the early phases. Case reports describe elevated right-sided pressures with right ventricular failure.[46,47] Animal studies show an increase in pulmonary artery pressure shortly after an AFE bolus.[48] After the initial transient vasospasm and rise in pulmonary artery pressures, blood pressure drops precipitously. With echocardiography and pulmonary artery catheters, left ventricular dysfunction has been shown to be present in the early and late phases of this syndrome.[49–52] Later in the course of the disease, a distributive "septic shock-like" physiology occurs with the development of noncardiogenic pulmonary edema.[53]

Disseminated intravascular coagulation may occur in 80% of patients and may be the first manifestation of AFE. Hemorrhage as a consequence of disseminated intravascular coagulation also may occur but rarely causes hypovolemic or hemorrhagic shock. This is likely related to the physiology of pregnancy, in which plasma volume is increased by nearly 50%, and the autotransfusion and redistribution of extravascular fluid that occurs during labor and delivery and the postpartum period.

The diagnosis of AFE is based on a high degree of suspicion and recognition of the constellation of signs and symptoms under the right circumstances. The presence of fetal squamous cells in the pulmonary vasculature is not a specific finding.[44] Although serologic assays and immunohistochemical staining using the monoclonal antibody TKH-2 to detect a common fetal antigen seem to have a high sensitivity for AFE,[54,55] these methods are not fully validated and cannot be recommended in routine practice. Treatment of AFE after the initial resuscitative effort is supportive. Goals of therapy should be early oxygenation, hemodynamic support, improving oliguria, and close monitoring for the development of coagulopathy.

OVARIAN HYPERSTIMULATION SYNDROME

Ovarian hyperstimulation syndrome (OHSS) is a rare but potentially life-threatening condition that tends to occur most commonly in association with assisted reproductive technologies but rarely occurs in association with spontaneous pregnancies. OHSS presents at approximately 3 to 8 weeks' gestation with ascites, dyspnea, severely enlarged polycystic ovaries, electrolyte imbalance, hemoconcentration, and hypercoagulability. OHSS occurs in 0.2% to 1% of all cycles that occur in assisted reproduction according to the World Health Organization estimates, but higher estimates have been reported in the literature.[56]

Luteinized granulosa cells express the mRNA of vascular endothelial growth factor among other factors.[57,58] Current findings suggest that vascular endothelial growth factor plays the most prominent role in increased vascular permeability and the development of hemoconcentration, fluid shifts, and electrolyte imbalance.[59] Vascular endothelial growth factor levels seem to correlate with disease severity.[60,61] Other factors, such as insulin-like growth factor and angiotensin-II, have been implicated in the pathophysiology.[56] Venous thromboembolism in patients with OHSS is thought to be caused by factors such as high serum estrogen levels and hemoconcentration. Some coagulation factors also may be affected in OHSS,[58,62] possibly predisposing patients to the development of thromboembolism. There have been multiple case reports of subclavian and internal jugular venous thrombosis in patients with OHSS.

The practice committee of the American Society of Reproductive Medicine[61] recognizes the difficulty in categorizing patients with OHSS according to severity because symptoms and signs represent a continuum that defies attempts at classifications of severity. Symptoms can vary from mild nausea, vomiting, and diarrhea to hemodynamic instability, acute renal failure, and acute respiratory distress syndrome. Ovarian torsion leading to an acute abdomen should not be missed because that risk increases with enlarged ovaries.

Patients with OHSS should be monitored frequently for worsening severity with daily weights and periodic laboratory measurements of electrolytes, analysis of renal and hepatic function, complete blood counts, and physical examinations. This follow-up is especially important if they are pregnant because the rising levels of human chorionic gonadotropic hormone may contribute further to the hyperstimulation. Intravenous fluids are needed to expand the intravascular volume, keeping in mind the increase in vascular permeability. Repeated paracenteses and thoracenteses are frequently needed in more severe cases. Thromboprophylaxis with anticoagulants such as unfractionated heparin or low molecular weight heparin and compression stockings or pneumatic compression should be strongly considered. Mechanical ventilation, invasive hemodynamic monitoring, and short-term hemodialysis are occasionally required. Treatment with dopamine of patients who have severe oliguric OHSS has been shown to dilate renal vessels and increase renal blood flow without significantly affecting blood pressure or heart rate.[63]

Some authors have recommended early termination of pregnancy in patients with critical complications of OHSS.[64] This decision should be made on an individual basis and with a multidisciplinary team, and it should be encouraged only if the termination is thought to positively impact the patient's condition.

PULMONARY EMBOLISM

Although not an obstetric disorder, pulmonary embolism (PE) remains the leading cause of nonobstetric maternal mortality in many countries around the world. Although mortality in the obstetric population from venous thromboembolism (VTE) is decreasing in some parts of the world,[65,66] PE continues to be a major cause of mortality in many other parts.[67,68] Therefore, a brief discussion of the salient features of this disorder in this population will be included.

Epidemiology

Pregnancy is an independent risk factor for venous thromboembolism (VTE), and retrospective cohort studies suggest that the incidence of VTE is 5 to 12 per 10,000 pregnancies in the antenatal period and 3 to 7 per 10,000 deliveries in the postpartum period[69–71] compared with an age and sex-adjusted incidence of 1.6 per 10,000 women and 0.2 per 10,000 women, respectively, in comparable time frames.[69] Hypercoagulability in pregnancy is a result of increased levels of procoagulant factors (increased factor V and VIII levels) and decreased fibrinolytic and anticoagulant activity (decreased protein S levels and increased activated protein C resistance).[72] Venous stasis is not only related to vascular compression by the gravid uterus but is also a consequence of progesterone, which starts rising early in the first trimester.[73] The risk of VTE in pregnancy is further increased in patients with additional risk factors, including prolonged bed rest,[74] advanced maternal age,[75] family history of thrombosis,[76] multiparity, previous thrombosis, thrombophilia, previous superficial phlebitis, pre-eclampsia, tobacco use, or operative delivery.[77]

Clinical Predictors

For the past two decades, clinical assessment has been used to stratify patients into risk categories using either clinical decision tools[78–81] or experienced clinician's assessment.[82] Because pregnancy is an independent risk factor for thrombosis, however, it is difficult to know how models of clinical prediction of PE would apply to a pregnant population. Clinical prediction is also complicated by the fact that physiologic dyspnea and an increase in heart rate occur commonly in pregnancy. It is likely that the distribution of physical findings, such as the presence of left leg swelling, may be more predictive of VTE in pregnant women than right leg swelling (because left-sided DVTs are much more common in pregnancy). Historical risk factors that include personal history of VTE or thrombophilia may be important determinants of pretest probability in the obstetric population. The performance of clinical assessment is more complicated in this subpopulation.

Diagnostic Tests

Some of the physiologic changes of pregnancy contribute to the diagnostic challenges in PE. For instance, alveolo-arterial gradient was found to be normal in more than 50% of pregnant patients diagnosed with a PE.[83] The need to make an accurate diagnosis and adequately treat PE certainly outweighs the risk of fetal radiation exposure that diagnostic testing for VTE entails. All of the imaging tests that involve ionizing radiation expose the fetus to a radiation dose that falls within the limits of what is considered "acceptable" in pregnancy. Protocol modifications may be used in a way that would limit radiation exposure without affecting diagnostic accuracy. Ventilation/

perfusion scans have the advantage of having some outcome data in the pregnant population but are limited by small numbers of patients and are retrospective.[84,85] The predictive value of ventilation perfusion scans depends heavily on the clinical presentation, and the positive predictive value ranges between 56% and 98% in nonpregnant patients with low versus high clinical suspicion.[82] Given the poor predictive value of the clinical presentation in pregnancy, the interpretation of ventilation perfusion scans is limited to some extent. Accuracy data of ventilation/perfusion scans are lacking in pregnancy. One of the major advantages of this test in pregnancy compared with the general population is the fact that the rate of intermediate/nondiagnostic scans is much lower in pregnancy—in the range of 3% to 25%.[84,86]

On the other hand, CT pulmonary angiograms (CTPAs) carry the advantage of exposing the fetus to a lower amount of radiation than ventilation/perfusion scans,[87] and they offer a different diagnosis (**Fig. 3**). The disadvantages of CTPAs are the amount of maternal breast radiation exposure, which is in the range of 2 to 5 rad.[88] Breast radiation may be minimized by the use of breast shields without significantly affecting image resolution.[88,89] Another disadvantage of CTPAs in pregnancy is the fact that plasma volume, cardiac output, and heart rate are increased, which dilute the contrast dye and result in a higher proportion of technically limited studies.[90] Accuracy and outcome data are lacking in pregnancy, but outcome trials are ongoing. One retrospective study that reviewed 78 patients with negative, technically adequate CTPAs found that 2 of 78 of those patients had concomitant positive ultrasound studies.[91] Iodinated contrast crosses the placenta, so there is a theoretic risk of fetal thyroid dysfunction.

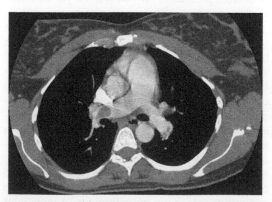

Fig. 3. 39-year-old G4P3 with mild chest discomfort and no hemodynamic instability. CTPA shows a large right pulmonary artery embolus.

Guidelines from the Contrast Media Safety Committee of the European Society of Urogenital Radiology released in 2005[92] stated that there is a paucity of information in the literature and encouraged the collection and publication of results of neonatal thyroid function results. After this statement, a small study by Atwell and colleagues[93] found no neonatal thyroid function abnormalities in newborns of 21 patients exposed to iodinated contrast during pregnancy. Larger studies are needed to shed light on this issue.

Many authors suggest the use of leg ultrasounds as an initial test in the evaluation of PE despite the negative data that suggest low sensitivity even in the general population (23%–52%)[94–97] and the fact that this approach is not validated in the pregnant or nonpregnant population. The positive predictive value of leg ultrasounds in patients without signs or symptoms of DVT is thought to be low. Leg ultrasounds are helpful as an adjunctive test to chest imaging studies in the evaluations of PE in pregnancy but cannot be recommended as initial tests.

MRI seems like an attractive alternative to ventilation/perfusion scans or CTPA because it does not involve any ionizing radiation. Most commonly used techniques involve the use of gadolinium, which is known to cross the placenta and has produced limited data in human pregnancies. Techniques such as real-time MRI do not necessitate the use of contrast agents. Real-time MRI is gated to a patient's respiration and shows clots on T2-weighted images. Further studies are needed before this test can be recommended for use in this population. Other diagnostic techniques such as D-dimers have not been studied sufficiently in pregnancy, and the fact that those levels rise during gestation complicates their use. The use of D-dimers is further complicated by the fact that they should be used in conjunction with clinical models of pretest probability, which are not yet validated in pregnancy.

Pregnant women with PE are treated with unfractionated heparin or low molecular weight heparin, neither of which crosses the placenta. Warfarin is rarely used in pregnant women because of its teratogenic effects. Compared with unfractionated heparin, low molecular weight heparin has the advantage of a lower rate of heparin-induced thrombocytopenia, less painful injection site, and a lower rate of osteopenia.[98] Heparin requirements are usually increased in pregnancy and bioavailability is reduced, likely in relation to pregnancy-related pharmacokinetics. Patients on low molecular weight heparin are best monitored with periodic anti-Xa levels given the weight changes in pregnancy and the possible changes in medication redistribution. Pregnant patients on therapeutic anticoagulation should have a detailed labor and delivery plan to minimize the risk of bleeding during vaginal or cesarean deliveries; however, this discussion is outside the scope of this article.

Thrombolysis has been described in more than 170 cases in pregnant patients worldwide. When these cases are combined, the maternal mortality rate is 1.2%, the bleeding rate is 8.1%, and the incidence of fetal loss is 5.8%.[99] Streptokinase at therapeutic doses was not associated with a fibrinolytic effect in cord blood, and neither streptokinase nor urokinase seems to be teratogenic. Hemorrhagic complications mostly occur intrapartum or postpartum when fibrinolytic therapy has been given near delivery. Tissue plasminogen activator is more frequently used, is not teratogenic, and is likely the safest fibrinolytic drug in pregnancy. Indications for the use of thrombolysis are not different in the pregnant population, and thrombolytic drugs should be strongly considered in the presence of a life-threatening PE remote from delivery.

PERIPARTUM CARDIOMYOPATHY

Peripartum cardiomyopathy is a dilated cardiomyopathy of uncertain cause. The true incidence is unknown, with reported rates ranging from 1 in 1500 to 1 in 15,000. This wide variation may reflect differences in geographic regions, referral bias, and individual practice patterns. Diagnostic criteria for peripartum cardiomyopathy have been established by the National Heart, Lung and Blood Institute:

- Development of cardiac failure in the last month of pregnancy or within 5 months after delivery
- The absence of a determinable cause of cardiac failure
- The absence of demonstrable heart disease before the last month of pregnancy
- Left ventricular dysfunction as demonstrated by echocardiography[100]

Risk factors for peripartum cardiomyopathy include advanced maternal age, multiple gestation, pre-eclampsia, gestational hypertension, and African descent. Several possible causes have been proposed, including myocarditis, abnormal immune response to pregnancy, maladaptive response to the hemodynamic stress of pregnancy, stress-activated cytokines, and prolonged tocolysis. There have also been some reports of familial peripartum cardiomyopathy.

Medical treatment of peripartum cardiomyopathy is similar to the treatment of other forms of congestive heart failure. Although no studies have compared therapeutic approaches, standard therapy with sodium restriction, diuretics, and vasodilators should be initiated. Loop diuretics seem to be safe in pregnancy and may be used in breastfeeding mothers. Angiotensin-converting enzyme inhibitors are contraindicated in pregnancy because of teratogenicity, but some are compatible with breastfeeding and should be initiated immediately after delivery. Hydralazine and nitrates are safer alternatives in pregnancy. Beta blockers may be useful primarily in the postpartum period for women who continue to have symptoms and left ventricular dysfunction despite more than 2 weeks of standard heart failure therapy. Anticoagulation should be considered in patients with peripartum cardiomyopathy because of a high rate of thromboembolic disease, especially in women with an ejection fraction less than 35%, atrial fibrillation, or mural thrombus.[101] The higher likelihood of thromboembolic disease is likely secondary to the hypercoagulable state of pregnancy and stasis of blood in the left ventricle. In the United States, mortality estimates from peripartum cardiomyopathy range from 25% to 50%. Approximately 50% of women recover to baseline ventricular function within 6 months of delivery. The other 50% of women have varying degrees of persistent dysfunction ranging from mild, compensated heart failure to deterioration and death, with most deaths occurring in the first 3 months postpartum.

REFERENCES

1. Rizk NW, Kalassian KG, Gilligan T, et al. Obstetric complications in pulmonary and critical care medicine. Chest 1996;110:791–809.
2. Karnad DR, Lapsia V, Krishman A, et al. Prognostic factors in obstetric patients admitted to an Indian intensive care unit. Crit Care Med 2004;32:1294–9.
3. Kaaja RJ, Greer IA. Manifestations of chronic disease during pregnancy. JAMA 2005;294(21): 2751–7.
4. Panchal S, Arria AM, Harris AP. Intensive care utilization during hospital admission for delivery. Anesthesiology 2000;92:1527–44.
5. Rochat RW, Koonin LM, Atrash HK, et al. The Maternal Mortality Collaborative 2 Maternal mortality in the United States: report from the Maternal Mortality Collaborative. Obstet Gynecol 1988;72(1):91–7.
6. Lewis G, editor. The Confidential Enquiry into Maternal and Child Health (CEMACH). Saving mothers' lives: reviewing maternal deaths to make motherhood safer-2003–2005. The seventh report on confidential enquiries into maternal deaths in the United Kingdom. London: CEMACH; 2007.
7. Tuffnell DJ, Jankowicz D, Lindow SW, et al. Outcomes of severe pre-eclampsia/eclampsia in Yorkshire 1999/2003. BJOG 2005;112:875–80.
8. Meekins JW, Pijnenborg R, Hanssens M, et al. A study of placental bed spiral arteries and trophoblast invasion in normal and severe pre-eclamptic pregnancies. BJOG 1994;101(8):669–74.
9. Magee LA, Helewa M, Moutquin JM, et al. Diagnosis, evaluation and management of the hypertensive disorders of pregnancy. J Obstet Gynaecol Can 2008;30(3 Suppl 1):1–48.
10. Which anticonvulsant for women with ecclampsia? Evidence from the collaborative ecclampsia trial. Lancet 1995;345:1455.
11. Sibai BM, Mabie BC, Harvey CJ, et al. Pulmonary edema in severe preeclampsia-eclampsia: analysis of thirty-seven consecutive cases. Am J Obstet Gynecol 1987;156(5):1174–9.
12. Rackow EC, Fein AI, Lippo J. Colloid osmotic pressure as a prognostic indicator of pulmonary edema and mortality in the critically ill. Chest 1977;79:709.
13. Oian P, Maltau JM. Transcapillary forces in normal pregnant women. Acta Med Scand Suppl 1985; 693:19–22.
14. Benedetti TJ, Starzyk P, Frost F. Maternal deaths in Washington State. Obstet Gynecol 1985;66(1): 99–101.
15. Barton JR, Sibai BM. Life-threatening emergencies in PEC-eclampsia. J Ky Med Assoc 2006;104(9): 410–8.
16. Yeast JD, Halberstadt C, Meyer BA, et al. The risk of pulmonary edema and colloid osmotic pressure changes during magnesium sulfate infusion. Am J Obstet Gynecol 1993;169:1566–71.
17. Easterling TR, Benedetti TJ, Schmucker BC, et al. Maternal hemodynamics in normal and preeclamptic pregnancies: a longitudinal study. Obstet Gynecol 1990;76(6):1061–9.
18. Bosio PM, McKenna PJ, Conroy R, et al. Maternal central hemodynamics in hypertensive disorders of pregnancy. Obstet Gynecol 1999;94(6):978–84.
19. Hjertberg R, Belfrage P, Hagnevik K. Hemodynamic measurements with Swan-Ganz catheter in women with severe proteinuric gestational hypertension (pre-eclampsia). Acta Obstet Gynecol Scand 1991;70(3):193–8.
20. Penny JA, Anthony J, Shennan AH, et al. A comparison of hemodynamic data derived by pulmonary artery flotation catheter and the esophageal Doppler monitor in PEC. Am J Obstet Gynecol 2000; 183(3):658–61.
21. Gilbert WM, Towner DR, Field NT, et al. The safety and utility of pulmonary artery catheterization in severe PEC and eclampsia. Am J Obstet Gynecol 2000;182:1397–403.

22. Rang S, van Montfrans GA, Wolf H. Serila hemodynamic measurement in normal pregnancy, PEC and fetal growth restriction. Am J Obstet Gynecol 2008;198(5):519e1–9.

23. Magee LA, Cahm C, Waterman EJ, et al. Hydralazine for treatment of severe hypertension in pregnancy: meta-analysis. BMJ 2003;327:955–60.

24. Duley L, Henderson-Smart DJ, Meher S. Drugs for treatment of very high blood pressure during pregnancy. Cochrane Database Syst Rev 2006 Jul 19;3: CD001449.

25. Magee LA, Miremadi S, Li J, et al. Therapy with both magnesium sulfate and nifedipine does not increase the risk of serious magnesium-related maternal side effects in women with PEC. Am J Obstet Gynecol 2005;193:153–63.

26. Sibai BM, Ramadan MK, Usta I, et al. Maternal morbidity and mortality in 442 pregnancies with hemolysis, elevated liver enzymes, and low platelets (HELLP syndrome). Am J Obstet Gynecol 1993; 169(4):1000–6.

27. Sibai BM. Diagnosis, controversies, and management of the syndrome of hemolysis, elevated liver enzymes, and low platelet count. Obstet Gynecol 2004;103(5 Pt 1):981–91.

28. Matchaba P, Moodley J. Corticosteroids for HELLP syndrome in pregnancy. Cochrane Database Syst Rev 2004;(1):CD002076.

29. Fonseca JE, Mendez F, Catano C, et al. Dexamethasone treatment does not improve the outcome of women with HELLP syndrome: a double-blind, placebo-controlled, randomized clinical trial. Am J Obstet Gynecol 2005;193(5):1591–8.

30. Riely CA. Acute fatty liver of pregnancy. Semin Liver Dis 1987;7:47.

31. King JF, Grant A, Keirse MJ, et al. Beta-mimetics in preterm labour: an overview of the randomized controlled trials. Br J Obstet Gynaecol 1988;95(3): 211–22.

32. Perry KG Jr, Morrison JC, Rust OA, et al. Incidence of adverse cardiopulmonary effects with low-dose continuous terbutaline infusion. Am J Obstet Gynecol 1995;173(4):1273–7.

33. Gabriel R, Harika G, Saniez D, et al. Prolonged intravenous ritodrine therapy: a comparison between multiple and singleton pregnancies. Eur J Obstet Gynecol Reprod Biol 1994;57:65–71.

34. Bax A, Middeldorp AM, Harinck B, et al. Unilateral pulmonary edema as a life-threatening complication of ritodrine. Acta Obstet Gynecol Scand 1999;78(10):915–6.

35. Sciscione AC, Ivester T, Largoza M, et al. Acute pulmonary edema in pregnancy. Obstet Gynecol 2003;101(3):511–5.

36. Nassar AH, Ghazeeri G, Usta IM. Nifedipine-associated pulmonary complications in pregnancy. Int J Gynaecol Obstet 2007;97(2):148–9.

37. Carbonne B, Papatsonis DN, Flenady VJ, et al. Comment on the article "Acute pulmonary oedema during nicardipine therapy for premature labour. Report of five cases" by Vaast P, et al. Eur J Obstet Gynecol Reprod Biol 2005;120(1):119 [author reply 119–20].

38. Samol JM, Lambers DS. Magnesium sulfate tocolysis and pulmonary edema: the drug or the vehicle? Am J Obstet Gynecol 2005;192(5):1430–2.

39. Steiner PE, Lushbaugh CC. Landmark article, Oct. 1941: maternal pulmonary embolism by amniotic fluid as a cause of obstetric shock and unexpected deaths in obstetrics. By Paul Steiner and C.C. Lushbaugh. JAMA 1986;255(16):2187–203.

40. Clark SL, Hankins GD, Dudley DA, et al. Amniotic fluid embolism: analysis of the national registry. Am J Obstet Gynecol 1995;172(4 Pt 1):1158–67.

41. Tuffnell DJ, Johnson H. Amniotic fluid embolism: the UK register. Hosp Med 2000;61(8):532–4.

42. Tuffnell DJ. Amniotic fluid embolism. Curr Opin Obstet Gynecol 2003;15:119–22.

43. Gilbert WM, Danielsen B. Amniotic fluid embolism: decreased mortality in a population based study. Obstet Gynecol 1999;93:973–7.

44. Clark SL, Pavlova Z, Greenspoon J, et al. Squamous cells in the maternal circulation. Am J Obstet Gynecol 1986;154:104–6.

45. Aurangzeb I, George L, Roof S. Amniotic fluid embolism. Crit Care Clin 2004;20:643–50.

46. Shechtman M, Ziser A, Markovits R, et al. Amniotic fluid embolism: findings on transesophageal echocardiography. Anesth Analg 1999;89:1456.

47. Stanten RD, Iverson LI, Daugharty TM, et al. Amniotic fluid embolism causing catastrophic pulmonary vasoconstriction: diagnosis by transesophageal echocardiogram and treatment by cardiopulmonary bypass. Obstet Gynecol 2003;102:496.

48. Hankins GD, Snyder RR, Clark SL, et al. Acute hemodynamic and respiratory effects of amniotic fluid embolism in the pregnant goat model. Am J Obstet Gynecol 1993;168(4):1113–29.

49. Dib N, Bajwa T. Amniotic fluid embolism causing severe left ventricular dysfunction and death: case report and review of the literature. Cathet Cardiovasc Diagn 1996;39:177–80.

50. Fletcher SJ, Parr M. Amniotic fluid embolism: a case report and review. Resuscitation 2000;43:141–6.

51. Clark SL, Cotton DB, Gonik B, et al. Central hemodynamic alterations in amniotic fluid embolism. Am J Obstet Gynecol 1988;158:1124–6.

52. Girard P, Mal H, Laine JF, et al. Left heart failure in amniotic fluid embolism. Anesthesiology 1986;64: 262–5.

53. Moore J, Baldisseri MR. Amniotic fluid embolism. Crit Care Med 2005;33(10):S279–85.

54. Oi H, Kobayashi H, Hirashima Y, et al. Serological and immunohistochemical diagnosis of amniotic

fluid embolism. Semin Thromb Hemost 1998;24(5): 479–84.

55. Kobayashi H, Oi H, Hayakawa H, et al. Histological diagnosis of amniotic fluid embolism by monoclonal antibody TKH-2 that recognizes NeuAc alpha 2-6GalNAc epitope. Hum Pathol 1997;28(4):428–33.

56. The practice committee of the American Society of Reproductive Medicine. Ovarian hyperstimulation syndrome. Fertil Steril 2004;82(Suppl 1):S81–6.

57. Wang TH, Horng SG, Chang CL, et al. Human chorionic gonadotropin –induced ovarian hyperstimulation syndrome: two distinct entities with up-regulation of vascular endothelial growth factor. J Clin Endocrinol Metab 2002;87:3300–8.

58. Binder H, Dittrich R, Einhaus F, et al. Update on ovarian hyperstimulation syndrome: part I-incidence and pathogenesis. Int J Fertil 2007;52(1): 11–26.

59. Agrawal R, Conway G, Sladkevicius P, et al. Serum vascular endothelial growth factor and Doppler blood flow velocities In in-vitro fertilization: relevance to ovarian hyperstimulation syndrome and polycystic ovaries. Fertil Steril 1998;70:651–8.

60. Levin ER, Rosen FG, Cassidenti DL, et al. Role of vascular endothelial cell growth factor in ovarian hyperstimulation syndrome. J Clin Invest 1998; 102:1978–85.

61. Practice committee for the American Society of Reproductive Medicine. Ovarian Hyperstimulation syndrome. Fertil Steril 2006;86(5 Suppl 1): S178–83.

62. Biron C, Galtier-Dereure F, Rabesandratana H, et al. Hemostasis parameters during ovarian stimulation for in vitro fertilization: results of a prospective study. Fertil Steril 1997;67(1):104–9.

63. Ferraretti AP, Gianaroli L, Diotallevi L, et al. Dopamine treatment for severe ovarian hyperstimulation syndrome. Humanit Rep 1992;7(2):180–3.

64. Vlahos NF, Gregoriou O. Prevention and management of ovarian hyperstimulation syndrome. Ann N Y Acad Sci 2006;1092:247–64.

65. Biaggi A, Paradisi G, Ferrazzani S, et al. Maternal mortality in Italy, 1980-1996. Eur J Obstet Gynecol Reprod Biol 2004;114:144–9.

66. Samuelsson E, Hellgren M, Hogberg U. Pregnancy related deaths due to pulmonary embolism in Sweden. Acta Obstet Gynecol 2007;86:435–43.

67. Panting-Kemp A, Geller SE, Ngyen T, et al. Maternal deaths in an urban perinatal network, 1992–1998. Am J Obstet Gynecol 2000;183(5): 207–1212.

68. Sullivan EA, Ford JB, Chambers G, et al. Maternal mortality in Australia, 1973-1996. Aust N Z J Obstet Gynaecol 2004;44:452–7.

69. Andersen BS, Steffensen FH, Sorensen HT, et al. The cumulative incidence of venous thromboembolism during pregnancy and puerperium. An 11 year Danish population–based study of 63,300 pregnancies. Acta Obstet Gynecol Scand 1998;77:170–3.

70. Gherman RB, Goodwin TM, Leung B, et al. Incidence, clinical characteristics, and timing of objectively diagnosed venous thromboembolism during pregnancy. Obstet Gynecol 1999;94:730–4.

71. Simpson EL, Lawrenson RA, Nightingale AL, et al. Venous thromboembolism in pregnancy and the puerperium: incidence and additional risk factors from a London perinatal database. BJOG 2001; 108:56–60.

72. Clark P, Brennand J, Conkie JA, et al. Activated protein C sensitivity, protein C, protein S and coagulation in normal pregnancy. Thromb Haemost 1998;79:1166–70.

73. Macklon NS, Greer IA, Bowman AW. An ultrasound study of gestational and postural changes in the deep venous system of the leg in pregnancy. Br J Obstet Gynaecol 1997;104:191–7.

74. Blanco-Molina, Trujillo-Santos J, Criado J, et al. Venous thromboembolism during pregnancy or postpartum: findings from the RIETE registry. Thromb Haemost 2007;97(2):186–90.

75. Macklon NS, Greer IA. Venous thromboembolic disease in obstetrics and gynaecology: the Scottish experience. Scott Med J 1996;41:83–6.

76. McColl MD, Ramsay JE, Tait RC, et al. Risk factors for pregnancy associated venous thromboembolism. Thromb Haemost 1997;78:1183–8.

77. Danilenko-Dixon DR, Heit JA, Silverstein MD, et al. Risk factors for deep vein thrombosis and pulmonary embolism during pregnancy or post partum: a population-based, case-control study. Am J Obstet Gynecol 2001;184:104–10.

78. Wicki J, Perneger TV, Junod AF, et al. Assessing clinical probability of pulmonary embolism in the emergency ward: a simple score. Arch Intern Med 2001;161(1):92–7.

79. Wells PS, Anderson DR, Rodger MA, et al. Excluding pulmonary embolism at the bedside without diagnostic imaging: management of patients with suspected pulmonary embolism presenting to the emergency department by using a simple clinical model and D-dimer. Ann Intern Med 2001;135: 98–107.

80. Wells PS, Anderson DR, Rodger MA, et al. Derivation of a simple clinical model to categorize patients probability of pulmonary embolism: increasing the models utility with the SimpliRED D-dimer. Thromb Haemost 2000;83:416–20.

81. Perrier A, Desmarais S, Miron MJ, et al. Non-invasive diagnosis of venous thromboembolism in outpatients. Lancet 1999;353:190–5.

82. PIOPED Investigators. Value of the ventilation/perfusion scan in acute pulmonary embolism. Results of the prospective investigation of pulmonary embolism diagnosis (PIOPED). JAMA 1990;263:2753–9.

83. Powrie RO, Larson L, Rosene-Montella K, et al. Alveolar-arterial oxygen gradient in acute pulmonary embolism in pregnancy. Am J Obstet Gynecol 1998;178(2);394–6.

84. Chan WS, Ray JG, Murray S, et al. Suspected pulmonary embolism in pregnancy: clinical presentation, results of lung scanning, and subsequent maternal and pediatric outcomes. Arch Intern Med 2002;162(10):1170–5.

85. Balan KK, Critchley M, Vedavathy KK, et al. The value of ventilation-perfusion imaging in pregnancy. Br J Radiol 1997;70(832):338–40.

86. Yoo D, Lazarus E, Khalil H, et al. Diagnostic yield of ventilation perfusion (V/Q) scans in pregnancy: review of the findings in 315 consecutive pregnant patients from 1999 through 2006. Presented at RSNA meeting, Chicago, IL, November 25–30, 2007.

87. Winer-Muram HT, Boone JM, Brown HL, et al. Pulmonary embolism in pregnant patients: fetal radiation dose with helical CT. Radiology 2002;224(2):487–92.

88. Hopper KD, King SH, Lobell ME, et al. The breast: in-plane x-ray protootion during diagnostic thoracic CT–shielding with bismuth radioprotective garments. Radiology 1997;205(3):853–8.

89. Parker MS, Hui FK, Camacho MA, et al. Female breast radiation exposure during CT pulmonary angiography. AJR Am J Roentgenol 2005;185:1228–33.

90. Khalil H, Bourjeily G, Lazarus E, et al. Multidetector CT pulmonary angiograms in pregnant patients: the "limited, no central PE"—how limited? Presented at RSNA meeting, Chicago, IL, November 25–30, 2007.

91. Bourjeily G, Khalil H, Habr F, et al. Multidetector-row computed tomography in the detection of pulmonary embolism in pregnancy. Chest 2007;132(4):500S.

92. Webb JA, Thomsen HS, Morcos SK. Members of the contrast media safety committee of the european society of urogenital radiology. The use of iodinated and gadolinium contrast media during pregnancy and lactation. Eur Radiol 2005;15:1234–40.

93. Atwell TD, Lteif AN, Brown DL, et al. Neonatal thyroid function after administration of IV iodinated contrast agents to 21 pregnancy patients. AJR 2008;191:268–71.

94. Torres JA, Aracil E, Puras E, et al. Role of venous duplex imaging of lower extremity for pulmonary embolism diagnosis. Angiologia 1999;51:71–6.

95. MacGillavry M, Sanson B, Buller H, et al. Compression ultrasonography of the leg veins in patients with clinically suspected pulmonary embolism: is a more extensive assessment of compressibility useful? Thromb Haemost 2000;884:973–6.

96. Turkstra F, Kuijer PM, van Beek EJ, et al. Diagnostic utility of ultrasonography of leg veins in patients suspected of having pulmonary embolism. Ann Intern Med 1997;126(10):775–81.

97. Barrelier M, Lezin B, Landy S, et al. Prevalence of duplex ultrasonography detectable venous thrombosis in patients with suspected or acute pulmonary embolism. J Mal Vasc 2001;26:23–30.

98. Pettila V, Leinonen P, Markkola A, et al. Postpartum bone mineral density in women treated for thromboprophylaxis with unfractionated heparin or LMW heparin. Thromb Haemost 2002;87:182–6.

99. Turrentine MA, Braems G, Ramirez MM. Use of thrombolytics for the treatment of thromboembolic disease during pregnancy. Obstet Gynecol Surv 1995;50:534–41.

100. Pearson GD, Veille JC, Rahimtoola S, et al. Peripartum cardiomyopathy: national heart, lung, and blood institute and office of rare diseases (National Institutes of Health) workshop recommendations and review. JAMA 2000;283(9):1183–8.

101. Task Force on the Management of Cardiovascular Diseases during Pregnancy of the European Society of Cardiology. Expert consensus document on management of cardiovascular diseases during pregnancy. Eur Heart J 2003;24:761–81.

Critical Care Management of Subarachnoid Hemorrhage and Ischemic Stroke

David B. Seder, MD[a],*, Stephan A. Mayer, MD[b,c]

KEYWORDS
- Subarachnoid hemorrhage • Ischemic stroke
- Cerebral infarction • Multimodality monitoring
- Medical complications • ICU management

For decades, therapeutic nihilism has dominated the care of patients with severe brain injury, but large case series and clinical trial data suggest that poor neurologic outcomes after severe aneurysmal subarachnoid hemorrhage (SAH) or massive ischemic stroke are by no means certain. When aggressive critical care, surgical, and endovascular treatments are used, functional independence can be expected in 40% to 60% of patients with Hunt and Hess grade 4 and 5 SAH,[1–3] 22% to 45% of patients with acute basilar thrombosis,[4–9] and 40% to 45% of patients with malignant middle cerebral artery (MCA) infarction[10,11]—diseases previously considered almost uniformly fatal. Furthermore, stroke survivors with severe neurologic disability but adequate social resources, such as the locked-in survivors of basilar occlusion, may rate their quality of life as acceptable, and preferable to death (**Fig. 1**).[12,13] In the face of these data, intensivists, surgeons, and neurologists should begin to question withholding aggressive care based on the perception of futility, gain awareness of our own biases regarding outcome after severe brain injury, and be honest about uncertainty with patients and their families.

EPIDEMIOLOGY

Ischemic cerebral infarction accounts for 80% of all stroke in the United States,[14] but most patients will not require ICU admission. SAH is a generally more morbid disease, with a 30% to 50% overall mortality rate,[15] and virtually all patients at least briefly require ICU admission. Therefore, intensivists are likely to care for similar numbers of patients with ischemic stroke and SAH.

Catastrophic ischemic stroke syndromes are listed in **Table 1**. Typically, life-threatening ischemic strokes fall into one of several categories: occlusion of the internal carotid artery (ICA) or proximal MCA, causing a large-territory hemispheric infarction; acute basilar artery occlusion leading to posterior circulation infarctions; and large cerebellar infarction that causes compression of vital structures in the posterior fossa. Additionally, intensivists may be required to resuscitate patients with "flow-failure" states, caused by large-territory ischemia from high-grade cervical or intracranial atherosclerosis, by augmenting blood flow to areas at risk. Many patients with ischemic stroke have secondary

a Division of Pulmonary and Critical Care Medicine, Maine Medical Center, Portland, ME 04102, USA
b Clinical Neurology and Neurosurgery, Columbia University, New York, NY, USA
c Neurological Intensive Care Unit, Milstein Hospital, 8th Floor, Suite 300, Columbia University Medical Center, 177 Fort Washington Avenue, New York, NY 10032, USA
* Corresponding author.
E-mail address: sederd@mmc.org (D.B. Seder).

Clin Chest Med 30 (2009) 103–122
doi:10.1016/j.ccm.2008.11.004
0272-5231/08/$ – see front matter © 2009 Elsevier Inc. All rights reserved.

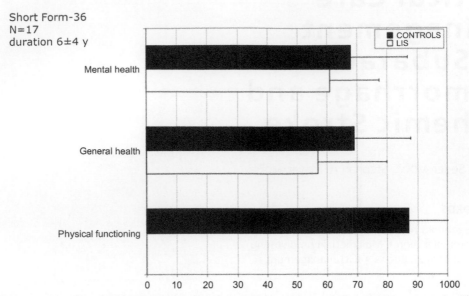

Short Form-36
N=17
duration 6±4 y

Fig. 1. Self-reported quality of life (QOL) in 15 chronic locked-in syndrome (LIS) patients compared with healthy age-matched controls. Scores range from 0 to 100, with higher scores indicating better QOL and functional status of patients with LIS. Although physical functioning was recorded as zero in all LIS patients, mental and personal general health were rated as similar to those of the control patients. (*From* Laureys S, Pellas F, Van Eeckhout P, et al. The locked-in syndrome: what is it like to be conscious but paralyzed and voiceless? Prog Brain Res 2005;150:495–511; with permission.)

neurologic decline from cytotoxic cerebral edema, maximal at 2 to 7 days after infarction,[16] and with careful ICU management, intensivists can prevent the devastating secondary neurologic injury caused by herniation syndromes during this critical period.

SAH follows a fairly reliable chronology, with management in the early phase dominated by cardiopulmonary stabilization, prevention of rebleeding, and the management of hydrocephalus and elevated intracranial pressure (ICP). This is followed by the vasospasm period, during which patients require intensive monitoring and treatment to prevent delayed cerebral ischemia (DCI) and infarction, and the late period when medical and neurologic complications of the disease and its therapies predominate. The intensity of ICU management is typically predicted by the severity of neurologic dysfunction of the patient at the time of presentation,[17] and other factors such as size and location of the aneurysm, severity of "ictus"—the acute episode of arterial rupture itself; amount and location of clot around the brain;[18,19] and the medical, surgical, and neurologic complications of the bleed. These factors are discussed in detail in this article.

GENERAL CONSIDERATIONS

Like all critical illnesses, the management of stroke begins with assessment of the airway, breathing,

and circulation. Many patients present with an acute decrease in level of arousal, poor tone in the posterior pharynx, and dulling of airway protective reflexes. These patients are at immediate risk for aspiration, hypoventilation, hypoxia, and respiratory failure. Patients in the acute phase of neurologic decline with moderate to severe respiratory compromise should be intubated without delay. These patients will undergo transfers within and between hospitals, brain and vascular imaging requiring them to lie flat, and multiple transitions of caregivers, predisposing to large-volume aspiration and exacerbation of the primary brain injury. Furthermore, acute stroke patients are clinically unstable, and thrombosis or bleed expansion may lead to an acute decrease in neurologic status, or even cardiopulmonary arrest. Conversely, once patients have stabilized clinically and neurologically, many can be extubated safely despite a decreased level of arousal as long as airway protective mechanisms are intact.[20]

Intubation of patients with intracranial mass effect should be performed cautiously (**Fig. 2**). Patients should be laid flat only for a brief period, and then immediately returned to a 30-degree angle of head positioning. Care must be taken not to cause significant hypotension during or after induction, which can trigger reflex cerebral vasodilation and subsequent ICP crisis, or hypoperfusion of the ischemic penumbra and an increase in

Table 1
Ischemic stroke syndromes requiring ICU care

Ischemic Stroke Syndrome	Acute Interventions	Time Window for Reperfusion Therapy	Reason for ICU Care	Duration of ICU Care/Placement Issues
Routine monitoring after fibrinolytic therapy	-IV tPA -IA tPA	3 hours 6 Hours	Neurologic monitoring for hemorrhagic conversion	-24 hours
Acute basilar artery occlusion	-IV tPA -IA tPA -Mechanical clot disruption, retrieval	12–24 hours	-Respiratory failure -Post-tPA monitoring -Monitor for progression, re-occlusion, hemorrhage -Cerebellar infarction (see below)	-3–10 days -Feeding tube -Possible tracheostomy
Holo-MCA or hemispheric infarction	-IV tPA -IA tPA -Mechanical clot disruption, retrieval -hemicraniectomy	6–8 hours	-Post-infarction edema leads to herniation syndromes -Consideration of hemicraniectomy -Respiratory failure	-3–10 days -Feeding tube -Possible tracheostomy
Flow failure syndromes	-Angioplasty, CEA, or carotid stenting -Rarely, intracranial stenting or bypass surgery	Variable	-Invasive BP monitoring and hemodynamic augmentation -Monitor for reperfusion-associated hemorrhage after endovascular therapy	1–4 days
Cerebellar infarction with edema	-Surgical decompression -EVD placement	N/A	-Edema may cause posterior fossa herniation syndrome, occlusion of the 4th ventricle	2–5 days

Abbreviations: CEA, carotid endarterectomy; IV tPA, intravenous tissue plasminogen activator; IA tPA, intra-arterial tissue plasminogen activator; MCA, middle cerebral artery; EVD, external ventricular drain.

infarct size. It is prudent to moderately hyperventilate most patients with CNS mass lesions before attempting intubation, because any delay in endotracheal tube placement will cause elevation of partial pressure of arterial carbon dioxide and a corresponding rise in ICP. Finally, succinylcholine is known to cause an acute elevation in ICP, which may be blunted with precurization.[21] The spike in ICP associated with direct laryngoscopy itself can be reduced by 1 mg/kg intravenous (IV) lidocaine administered immediately before the procedure.[22] Patients should receive IV fluids before and during intubation, anticipating a drop in cardiac preload associated with the initiation of positive pressure mechanical ventilation and the administration of vasodilator anaesthetic agents.

Generous IV access should be established early, with the recognition that vasopressors, osmotically

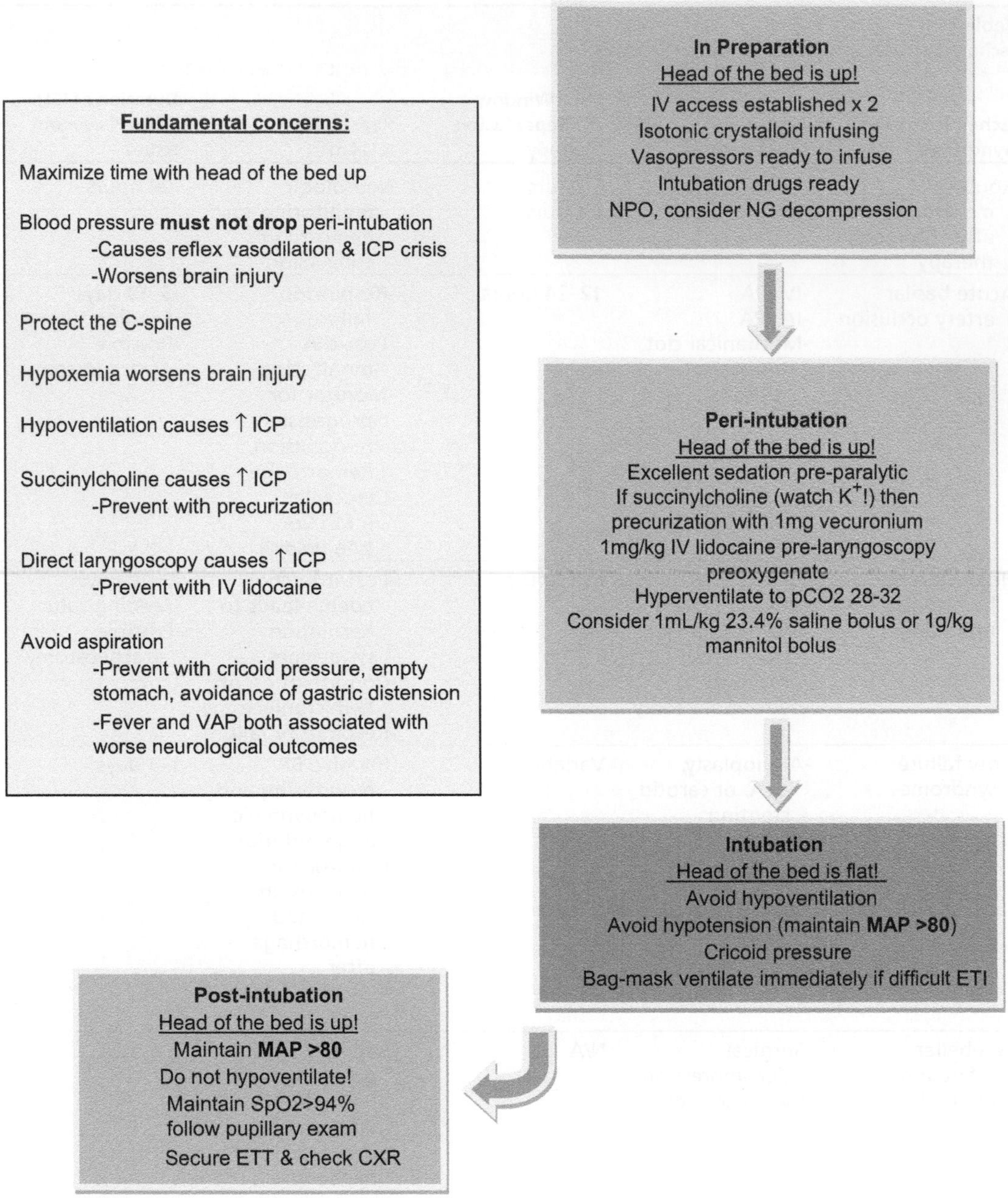

Fundamental concerns:

Maximize time with head of the bed up

Blood pressure **must not drop** peri-intubation
     -Causes reflex vasodilation & ICP crisis
     -Worsens brain injury

Protect the C-spine

Hypoxemia worsens brain injury

Hypoventilation causes ↑ ICP

Succinylcholine causes ↑ ICP
     -Prevent with precurization

Direct laryngoscopy causes ↑ ICP
     -Prevent with IV lidocaine

Avoid aspiration
     -Prevent with cricoid pressure, empty
     stomach, avoidance of gastric distension
     -Fever and VAP both associated with
     worse neurological outcomes

In Preparation
Head of the bed is up!
IV access established x 2
Isotonic crystalloid infusing
Vasopressors ready to infuse
Intubation drugs ready
NPO, consider NG decompression

Peri-intubation
Head of the bed is up!
Excellent sedation pre-paralytic
If succinylcholine (watch K$^+$!) then
precurization with 1mg vecuronium
1mg/kg IV lidocaine pre-laryngoscopy
preoxygenate
Hyperventilate to pCO2 28-32
Consider 1mL/kg 23.4% saline bolus or 1g/kg
mannitol bolus

Intubation
Head of the bed is flat!
Avoid hypoventilation
Avoid hypotension (maintain **MAP >80**)
Cricoid pressure
Bag-mask ventilate immediately if difficult ETI

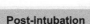

Post-intubation
Head of the bed is up!
Maintain **MAP >80**
Do not hypoventilate!
Maintain SpO2>94%
follow pupillary exam
Secure ETT & check CXR

Fig. 2. Intubation of the patient with elevated ICP.

active agents like hypertonic saline solution, IV sedation and analgesia, and the need to monitor cardiac hemodynamic function may require central venous access. The internal jugular site is best avoided when possible, because of the potential for interference with venous drainage of the head, and the potentially deleterious effects of internal jugular vein thrombosis on ICP.[23] Given the frequent need for arterial blood gas assessment and the rapid titration of vasoactive drips, arterial catheterization is preferred to noninvasive blood pressure monitoring. Because the femoral arteries are ideal access points for cerebral angiography and endovascular intervention, they should be used for blood pressure monitoring only in emergencies, or after communication with the interventional neuroradiologist, with radial and axillary arteries being preferred sites of monitoring.[24]

Tracheostomy and feeding tube placement are often required in patients with brainstem or cerebellar infarction, poor-grade SAH, or massive hemispheric infarction. These critical interventions facilitate care in the ICU, and ease the transition into rehabilitation by allowing earlier physical therapy, ventilator weaning, and transfer out of the ICU environment. When performed early for patients in whom long-term ventilator support is anticipated, tracheostomy is associated with less sedation and analgesia requirements, shorter duration of mechanical ventilation, and decreased mortality.[25–27] Bedside tracheostomy in the ICU, however, should be carefully timed and cautiously performed. Tracheostomy should not be performed before the aneurysm is secured, during the peak vasospasm period, or during ICP crisis when a high-amplitude pressure waveform suggests poor intracranial compliance. Both hypoventilation and hypotension will cause ICP elevation, and must be prevented during the procedure. Many patients with severe neurologic injury have normal respiratory function, and a comatose patient with tracheostomy can often be safely detached from mechanical ventilation entirely, preventing diaphragmatic atrophy[28] and the development of chronic respiratory failure. Feeding tubes placed in neurologic patients should include a postpyloric limb whenever possible to minimize regurgitation and the aspiration of tube feedings.

ANEURYSMAL SUBARACHNOID HEMORRHAGE

Hunt and Hess grades 1 to 3 (**Table 2**) carry a favorable prognosis, and almost always warrant aggressive treatment. Although patients may suffer complications such as hydrocephalus, vasospasm, or delayed cerebral ischemia (DCI), the outcome of their care is expected to be good, with most patients experiencing good or complete neurologic recovery.[29] Conversely, "poor-grade" subarachnoid hemorrhage is a catastrophic disease, and without aggressive neurosurgical and medical therapy, most patients will die. Because traditional outcomes in this population were poor, many clinicians have advocated placement of an external ventricular drain (EVD),[30] and in the cases where patients did not regain consciousness, have advocated for a "watchful waiting" or "expectant management" approach. Unfortunately, failure to pursue early aggressive treatment decreases the chance of a good outcome—a case of self-fulfilling prophecy. Failure to immediately diagnose and repair a ruptured intracranial aneurysm increases the risk of rebleeding, which is greatest in the first few days after presentation, and obviates the ability to treat with hypertensive hypervolemic therapy (HHT) should DCI develop. Recent data show that poor-grade SAH is in fact a treatable disease, and aggressive therapy is warranted during the acute phase (days 1 to 3) of hospitalization, unless brain death is imminent, or advance directives specify otherwise. Only after several days of medical and surgical stabilization is accurate long-term prognostication possible.[31]

Spontaneous subarachnoid hemorrhage typically results from the rupture of an intracranial aneurysm, although occasionally spontaneous SAH may be caused by venous bleeding (perimesencephalic SAH),[32] rupture of dural AVM, arterial dissection, mycotic aneurysm, or other vascular anomalies.[33] Subarachnoid hemorrhage is a neurosurgical and medical emergency, and the disease course often follows a predictable

Table 2
Hunt and Hess grades: neurologic status on presentation

Grade	Description	% Mortality (Hunt and Hess, 1968) n = 275	Mortality (Columbia Presbyterian, 1996–2002) n = 580
Grade I	Asymptomatic or mild HA	11	5
Grade II	Moderate to severe HA, or occulomotor palsy	26	5
Grade III	Confused, drowsy, or mild focal signs	37	10
Grade IV	Stupor (localizes pain)	71	34
Grade V	Coma (posturing or no motor response to pain)	100	52

Abbreviation: HA, headache.

From Mayer SA, Bernardini GL, Solomon RA, et al. Subarachnoid hemorrhage. In: Rowland LP, editor. Merritt's textbook of neurology. 11th edition. Baltimore, (MD): Lippincott, Williams, and Wilkins; 2005. p. 328–38; with permission.

chronology (**Fig. 3**). The onset of the classic SAH headache is often accompanied by loss of consciousness and is characterized by a surge in ICP, which temporarily equilibrates with mean arterial pressure (MAP) as the hemorrhage is tamponaded. Because cerebral perfusion pressure (CPP), defined as MAP minus ICP, is temporarily near zero, there is global circulatory arrest of blood flow within the cranium, resulting in loss of consciousness. This ICP surge rapidly abates, as spasm of the ruptured vessel occurs, clot forms, and arterial blood is shunted into and through the venous drainage.[34] Prolonged intracranial circulatory arrest may result in global cerebral edema after the brain is reperfused,[35] and depending on its severity and duration, sympathetic nervous

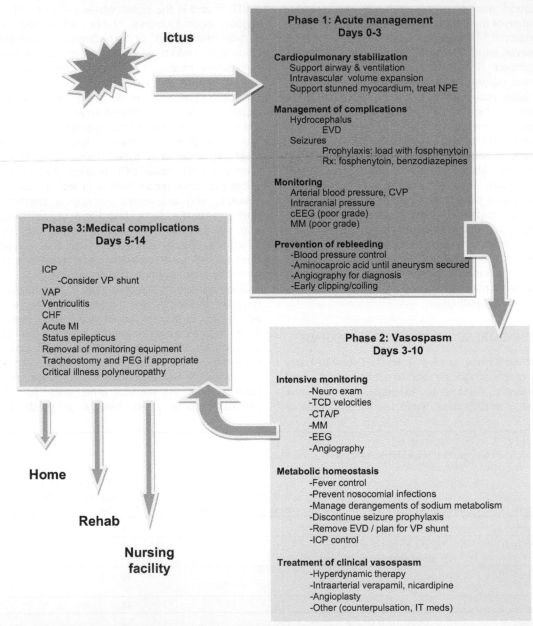

Fig. 3. Chronology of ICU care of patients with aneurismal subarachnoid hemorrhage. NPE, neurogenic pulmonary edema; EVD, external ventricular drainage; CVP, central venous pressure; cEEG, continuous electroencephalography; MM, multimodal monitoring; VP, venticuloperitoneal; CHF, congestive heart failure; MI, myocardial infarction; PEG, percutaneous enterogastrostomy tube; TCD, transcranial Doppler; CTA/P, computed tomography angiography with perfusion images; ICP, intracranial pressure; IT, intrathecal.

system and catecholamine-mediated cardiopulmonary abnormalities may occur, including neurogenic pulmonary edema,[36] neurogenic stunned myocardium,[37–39] and even cardiopulmonary arrest. In patients with inadequate collateral circulation, acute and focal vasospasm of the ruptured vessel may result in "ictal infarction," seen on MRI exclusively in poor-grade patients as infarction in the vascular territory of the aneurysm that is present on hospital admission.[40] This infarction is distinguished from that caused by "delayed cerebral ischemia" (DCI) that occurs in the setting of subacute (usually global) vasospasm, several days or longer after ictus.

Acute Management

On presentation, noncontrast head CT and careful neurologic examination should be immediately performed. Patients with a decreased level of arousal warrant urgent placement of an EVD.[30,41] IV fluids and oxygen are administered, and the standard measures of resuscitation are performed, including intravascular volume expansion, preservation of cerebral perfusion pressure, maintenance of a normal systemic blood pressure (by convention, systolic BP less than 140 mm Hg until the aneurysm is secured), and control of seizures, pain, and agitation that might trigger a BP surge and hemorrhage. It is appropriate to administer IV fosphenytoin, 15 to 20 mg/kg IV bolus on presentation, followed by a traditional maintenance dose until the aneurysm is secured. In patients without known or suspected acute thromboembolic disease or myocardial ischemia, aminocaproic acid 4 g IV load followed by infusion of 1 g/h until the aneurysm is secured can reduce the risk of early rebleeding.[42] Patients must be urgently transferred to a center with neurosurgical and endovascular expertise in the treatment of spontaneous SAH,[43,44] and when elevated ICP is known or suspected, 20% mannitol 1 g/kg, or 23.4% saline 1 mL/kg should be administered.[45–47] Patients with elevated ICP, with neurologic worsening, or with coma should be intubated, and ventilated to a pCO2 of approximately 30 to 35 mm Hg.

Subarachnoid blood often interferes with normal drainage of the cerebrospinal fluid, and hydrocephalus is the most common reason for acute neurologic decline in the hours immediately following the ictus. When a previously interactive patient with acute SAH becomes progressively obtunded, with increased tone and reflexes in the lower extremities and tonic downgaze deviation, hydrocephalus should be strongly suspected,[48–50] and an EVD placed. Conversely, an abrupt loss of consciousness with hemodynamic instability and a surge in ICP and bright red blood from the EVD suggests aneurysmal rebleeding.[51]

Aneurysm Repair

The ruptured aneurysm must be identified and secured as soon as possible after medical stabilization, as rebleeding will occur in 5% to 10% of patients within 72 hours, and is strongly associated with poor outcome.[52,53] Clipping or coiling of ruptured cerebral aneurysms, sometimes in highly inaccessible locations, is an extremely challenging technical neurosurgical and endovascular problem requiring skill and extensive operator experience. Endovascular and surgical treatment of ruptured aneurysms are both acceptable alternatives; in some vascular locations, particularly the posterior circulation, coiling is preferred for technical reasons, whereas other aneurysms require surgical clipping because of morphology or difficult endovascular access.[54] In the International Subarachnoid Aneurysm Trial (ISAT), a randomized clinical trial of 2143 good-grade patients with anterior circulation aneurysms suitable for endovascular or surgical therapy, patients treated with coiling had a lower incidence of the combined primary end point of death or dependency at 1 year (23.7% versus 30.6%, P = .0019).[55] This difference was primarily because of a lower incidence of disability in the coiling group, suggesting that, all else being equal, coiling might be safer than clipping. The clipping versus coiling of poor-grade SAH has not been studied, but there has been increasing reluctance to perform open craniotomy in patients with poor-grade SAH because of the high risk of perioperative complications, and in many centers these patients uniformly receive endovascular therapy. Nonetheless, critical care management of poor grade SAH is nearly impossible without aneurysm securing, and clipping is clearly preferable to no treatment at all.[31]

Vasospasm

During the subacute phase following medical and surgical stabilization, patients may suffer vasospasm and delayed cerebral ischemia (DCI). Despite minor improvements in prevention and therapy, vasospasm is poorly understood, and remains an important cause of morbidity after SAH.[56] The pathophysiology of vasospasm is poorly understood, but most evidence indicates that hemoglobin breakdown products and other spasmogenic factors in the blood reabsorbed from the subarachnoid space causes a sustained inflammatory vasculopathy.[57] Vasospasm typically progresses between postbleed days 3 and 12, although both early and late spasm have reported. The most important screening test for symptomatic vasospasm is a focused and careful neurologic examination. For this reason, routine interruption of sedation several times daily is essential in intubated poor-grade patients. Limb weakness, aphasia, or neglect may be signs of MCA ischemia, but attention must also be paid to subtle changes in mood and level of interaction, which are hallmarks of ACA ischemia. Transcranial Doppler ultrasonography is reasonably specific for detecting significant spasm of the MCA and other proximal cerebral arteries, but is insensitive to distal vasospasm and is not particularly useful for predicting symptomatic DCI.[58]

Once ischemia due to vasospasm is suspected in a patient whose aneurysm has been secured, hyperdynamic therapy is initiated by increasing IV fluids or colloids, and driving up the systolic arterial pressure to levels in the range of 160 to 220 mm Hg, with repeat neurologic examination to evaluate the clinical response (**Table 3**). CT angiography with perfusion images[59,60] or traditional cerebral angiography are then performed, although MR perfusion imaging may also be useful when available.[61] Vasospasm in the proximal

vessels is easily seen with angiography, but distal small vessel vasospasm is subtle, and easily missed. It is common practice to inject vasodilators, commonly paperavine, verapamil, or nicardipine, into vessels in spasm at the time of angiography.[62] Although effective, this therapy is infrequently durable,[63] and patients may require repeat injections. Alternatively, angioplasty of proximal vessels can be performed, which carries a 5% to 10% risk of major complications,[64–66] but has a more durable effect than vasodilators.[63] New protocols with aortic counterpulsation devices[67] and intrathecal therapeutics[68] are in development, and show promise for patients with refractory spasm.

Neuromonitoring

Patients with poor-grade SAH have a more challenging ICU course. Because these patients may have prolonged coma, and are typically at high risk of vasospasm, the neurologic examination is considered insufficiently sensitive to detect impending spasm, and more intensive monitoring is required (**Table 4**). In this role, continuous EEG, brain parenchymal oximetry, and cerebral microdialysis are alternatives to be considered. When

Table 3
Standard blood pressure and CVP goals in SAH and ischemic stroke

	BP Goal	CVP Goal	Therapeutic Goal
SAH—before aneurysm secure	MAP above 65, SBP<140	≥6	Prevent rebleeding
SAH—after aneurysm secure and low concern for vasospasm	MAP 70–90	≥6	Maintain good cerebral perfusion pressure
SAH—after aneurysm secure, vasospasm, or elevated ICP	Variable – manipulate to effect	>8	Hyperdynamic therapy
Ischemic stroke—no tPA	Autoregulate, if malignant MCA keep SBP<220	≥6	Perfuse ischemic penumbra
Ischemic stroke – before or after tPA	SBP < 185, DBP<105	≥6	Prevent hemorrhagic transformation
Ischemic stroke—after IA tPA and/or mechanical clot removal, angioplasty, or stenting	SBP <160	≥6	Prevent hemorrhagic transformation, reperfusion injury
Flow failure stroke with active or ongoing ischemia	SBP >160, titrate to symptomatic improvement	>8	Maintain flow in ischemic system, prevent thrombosis
Elevated ICP (requires ICP monitor)	CPP >60	≥6	Prevent reflex vasodilation and ICP surge

Abbreviations: CVP, central venous pressure; SAH, subarachnoid hemorrhage; MAP, mean arterial pressure; SBP, systolic blood pressure; DBP, diastolic blood pressure; ICP, intracranial pressure; CPP, cerebral perfusion pressure; IA tPA, intra-arterial tissue plasminogen activator.

Table 4
Neuromonitoring of poor-grade SAH for vasospasm

Modality	Ischemic Findings	Advantages	Disadvantages
Transcranial Doppler	Mean velocity >140 or Lindegaard ratio >3.0	Noninvasive, widely available, good NPV for MCA spasm	Insensitive, falsely reassuring
CTA/perfusion	Proximal spasm or hypoperfusion of vascular territory	Noninvasive vascular images correlate well with proximal angiographic spasm	IV contrast Transport to scanner False positives
MRA/perfusion	Hypoperfusion of vascular territory	Perfusion images without contrast, incidental MRI findings	Slow Transport to scanner Poor-quality vascular images
Cerebral angiography	Proximal vessel spasm or poor distal flow	Gold standard for vasospasm	Invasive IV contrast Distal spasm hard to see
Continuous EEG	Increased alpha-delta ratio	Noninvasive	Requires monitoring by EEG-trained physician
PbtO2	<20 mm Hg	Widely available Direct measure of brain metabolism	Invasive Nonspecific for spasm
Brain glucose	<20 mg/dL	Direct measure of brain metabolism	Invasive Nonspecific for spasm
Lactate/pyruvate ratio	>40 or rising	Direct measure of brain metabolism	Invasive Nonspecific for spasm Technically challenging

Abbreviations: SAH, subarachnoid hemorrhage; NPV, negative predictive value; MCA, middle cerebral artery; CTA, computed tomography angiogram; MRA, magnetic resonance angiography; MRI, magnetic resonance imaging; IV, intravenous; EEG, electroencephalography; PbrO2, parenchymal brain oxygen.

continuous EEG is used, a fall in the ratio of alpha/delta wave electrical activity may suggest vasospasm in the monitored region,[69] and has been used to help determine the need for angiography, and to titrate therapy.[70] Brain tissue oxygen monitoring (PbtO2) is widely available, and can be placed in an area of white matter at risk. Low brain parenchymal oxygen levels suggest ischemia, inadequate oxygen delivery at the tissue level, or increased cerebral metabolism.[71] PbtO2 is normally 40 mm Hg; sustained levels below 15 mm Hg are associated with an increased risk of death or poor functional outcome. Cerebral microdialysis makes use of a semipermeable microcapillary tube placed through a craniotomy (typically in conjunction with an ICP monitor and PbtO2 probe), and allows for hourly sampling of parenchymal brain metabolites. Glucose, lactate, and pyruvate, glycerol, and glutamate and other small molecules may be analyzed, with a low brain glucose level and high lactate/pyruvate ratio concerning for ischemia.[72] These modalities are all useful monitoring devices for vasospasm, but require a great deal of technical expertise and

a reliable algorithm upon which to base interventions.[73,74]

Medical Complications

Medical complications of SAH and their management are summarized in **Table 5**. These include fever, seizures, elevated intracranial pressure, ventilator-associated pneumonia, bacterial or chemical ventriculitis, electrolyte imbalances, and a host of other intrinsic or iatrogenic medical complications.[75–80] Of these complications, fever, anemia, and hyperglycemia are associated with worse neurologic outcomes, reinforcing the concept of secondary neurologic injury, and reflecting an opportunity for intensivists to impact on neurologic recovery with outstanding day-to-day ICU care.

ISCHEMIC STROKE

Ischemic stroke is a heterogeneous group of diseases with extremely variable prognosis, acute management, and critical care concerns. Intensivists must rapidly distinguish between potentially

Table 5
Medical complications of SAH

Complication	Incidence, %	Effect on Outcome	Management
Fever	54	Poor outcome, RR 4.4	Therapeutic normothermia
Anemia	36	Poor outcome, RR 1.8	Minimize blood draws
Hyperglycemia	30	Poor outcome, RR 1.8	IV insulin to goal 100–140g/dL
VAP	20	Death or disability, OR 2.04, 7-d increased hospital LOS	Standard measures
Bloodstream infection	8	Death or disability, OR 2.51, 4-d increased hospital LOS	Strict central line insertion policies and maintenance, early enteral feeds
Hypernatremia	22	Pulmonary edema, RR 4.1, elevated troponin, RR 3.7, decreased LVEF, RR 4.7	Hypertonic saline only in response to ICP crisis
Hypotension requiring vasopressors	18		Transthoracic echocardiogram Norepinephrine if normal LVEF Dobutamine if LVEF < 50%
Hyponatremia	14		Maintain Na+ ≥ 135 SiADH—conivaptan CSW—sodium replacement
Pulmonary edema	14		Dobutamine if low LVEF Prevent sodium overload Cautious diuresis—monitor CVP
UTI	13	3-d increased hospital LOS	Standard measures
Ventriculitis	5	5-d increased hospital LOS	Early removal of EVD
Arrhythmia (primarily AF)	5	Death or disability RR 8.0, 5-d increased hospital LOS	
Seizures	5		Prophylaxis until aneurysm secure, then discontinue cEEG in comatose patients

Abbreviations: RR, relative risk; OR, odds ratio; IV, intravenous; LOS, length of stay; VAP, ventilator-associated pneumonia; UTI, urinary tract infection; AF, atrial fibrillation or flutter; ICP, intracranial pressure; cEEG, continuous electroencephalography; SiADH, syndrome of inappropriate antidiuretic hormone; CSW, cerebral salt wasting; LVEF, left ventricular ejection fraction; EVD, external ventricular drain; Na+, serum sodium level; CVP, central venous pressure.
Data from Refs.[75–80]

catastrophic large vessel or posterior circulation strokes, and smaller lacunar or embolic events. The intensive care of patients with large or critical ischemic strokes is based on four goals: (1) reperfusion; (2) the prevention of infarct expansion, recurrence, or hemorrhagic conversion; (3) the prevention and treatment of malignant edema; and (4) prevention of medical complications.

Intravenous Thrombolysis

Because critical brain tissue hypoperfusion progresses rapidly to infarction, reperfusion therapy for ischemic stroke requires a high level of acuity and preparedness. Current American Heart Association (AHA) guidelines[81] are based primarily on results of the National Institute of Neurological Disorders and Stroke tissue plasminogen activator (t-PA) stroke study, which randomized patients with definitive onset of symptoms within 3 hours to IV fibrinolytic therapy or placebo.[82] Although most stroke centers have used a strict 3-hour window for the administration of IV tPA,[83,84] a more recent trial suggests that benefit may exist for up to 4.5 hours after the onset of symptoms.[85] Clinicians must determine the exact time of the onset of symptoms, perform rapid neurologic examination including the National Institute of Health Stroke Scale (NIHSS), obtain and review noncontrast head CT or MRI,[86] review inclusion and exclusion criteria for t-PA administration, obtain informed consent from the patient and family, and administer the drug within the time period. After the administration of IV t-PA, patients should be monitored in an ICU, with strict control of blood pressure to below 185/105 mm Hg and control of hyperglycemia to prevent hemorrhagic conversion.[81] Patients with suspected large vessel infarctions are often referred urgently for cerebral angiography after IV thrombolytic therapy is given to diagnose and treat persistent large vessel occlusions, a management strategy referred to as "bridging therapy."[87,88]

Multimodality Imaging

Newer neuroimaging techniques can demonstrate the state of vessel patency and tissue perfusion and viability. It can clarify prognosis and help determine the most appropriate course of treatment,[86,89,90] but should *never* delay an acute reperfusion intervention. Choice of neuroimaging for patients with suspected large vessel syndromes depends on renal function, local practice patterns, and rapid availability of interventional neuroradiology expertise. CT angiography of the head and neck can be performed quickly, and will identify large-vessel occlusion in vessels near the Circle of Willis almost as reliably as conventional cerebral angiography.[91] Furthermore, when flow-failure is suspected in a patient with waxing and waning symptoms, CT perfusion images reveal vascular territory at risk that remains uninfarcted.[92] Magnetic resonance (MR) imaging is extremely useful in managing patients with large-vessel occlusion.[93] Diffusion-weighted imaging (DWI) reveal ischemic tissue tissues long before infarction occurs,[94] fluid inversion recovery (FLAIR) sequences determine the extent of infarction, gradient echo images reveal areas of hemorrhagic transformation,[95] and MR angiography demonstrates the patency of large vessels and clarifies the presence and anatomy of collateral blood flow. MR perfusion imaging is used in some centers to investigate "diffusion/perfusion" mismatch, also indicative of ischemic territory at risk[94,96] that might be salvaged with reperfusion.

Intra-Arterial Reperfusion

Endovascular reperfusion of acutely occluded large cerebral arteries should be performed as soon as possible. The maximal time window for successful clinical recovery after reperfusion is within 6 to 8 hours for MCA or ICA occlusions,[97,98] or 12 to 24 hours for basilar artery occlusions.[99] "Bridging therapy," in which the initial IV t-PA bolus is followed by a local intra-arterial (IA) t-PA infusion[100-102] or embolism removal with a clot retractor device,[103-106] is particularly appealing in large-vessel cases where endovascular treatment is available. Good outcome with these interventional approaches is highly correlated with whether or not the occluded vessel can be recanalized in a timely fashion. Although anecdotal evidence for this approach is striking, this intensity of care requires a high state of preparedness, and the efficacy of the approach remains to be conclusively proven.[81] Many centers will provide endovascular treatment to younger and less medically complicated patients with potentially catastrophic strokes, after thoughtful discussion with family members to discuss the risks and benefits of this type of intervention.[87,88]

Infarct Expansion

Infarct expansion is prevented by assuring adequate cerebral blood flow (CBF) into the ischemic penumbra, an area typically perfused by maximally vasodilated collateral vessels. Many patients achieve this collateral perfusion on their own by regional vasodilation and systemic autohypertension, and clinicians should be cautious not to interfere with these intrinsic compensatory mechanisms. Blood pressure goals for patients with ischemic stroke are outlined in **Table 3**. Patients should be mildly volume-expanded with isotonic crystalloid formulations. Occasionally, blood flow augmentation with vasopressors or inotropes and aggressive volume resuscitation is necessary, such as when sepsis or the systemic inflammatory response syndrome (SIRS) cause inappropriate vasodilation, or when cardiomyopathy is present. In selected patients with large-vessel steno-occlusive disease and a fluctuating deficit suggestive of "misery perfusion" from flow-failure, a 30-minute trial of induced hypertension with phenylephrine (10–50 µg/min to raise MAP 20%) has been shown to lead to immediate clinical improvement in 20% of patients.[107] Fever is clearly associated with infarct expansion, probably because of its effect in increasing cerebral metabolic rate for oxygen (CMRO2) and worsening demand/perfusion relationships, and should be actively suppressed for the first several days after the stroke.[81,108,109]

Stroke Recurrence

Prevention of recurrent cerebral infarction requires that an accurate diagnosis of the etiology of the stroke be made shortly after hospitalization, and appropriate treatment begun. The highest 30-day risk for stroke recurrence, in the range of 5% to

10%, occurs in patients with symptomatic high-grade carotid stenosis, and to a lesser extent in patients with cardiac embolism. It is important to consider less common diagnoses, such as carotid or vertebral artery dissection, inflammatory vasculitis, bacterial or inflammatory endocarditis, and dural sinus thrombosis. All patients with acute ischemic stroke should receive 160 to 325 mg aspirin within 48 hours of the event, an intervention that decreases both the rate of recurrent stroke and mortality at 14 and 30 days.[110–112] IV heparin may be considered as an option on a case-by-case basis in patients with mobile intracardiac thrombi, active high-grade atherothrombosis, or other high-risk situations, but in general is not effective for reducing the risk of recurrent stroke.

Hemorrhagic Transformation

Hemorrhagic transformation resulting in parenchymal hematoma formation is strongly associated with poor outcome, occurring in 3% to 9% of ischemic strokes overall.[113–115] Hemorrhagic conversion should always be considered when a patient with large territorial infarction, cardioembolic source, systemic anticoagulation, recent thrombolytic therapy, or uncontrolled hypertension suffers acute, unexplained neurologic decline.[114,115] Full-dose anticoagulation should be avoided if possible for the first 2 weeks after territorial infarction, unless atrial fibrillation or an established and persistent high-risk embolic source is identified.[81] After IV t-PA, risk factors for hemorrhagic conversion include a large area of established infarction, increasing age, hyperglycemia, uncontrolled hypertension, congestive heart failure, and prior treatment with aspirin.[116]

Infarct-Related Edema

Patients with large cortical or cerebellar infarctions are at high risk of developing malignant cytotoxic edema in the zone of infarcted tissue. In the case of complete MCA artery territory infarction, patients may develop compartmentalized ICP elevation and suffer secondary infarction of the anterior or posterior cerebral arteries due to subfalcine herniation, or become brain dead if prolonged transtentorial herniation occurs. In the posterior fossa, intercompartment pressure rises rapidly if the cerebellum swells, leading to brainstem and fourth ventricular compression, hydrocephalus, and rapid progression to coma. The peak of brain edema typically occurs at day 2 to 7 after an MCA infarction, but can occur as late as day 14. Medical treatment for large cortical infarctions includes bolus osmolar therapy with 20% mannitol (0.5–1.5 g/kg hourly as needed) or

23.4% hypertonic saline solution (0.5–2.0 mL/kg); maintenance of the angle of the head of the bed greater than 30 degrees; maintenance of adequate cerebral perfusion pressure; and the avoidance of dehydration or hypovolemia, hypoventilation, hypoxia, fever, seizures, and fluctuations in serum glucose levels (see **Table 5**).[117–120] Despite rigorous adherence to these measures, it often is impossible to prevent herniation in patients with hemispheric infarction using medical therapy alone, and patients with significant cardiopulmonary or renal disease are unlikely to tolerate aggressive manipulation of serum osmolarity, blood pressure, and intravascular volume status.

Basilar Artery Occlusion

Acute occlusion of the basilar artery can result in bilateral infarction of the pons, midbrain, thalami, cerebellum, occipital lobes, or the posterior aspect of the medial temporal lobes. The clinical syndrome is of cranial nerve deficits, hemi or quadriparesis, dizziness, visual loss, incoordination, acute changes in the level of consciousness, and respiratory failure. Without reperfusion, acute basilar occlusion is fatal in 85% to 95% of cases,[6,121] and mortality remains in the range of 70% even with the most aggressive treatment.[4] The major risk factors for death are failure to recanalize the basilar artery and coma at the time of presentation,[9] and earlier administration of fibrinolytic therapy is strongly associated with better functional outcome.[7] Basilar artery occlusion not infrequently results in bilateral pontine infarction causing the "locked-in" syndrome, in which a fully conscious patient is paralyzed and mute, with only vertical gaze preserved for communication with caregivers and family. When clots in the basilar artery embolize to the top of the basilar or posterior cerebral arteries, cortical blindness and variably decreased levels of arousal may result.

Because outcomes without recanalization are so poor, IV or IA tPA are often considered for up to 24 hours after the onset of symptoms,[4] and multiple case reports suggest that success may be possible with late recanalization.[122–125] One recent case series of mechanical thrombectomy in the basilar system reported 44% good outcomes, a dramatic improvement over historical controls.[126] It is important to remember that retrograde collateral flow from the anterior circulation through the posterior communicating arteries can often supply the posterior circulation when the basilar artery itself is occluded, and that much of the basilar territory may be ischemic but not infarcted in the hours after acute occlusion. The most severe and devastating injury is often caused

Table 6
Medical therapy for mass effect from edema after stroke

Therapy	Indication	Mechanism	Limitations
Absolute avoidance of free water and hypotonic solutions	Initiate immediately	Limits water entry down osmotic gradient into infarcted tissue	None
Maintenance of normal or mildly elevated serum osmolarity	Initiate immediately	Osmotic gradient favors efflux of interstitial and intracellular fluid into capillaries	Heart failure Na>165 associated with poor outcomes
CPP optimization	Initiate immediately	Prevents reflex vasodilation and elevated ICP	Requires ICP monitoring
Maintenance of ≥ 30° bed positioning	Initiate immediately	Minimizes ICP	None
Avoidance of hypovolemia	Initiate immediately	Prevents brain hypoperfusion	None
Avoidance of hypoventilation	Initiate immediately	Prevents CO_2-mediated vasodilation and ICP surge	May require intubation
Normoxia and normoglycemia	Initiate immediately	Maximizes oxygen delivery to brain, normalizes metabolism	None—avoid hypoglycemia!
Avoidance of seizures	Treat seizures but do not give prophylaxis	Seizures cause ICP crisis, increased cerebral metabolism, and excitotoxicity	Phenytoin associated with worse cognitive outcomes
Avoidance of fever	T ≥ 38.3°C	Fevers increase ICP, aggravate ischemia, and are associated with poor outcome	Uncontrolled shivering increases systemic and cerebral metabolic stress
20% mannitol 1 g/kg IV	Clinical signs of herniation: ↓ LOC attributed to edema, pupillary abnormalities	Osmotic diuretic	Do not give to dehydrated patients; use 23.4% NaCl instead. Can cause electrolyte depletion
23.4% NaCl 1–2 mL/kg IV push over 5 min	Clinical signs of herniation: ↓ LOC attributed to edema, pupillary abnormalities	Osmotic agent and intravascular volume expander	Volume overload, may be aggravate pulmonary edema or ALI
Hyperventilation	Acute herniation syndrones, critical elevated ICP	Extremely rapid cerebral vasoconstriction-reduces ICP by reducing CBF	Excessive hyperventilation (PCO2 <30 mm Hg) may aggravate brain ischemia
Therapeutic hypothermia	Refractory elevated ICP and/or herniation	Decreases cerebral metabolism, reduces secondary brain injury	Increased risk of infection, side effects of antishivering regimen
Pentobarbital coma	Refractory ICP crisis	Decreases $CMRO_2$ and CBF	Infection, myocardial suppression, loss of neurologic examination

Abbreviations: Na, serum sodium level; ICP, intracerebral pressure; CPP, cerebral perfusion pressure; TTM, therapeutic temperature management; LOC, level of consciousness; VAP, ventilator-associated pneumonia; CBF, cerebral blood flow; $CMRO_2$, cerebral metabolic rate for oxygen.

by occlusion of small pontine penetrator arteries off the lower and mid basilar, and by emboli to the thalami. Urgent MRI may help to distinguish between futile and viable cases, with hyperintense DWI suggesting injury, and hyperintense FLAIR lesions suggesting completed infarction.[127,128] Clinicians must be careful never to delay recanalization by unnecessary imaging, however, because delay in recanalization decreases the chances of tissue survival.

After the reperfusion period, patients with extensive cerebellar infarctions are at high risk of edema and mass effect in the posterior fossa, and may require urgent occipital craniotomy to prevent herniation and brain death. Although unproven, the initiation of a prophylactic anti-edema strategy at this juncture (**Table 6**) may be appropriate to prevent the need for surgical decompression. Patients should be closely observed, with interval head CT scans, to evaluate the progression of posterior fossa edema and evaluate for fourth ventricle obstruction and hydrocephalus. Although the presence of a large cerebellar infarction poses the risk of secondary brainstem injury as a result of swelling and mass effect, many patients with cerebellar strokes make excellent functional recovery if the critical phase of swelling can be minimized. Conversely, moderate-sized infarctions in the brainstem itself or the thalami may be neurologically devastating, because of the close proximity of respiratory centers, cranial nerve nuclei, motor and sensory pathways, and arousal centers.

Massive Hemispheric Infarction

Most massive hemispheric infarctions are caused by emboli to the distal internal carotid or proximal middle cerebral arteries, and without aggressive management as many as 78% will die.[16] Clinically, these strokes often result in an acute and dense contralateral hemiplegia, gaze deviation toward the affected hemisphere, a visual field cut opposite the side of infarction, and neglect or aphasia syndromes. Because the initial noncontrast head CT will rarely differentiate between a large cortical stroke and lacunar syndrome in patients with acute hemiplegia, noting the presence of "cortical findings" on neurologic examination is crucial in making the early diagnosis of a large-vessel anterior circulation stroke, and identifying patients at risk for the "malignant MCA syndrome." Malignant MCA Infarction, in which cytotoxic cerebral edema causes subfalcine and uncal herniation, is more common in patients with more than 50% MCA territory affected, an NIHSS score above 20, age younger than 55, female gender, history of hypertension, and internal carotid occlusion.[129-131]

Because of the volume of tissue involved and inevitable swelling after infarction, patients with large territorial infarctions frequently develop

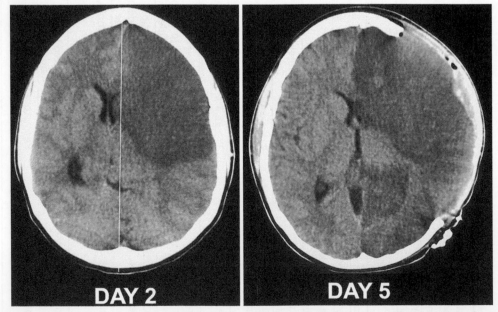

Fig. 4. Hemicraniectomy in a 35-year-old woman with malignant left MCA territory infarction. Note the addition of infarction involving the posterior MCA and posterior cerebral artery territories on the day 5 scan. Surgery was performed on day 3 after she progressed to bilaterally fixed pupils and extensor posturing. The midline structures were restored, the herniation syndrome was reversed, and the patient survived with moderate-to-severe disability.

elevated ICP and intercompartmental hernia-tion.[129,132–135] The medical treatment of cytotoxic brain edema is described in **Table 6**, but many patients, particularly those with large infarctions and minimal brain atrophy, require hemicraniec-tomy to prevent severe secondary neurologic injury. Hemicraniectomy with duroplasty allows the swelling brain to expand outward, preventing crush injury or infarction from elevated ICP or arte-rial compression (**Fig. 4**). Although many clinicians believe early hemicraniectomy before the deve-lopment of a herniation syndrome is most appro-priate,[136] the timing of hemicraniectomy is not clearly related to outcome.[10,137] Hemicraniectomy with duroplasty for the malignant MCA syndrome in patients younger than 60 years has been studied in three independent randomized clinical trials in Europe,[11,138,139] the results of which were pub-lished in a pooled analysis[11] and demonstrated a near-doubling of the number of patients with good neurologic outcome (mRs 0–3) from 23% to 43% at 6 months—a number-needed-to-treat (NNT) of four to prevent one poor outcome. Mortality was reduced by an even greater extent, from approximately 75% to 25%, a NNT of two to save one life. This overall improvement in survival and functional status was gained at the cost of a higher overall number of patients surviving but remaining partially or fully dependent on caregivers (mRs -5). Although many clinicians are hesitant to use hemicraniectomy in domi-nant-hemisphere infarctions, improved long-term functional outcome is not necessarily better with right compared with left-sided infarction,[140] and the potential for regaining language function after the procedure remains.[141]

SUMMARY

Patients with severe brain injury from SAH and ischemic stroke have seen an improvement in survival and long-term neurologic outcome over the past decade when aggressive surgical and medical neuroprotective measures are used. Many patients once considered to have a fatal brain injury can now be treated with the prospect of an acceptable recovery. The critical care management of these patients relies on rapid eval-uation and surgical triage, early and aggressive monitoring, and treatment of both neurologic and medical complications. When this multidiscplinary intensive care effort is used, secondary neurologic injury can be avoided, and patients have the best prospect for a good long-term functional recovery. Clinicians should resist the temptation to make unfounded early prognostic statements when evaluating brain injury, recognizing that negative prognostication is a major impediment to care, and that prognostication is most accurately and appropriately performed after medical and neuro-logic stabilization. Medical and neurologic inten-sivists must become familiar with long-term outcomes data regarding the quality of life of survi-vors of poor-grade subarachnoid hemorrhage and catastrophic ischemic stroke, so that they may provide correct, up-to-date information to patients and their families during the critical decision-making period. These clinicians must also become advocates for good-quality neuro-rehabilitation, so that the enormous initial outlay of ICU resources and efforts not be wasted by poor follow-up care.

REFERENCES

1. Mocco J, Ransom ER, Komotar RJ, et al. Preopera-tive prediction of long-term outcome in poor-grade aneurysmal subarachnoid hemorrhage. Neurosur-gery 2006;59(3):529–38.
2. Pereira AR, Sanchez-Peña P, Biondi A, et al. Predictors of 1-year outcome after coiling for poor-grade subarachnoid aneurysmal hemorrhage. Neurocrit Care 2007;7(1):18–26.
3. Weir RU, Marcellus ML, Do HM, et al. Aneurysmal subarachnoid hemorrhage in patients with Hunt and Hess grade 4 or 5: treatment using the Guglielmi detachable coil system. AJNR Am J Neuroradiol 2003;24(4):585–90.
4. Lindsberg PJ, Soinne L, Tatlisumak T, et al. Long-term outcome after intravenous thrombolysis of basilar artery occlusion. JAMA 2004;292(15): 1862–6.
5. Lindsberg PJ, Mattle. Therapy of basilar artery occlusion: a systematic analysis comparing intra-arterial and intravenous thrombolysis. Stroke 2006;37(3):922–8.
6. Brandt T, von Kummer R, Müller-Kuppers M, et al. Thrombolytic therapy of acute basilar artery occlu-sion: variables affecting recanalization and outcome. Stroke 1996;27:875–81.
7. Eckert B, Kucinski T, Pfeiffer G, et al. Endovascular therapy of acute vertebrobasilar occlusion: early treatment onset as the most important factor. Cere-brovasc Dis 2002;14:42–50.
8. Wijdicks E, Nichols DA, Thielen KR, et al. Intra-arte-rial thrombolysis in acute basilar artery thromboem-bolism: the initial Mayo Clinic experience. Mayo Clin Proc 1997;72:1005–13.
9. Levy EI, Firlik AD, Wisniewski S, et al. Factors affecting survival rates for acute vertebrobasilar artery occlusions treated with intra-arterial throm-bolytic therapy: a meta-analytical approach. Neuro-surgery 1999;45:539–45.

10. Gupta R, Connolly ES, Mayer S, et al. Hemicraniectomy for massive middle cerebral artery territory infarction: a systematic review. Stroke 2004;35(2): 539–43.

11. Vahedi K, Hofmeijer J, Juettler E, et al. Early decompressive surgery in malignant infarction of the middle cerebral artery: a pooled analysis of three randomised controlled trials. Lancet Neurol 2007;6(3):215–22.

12. Laureys S, Pellas F, Van Eeckhout P, et al. The locked-in syndrome: what is it like to be conscious but paralyzed and voiceless? Prog Brain Res 2005; 150:495–511.

13. Doble JE, Haig AJ, Anderson C, et al. Impairment, activity, participation, life satisfaction, and survival in persons with locked-in syndrome for over a decade: follow-up on a previously reported cohort. J Head Trauma Rehabil 2003;18(5):435–44.

14. Rosamond W, Flegal K, Furie K, et al. Heart disease and stroke statistics–2008 update: a report from the American Heart Association statistics committee and stroke statistics subcommittee. Circulation 2008;117:e25.

15. Hop JW, Rinkel GJ, Algra A, et al. Case-fatality rates and functional outcome after subarachnoid hemorrhage: a systematic review. Stroke 1997;28:660–4.

16. Hacke W, Schwab S, Horn M, et al. Malignant middle cerebral artery territory infarction: clinical course and prognostic signs. Arch Neurol 1996; 53(4):309–15.

17. Aulmann C, Steudl WI, Feldmann. Validation of the prognostic accuracy of neurosurgical admission scales after rupture of cerebral aneurysms. Zentralbl Neurochir 1998;59(3):171–80.

18. Juarez JL, Tarr RW, Selman. Aneurysmal subarachnoid hemorrhage. N Engl J Med 2006;354(4):387–96.

19. Claassen J, Bernardini GL, Kreiter K, et al. Effect of cisternal and ventricular blood on risk of delayed cerebral ischemia after subarachnoid hemorrhage: the Fisher scale revisited. Stroke 2001;32:2012–20.

20. Coplin WM, Pierson DJ, Cooley KD, et al. Implications of extubation delay in brain-injured patients meeting standard weaning criteria. Am J Respir Crit Care Med 2000;161(5):1530–6.

21. Clancy M, Halford S, Walls R, et al. In patients with head injuries who undergo rapid sequence intubation using succinylcholine, does pretreatment with a competitive neuromuscular blocking agent improve outcome? A literature review. Emerg Med J 2001;18(5):373–5.

22. Bilotta F, Branca G, Lam A, et al. Endotracheal lidocaine in preventing endotracheal suctioning-induced changes in cerebral hemodynamics in patients with severe head trauma. Neurocrit Care 2008;8(2):241–6.

23. Duke BJ, Ryu RK, Brega KE, et al. Traumatic bilateral jugular vein thrombosis: case report and review of the literature. Neurosurgery 1997;41(3): 680–3.

24. Scheer B, Perel A, Pfeiffer UJ. Clinical review: complications and risk factors of peripheral arterial catheters used for haemodynamic monitoring in anaesthesia and intensive care medicine. Crit Care 2002;6(3):199–204.

25. Nieszkowska A, Combes A, Luyt CE, et al. Impact of tracheostomy on sedative administration, sedation level, and comfort of mechanically ventilated intensive care unit patients. Crit Care Med 2005; 33:2527–33.

26. Griffiths J, Barber VS, Morgan L, et al. Systematic review and meta-analysis of the timing of tracheostomy in adult patients undergoing artificial ventilation. Br Med J 2005;330:1243.

27. Rumbak MJ, Newton M, Truncale T, et al. A prospective, randomized study comparing early percutaneous dilational tracheostomy to prolonged translaryngeal intubation (delayed tracheostomy) in critically ill medical patients. Crit care Med 2004;32:1689–94.

28. Levine S, Nguyen T, Taylor N, et al. Rapid disuse atrophy of diaphragm fibers in mechanically ventilated humans. N Engl J Med 2008;358(13):1327–35.

29. Mayer SA, Bernardini GL, Solomon RA, et al. Subarachnoid hemorrhage. In: Rowland LP, editor. Merritt's textbook of neurology. 11th edition. Baltimore (MD): Lippincott, Williams, and Wilkins; 2005. p. 328–38.

30. Ransom ER, Mocco J, Komotar RJ, et al. External ventricular drainage response in poor grade aneurysmal subarachnoid hemorrhage: effect on preoperative grading and prognosis. Neurocrit Care 2007;6(3):174–80.

31. Komotar RJ, Schmidt JM, Starke RM, et al. Resuscitation and critical care of poor grade subarachnoid hemorrhage. Neurosurgery in press.

32. Adams HP Jr, Gordon DL. Nonaneurysmal subarachnoid hemorrhage. Ann Neurol 1991;29:461–2.

33. Van Gijn J, Rinkel GJ. Subarachnoid haemorrhage: diagnosis, causes and management. Brain 2001; 124:249–78.

34. Sehba FA, Bederson JB. Mechanisms of acute brain injury after subarachnoid hemorrhage. Neurol Res 2006;28(4):381–98.

35. Mocco J, Prickett CS, Komotar RJ, et al. Potential mechanisms and clinical significance of global cerebral edema following aneurysmal subarachnoid hemorrhage. Neurosurg Focus 2007;22(5):E7.

36. Muroi C, Keller M, Pangalu A, et al. Neurogenic pulmonary edema in patients with subarachnoid hemorrhage. J Neurosurg Anesthesiol 2008;20(3): 188–92.

37. Mayer SA, Lin J, Homma S, et al. Myocardial injury and left ventricular performance after subarachnoid hemorrhage. Stroke 1999;30(4):780–6.

38. Lee VH, Connolly HM, Fulgham JR, et al. Tako-tsubo cardiomyopathy in aneurysmal subarachnoid hemorrhage: an underappreciated ventricular dysfunction. J Neurosurg 2006;105(2):264–70.

39. Naidech AM, Kreiter KT, Janjua N, et al. Cardiac troponin elevation, cardiovascular morbidity, and outcome after subarachnoid hemorrhage. Circulation 2005;112(18):2851–6.

40. Schmidt JM, Rincon F, Fernandez A, et al. Cerebral infarction associated with acute subarachnoid hemorrhage. Neurocrit Care 2007;7(1):10–7.

41. Sakowitz OW, Raabe A, Vucak D, et al. Contemporary management of aneurysmal subarachnoid hemorrhage in Germany: results of a survey among 100 neurosurgical departments. Neurosurgery 2006;58(1):137–45.

42. Starke RM, Kim GH, Fernandez A, et al. Impact of a protocol for acute antifibrinolytic therapy on aneurysm rebleeding after subarachnoid hemorrhage. Stroke 2008 Jul 24. EPub.

43. Suarez JI, Zaidat OO, Suri MF, et al. Length of stay and mortality in neurocritically ill patients: impact of a specialized neurocritical care team. Crit Care Med 2004;32:2311–7.

44. Bardach NS, Olson SJ, Elkins JS, et al. Regionalization of treatment for subarachnoid hemorrhage: a cost-utility analysis. Circulation 2004;109: 2207–12.

45. Koenig MA, Bryan M, Lewin JL 3rd, et al. Reversal of transtentorial herniation with hypertonic saline. Neurology 2008;70(13):1023–9.

46. Himmelseher S. Hypertonic saline solutions for treatment of intracranial hypertension. Curr Opin Anaesthesiol 2007;20(5):414–26.

47. Suarez JI, Qureshi AI, Bhardwaj A, et al. Treatment of refractory intracranial hypertension with 23.4% saline. Crit Care Med 1998;26(6):1118–22.

48. van Gijn J, Hijdra A, Wijdicks EFM, et al. Acute hydrocephalus after aneurysmal subarachnoid hemorrhage. J Neurosurg 1985;63:355–62.

49. Hasan D, Vermeulen M, Wijdicks EFM, et al. Management problems in acute hydrocephalus after subarachnoid hemorrhage. Stroke 1989;20:747–53.

50. van Gign J, Kerr RS, Rinkel GJE. Subarachnoid hemorrhage. Lancet 2007;369:306–18.

51. Ohkuma H, Tsurutani H, Suzuki S. Incidence and significance of early aneurysmal rebleeding before neurosurgical or neurological management. Stroke 2001;32:1176–80.

52. Naidech AM, Janjua N, Kreiter KT, et al. Predictors and impact of aneurysm rebleeding after subarachnoid hemorrhage. Arch Neurol 2005; 62(3):410–6.

53. Broderick JP, Brott TG, Duldner JE, et al. Initial and recurrent bleeding are the major causes of death following subarachnoid hemorrhage. Stroke 1994; 25:1342–7.

54. Komotar RJ, Zacharia BE, Mocco J, et al. Controversies in the surgical treatment of ruptured intracranial aneurysms: the first annual J. Lawrence Pool memorial research symposium—controversies in the management of cerebral aneurysms. Neurosurgery 2008;62(2):396–407.

55. Molyneux AJ, Kerr RS, Yu LM, et al. International Subarachnoid Aneurysm Trial (ISAT) of neurosurgical clipping versus endovascular coiling in 2143 patients with ruptured intracranial aneurysms: a randomised comparison of effects on survival, dependency, seizures, rebleeding, subgroups, and aneurysm occlusion. Lancet 2005;366:809–17.

56. Solenski NJ, Haley EC Jr, Kassell NF, et al. Medical complications of aneurysmal subarachnoid hemorrhage: a report of the multicenter, cooperative aneurysm study. Crit Care Med 1995;23:1007–17.

57. Pasqualin A. Epidemiology and pathophysiology of cerebral vasospasm following subarachnoid hemorrhage. J Neurosurg Sci 1998;42(Suppl 1):15–21.

58. Saqqur M, Zygun D, Demchuk A. Role of transcranial Doppler in neurocritical care. Crit Care Med 2007;35(Suppl 5):S216–23.

59. Chaudhary SR, Ko N, Dillon WP, et al. Prospective evaluation of multidetector-row CT angiography for the diagnosis of vasospasm following subarachnoid hemorrhage: a comparison with digital subtraction angiography. Cerebrovasc Dis 2008;25(1–2):144–50.

60. Laslo AM, Eastwood JD, Pakkiri P, et al. CT perfusion-derived mean transit time predicts early mortality and delayed vasospasm after experimental subarachnoid hemorrhage. Am J Neuroradiol 2008;29(1):79–85.

61. Rordorf G, Koroshetz WJ, Copen WA, et al. Diffusion- and perfusion-weighted imaging in vasospasm after subarachnoid hemorrhage. Stroke 1999;30(3):599–605.

62. Komotar RJ, Zacharia BE, Otten ML, et al. Controversies in the endovascular management of cerebral vasospasm after intracranial aneurysm rupture and future directions for therapeutic approaches. Neurosurgery 2008;62(4):897–905.

63. Elliott JP, Newell DW, Lam DJ, et al. Comparison of balloon angioplasty and papaverine infusion for the treatment of vasospasm following aneurysmal subarachnoid hemorrhage. J Neurosurg 1998;88: 277–84.

64. Zwienenberg-Lee M, Hartman J, Rudisill N, et al. Effect of prophylactic transluminal balloon angioplasty on cerebral vasospasm and outcome in patients with Fisher grade III subarachnoid hemorrhage: results of a phase II multicenter, randomized, clinical trial. Stroke 2008;39(6):1759–65.

65. Jestaedt L, Pham M, Bartsch AJ, et al. The impact of balloon angioplasty on the evolution of vasospasm-related infarction after aneurysmal

subarachnoid hemorrhage. Neurosurgery 2008; 62(3):610–7.

66. Brisman JL, Eskridge JM, Newell DW. Neurointerventional treatment of vasospasm. Neurol Res 2006;28(7):769–76.

67. Lylyk P, Vila JF, Miranda C. Partial aortic obstruction improves cerebral perfusion and clinical symptoms in patients with symptomatic vasospasm. Neurol Res 2005;27(Suppl 1):S129–35.

68. Hänggi D, Beseoglu K, Turowski B, et al. Feasibility and safety of intrathecal nimodipine on posthaemorrhagic cerebral vasospasm refractory to medical and endovascular therapy. Clin Neurol Neurosurg 2008 Jun 11; Epub.

69. Claassen J, Hirsch LJ, Kreiter KT, et al. Quantitative continuous EEG for detecting delayed cerebral ischemia in patients with poor-grade subarachnoid hemorrhage. Clin Neurophysiol 2004;115(12): 2699–710.

70. Claassen J, Mayer SA, Hirsch LJ. Continuous EEG monitoring in patients with subarachnoid hemorrhage. J Clin Neurophysiol 2005;22(2):92–8.

71. Oddo M, LeRoux P. Brain tissue oxygen monitors: more than an ischemia monitor. Crit Care Med 2008;36(6):1984–5.

72. Sarrafzadeh AS, Sakowitz OW, Kiening KL, et al. Bedside microdialysis: a tool to monitor cerebral metabolism in subarachnoid hemorrhage patients? Crit Care Med 2002;30(5):1062–70.

73. Rosenthal G, Hemphill JC III, Sorani M, et al. Brain tissue oxygen tension is more indicative of oxygen diffusion than oxygen delivery and metabolism in patients with traumatic brain injury. Crit Care Med 2008;36:1917–24.

74. Steifel MF, Spiotta AM, Gracias VH, et al. Reduced mortality in patients with severe traumatic brain injury in patients treated with brain tissue oxygen monitoring. J Neurosurg 2005;103:805–11.

75. Frontera JA, Fernandez A, Schmidt JM, et al. Impact of nosocomial infectious complications after subarachnoid hemorrhage. Neurosurgery 2008;62(1):80–7.

76. Naidech AM, Jovanovic B, Wartenberg KE, et al. Higher hemoglobin is associated with improved outcome after subarachnoid hemorrhage. Crit Care Med 2007;35(10):2383–9.

77. Wartenberg KE, Schmidt JM, Claassen J, et al. Impact of medical complications on outcome after subarachnoid hemorrhage. Crit Care Med 2006; 34(3):617–23.

78. Frontera JA, Fernandez A, Claassen J, et al. Hyperglycemia after SAH: predictors, associated complications, and impact on outcome. Stroke 2006; 37(1):199–203.

79. Frontera JA, Parra A, Shimbo D, et al. Cardiac arrhythmias after subarachnoid hemorrhage: risk factors and impact on outcome. Cerebrovasc Dis 2008;26(1):71–8.

80. Fisher LA, Ko N, Miss J, et al. Hypernatremia predicts adverse cardiovascular and neurological outcomes after SAH. Neurocrit Care 2006;5(3):180–5.

81. Adams HP Jr, del Zoppo G, Alberts MJ, et al. Guidelines for the early management of adults with ischemic stroke. Circulation 2007;115(20): e478–534.

82. The National Institute of Neurological Disorders and Stroke rt-PA Stroke Study Group. Tissue plasminogen activator for acute ischemic stroke. N Engl J Med 1995;333(24):1581–7.

83. Kent DM, Ruthazer R, Selker HP. Are some patients likely to benefit from recombinant tissue-type plasminogen activator for acute ischemic stroke even beyond 3 hours from symptom onset? Stroke 2003;34(2):464–7.

84. Clark WM, Wissman S, Albers GW, et al. Recombinant tissue-type plasminogen activator (Alteplase) for ischemic stroke 3 to 5 hours after symptom onset. The ATLANTIS Study: a randomized controlled trial. JAMA 1999;282(21):2019–26.

85. Hacke W, Kaste M, Bluhmki E, et al. Thrombolysis with alteplase 3 to 4.5 hours after acute ischemic stroke. N Engl J Med 2008;358:1317–29.

86. Chalela JA, Kidwell CS, Nentwich LM, et al. Magnetic resonance imaging and computed tomography in emergency assessment of patients with suspected acute stroke: a prospective comparison. Lancet 2007;369:293–8.

87. Choi JH, Bateman BT, Mangla S, et al. Endovascular recanalization therapy in acute ischemic stroke. Stroke 2006;37:419–24.

88. Janjua N, Brisman JL. Endovascular treatment of acute ischaemic stroke. Lancet Neurol 2007; 6(12):1086–93.

89. Kidwell CS, Chalela JA, Saver JL, et al. Comparison of MRI and CT for detection of acute intracerebral hemorrhage. JAMA 2004;292(15):1823–30.

90. Lee LJ, Kidwell CS, Alger J, et al. Impact on stroke subtype diagnosis of early diffusion-weighted magnetic resonance imaging and magnetic resonance angiography. Stroke 2000; 31(5):1081–9.

91. Katz DA, Marks MP, Napel SA, et al. Circle of Willis: evaluation with spiral CT angiography, MR angiography, and conventional angiography. Radiology 1995;195(2):445–9.

92. Tan JC, Dillon WP, Liu S, et al. Systematic comparison of perfusion-CT and CT-angiography in acute stroke patients. Ann Neurol 2007;61(6):533–43.

93. Heidenreich JO, Hsu D, Wang G, et al. Magnetic resonance imaging results can affect therapy decisions in hyperacute stroke care. Acta Radiol 2008; 49(5):550–7.

94. Sorensen AG, Copen WA, Ostergaard L, et al. Hyperacute stroke: simultaneous measurement of relative cerebral blood volume, relative cerebral

blood flow, and mean tissue transit time. Radiology 1999;210(2):519–27.

95. Fiebach JB, Schellinger PD, Gass A, et al. Stroke magnetic resonance imaging is accurate in hyperacute intracerebral hemorrhage: a multicenter study on the validity of stroke imaging. Stroke 2004;35(2):502–6.

96. Neumann-Haefelin T, Wittsack HJ, Wenserski F, et al. Diffusion- and perfusion-weighted MRI. The DWI/PWI mismatch region in acute stroke. Stroke 1999;30(8):1591–7.

97. Furlan A, Higashida R, Wechsler L, et al. Intra-arterial prourokinase for acute ischemic stroke: the PROACT II study: a randomized controlled trial. JAMA 1999;282:2003–11.

98. Inoue T, Kimura K, Minematsu K, et al. Japan multicenter stroke investigator's collaboration. A case-control analysis of intra-arterial urokinase thrombolysis in acute cardioembolic stroke. Cerebrovasc Dis 2005;19:225–8.

99. Macleod MR, Davis SM, Mitchell PJ, et al. Results of a multicentre, randomised controlled trial of intra-arterial urokinase in the treatment of acute posterior circulation ischaemic stroke. Cerebrovasc Dis 2005;20:12–7.

100. Lewandowski CA, Frankel M, Tomsick TA, et al. Combined intravenous and intra-arterial r-TPA versus intra-arterial therapy of acute ischemic stroke: emergency management of stroke (EMS) bridging trial. Stroke 1999;30:2598–605.

101. IMS Study Investigators. Combined intravenous and intra-arterial recanalization for acute ischemic stroke: the Interventional Management of Stroke Study. Stroke 2004;35:904–11.

102. Han MK, Kim SH, Ko SB, et al. Combined intravenous and intraarterial revascularization therapy using MRI perfusion/diffusion mismatch selection for acute ischemic stroke at 3–6 h after symptom onset. Neurocrit Care 2008;8:353–9.

103. Gobin YP, Starkman S, Duckwiler GR, et al. MERCI 1: a phase 1 study of mechanical embolus removal in cerebral ischemia. Stroke 2004;35:2848–54.

104. Sorimachi T, Fujii Y, Tsuchiya N, et al. Recanalization by mechanical embolus disruption during intra-arterial thrombolysis in the carotid territory. Am J Neuroradiol 2004;25:1391–402.

105. Smith WS, Sung G, Saver J, et al. Mechanical thrombectomy for acute ischemic stroke: final results of the multi MERCI trial. Stroke 2008;39:1205–12.

106. Brekenfeld C, Schroth G, El-Koussy M, et al. Mechanical thromboembolectomy for acute ischemic stroke: comparison of the catch thrombectomy device and the merci retriever in vivo. Stroke 2008;39:1213–9.

107. Rordorf G, et al. Pharmacological elevation of blood pressure in acute stroke. Clinical effects and safety. Stroke 1997;28:2133–8.

108. Azzimondi G, Bassein L, Nonino F, et al. Fever in acute stroke worsens prognosis: a prospective study. Stroke 1995;26:2040–3.

109. Diringer MN, Reaven NL, Funk SE, et al. Elevated body temperature independently contributes to increased length of stay in neurologic intensive care unit patients. Crit Care Med 2004;32:1489–95.

110. International Stroke Trial Collaborative Group. The International Stroke Trial (IST). A randomized trial of aspirin, subcutaneous heparin, both, or neither among 19,435 patients with acute ischemic stroke. Lancet 1997;349:1569.

111. Sandercock P, Gubitz G, Foley P, et al. Antiplatelet therapy for acute ischaemic stroke. Cochrane Database Syst Rev 2003;(2):CD000029.

112. Albers GW, Amarenco P, Easton JD, et al. Antithrombotic and thrombolytic therapy for ischemic stroke: the seventh ACCP conference on antithrombotic and thrombolytic therapy. Chest 2004; 126(Suppl 3):483S–512S.

113. Paciaroni M, Agnelli G, Micheli S, et al. Efficacy and safety of anticoagulant treatment in acute cardioembolic stroke. A meta-analysis of randomized controlled trials. Stroke 2007;38:423–30.

114. Khatri P, Wechsler LR, Broderick JP. Intracranial hemorrhage associated with revascularization therapies. Stroke 2007;38(2):431–40.

115. Hamann GF, del Zoppo GJ, von Kummer R. Hemorrhagic transformation of cerebral infarction—possible mechanisms. Thromb Haemost 1999;82:92–4.

116. Paciaroni M, Agnelli G, Corea F, et al. Early hemorrhagic transformation of brain infarction: rate, predictive factors, and influence on clinical outcome: results of a prospective multicenter study. Stroke 2008;39:2249–56.

117. Alvarez-Sabin J, Molina CA, Montaner J, et al. Effects of admission hyperglycemia on stroke outcome in reperfused tissue plasminogen activator–treated patients. Stroke 2003;34(5): 1235–41.

118. Ribo M, Molina C, Montaner J, et al. Acute hyperglycemia state is associated with lower tPA-induced recanalization rates in stroke patients. Stroke 2005;36(8):1705–9.

119. Alvarez-Sabin J, Molina CA, Ribo M, et al. Impact of admission hyperglycemia on stroke outcome after thrombolysis: risk stratification in relation to time to reperfusion. Stroke 2004;35(11):2493–8.

120. Roine RO, Lindsberg PJ. Editorial comment–prime time for proactive blood glucose control? Stroke 2004;35:2498–9.

121. Hacke W, Zeumer H, Ferbert A, et al. Intra-arterial thrombolytic therapy improves outcome in patients with acute vertebrobasilar occlusive disease. Stroke 1988;19:1216–22.

122. Veltkamp R, Jacobi C, Kress B, et al. Prolonged low-dose intravenous thrombolysis in a stroke

patient with distal basilar thrombus. Stroke 2006; 37(1):e9–11.

123. Grigoriadis S, Gomori JM, Grigoriadis N, et al. Clinically successful late recanalization of basilar artery occlusion in childhood: what are the odds? Case report and review of the literature. J Neurol Sci 2007;260:256–60.

124. Yu W, Kostanian V, Fisher M. Endovascular recanalization of basilar artery occlusion 80 days after symptom onset. Stroke 2007;38:1387–9.

125. Cross DT 3rd, Moran CJ, Akins PT, et al. Relationship between clot location and outcome after basilar artery thrombolysis. Am J Neuroradiol 1997;18:1221–8.

126. Lutsep HL, Rymer MM, Nesbit GM. Vertebrobasilar revascularization rates and outcomes in the MERCI and multi-MERCI trials. J Stroke Cerebrovasc Dis 2008;17:55–7.

127. Albers GW, Thijs VN, Wechsler L, et al. Magnetic resonance imaging profiles predict clinical response to early reperfusion: the diffusion and perfusion imaging evaluation for understanding stroke evolution (DEFUSE) study. Ann Neurol 2006;60:508–17.

128. Alexandrov AV, Hall CE, Labiche LA, et al. Ischemic stunning of the brain: early recanalization without immediate clinical improvement in acute ischemic stroke. Stroke 2004;35:449–52.

129. Jaramillo A, Gongora-Rivera F, Labreuche J, et al. Predictors for malignant middle cerebral artery infarctions: a postmortem analysis. Neurology 2006;66:815–20.

130. Agarwal P, Kumar S, Hariharan S, et al. Hyperdense middle cerebral artery sign: can it be used to select intra-arterial versus intravenous thrombolysis in acute ischemic stroke? Cerebrovasc Dis 2004;17:182–90.

131. Mattle HP, Arnold M, Georgiadis D, et al. Comparison of intraarterial and intravenous thrombolysis for ischemic stroke with hyperdense middle cerebral artery sign. Stroke 2008;39:379–83.

132. Von Kummer R, Meyding-Lamade U, Forsting M, et al. Sensitivity and prognostic value of early computed tomography in middle cerebral artery trunk occlusion. AJNR Am J Neuroradiol 1994;15:9–15.

133. Krieger DW, Demchuk AM, Kasner SE, et al. Early clinical and radiological predictors of fatal brain swelling in ischemic stroke. Stroke 1999;30: 287–93.

134. Kasner SE, Demchuk AM, Berrouschot J, et al. Predictors of fatal brain edema in massive hemispheric ischemic stroke. Stroke 2001;32: 2117–23.

135. Wijman CA. Editorial comment–can we predict massive space-occupying edema in large hemispheric infarctions? Stroke 2003;34:1899–900.

136. Chen CC, Cho DY, Tsai SC. Outcome of and prognostic factors for decompressive hemicraniectomy in malignant middle cerebral artery infarction. J Clin Neurosci 2007;14(4):317–21.

137. Rabinstein AA, Mueller-Kronast N, Maramattom BV, et al. Factors predicting prognosis after decompressive hemicraniectomy for hemispheric infarction. Neurology 2006;67(5):891–3.

138. Juttler E, Schwab S, Schmiedek P, et al. Decompressive surgery for the treatment of malignant infarction of the middle cerebral artery (DESTINY): a randomized, controlled trial. Stroke 2007;38: 2518–25.

139. Hemicraniectomy after MCA infarction with life-threatening edema trial (HAMLET). Ongoing trial at the time of this review – details. Available at: http://www.strokecenter.org/trials/trialDetail.aspx?tid=484. Accessed 12/23/2008.

140. Carter BS, Ogilvy CS, Candia GJ, et al. One-year outcome after decompressive surgery for massive nondominant hemispheric infarction. Neurosurgery 1997;40:1168–75.

141. Kastrau F, Wolter M, Huber W, et al. Recovery from aphasia after hemicraniectomy for infarction of the speech-dominant hemisphere. Stroke 2005;36: 825–9.

Coagulation Disorders in the ICU

Peter W. Marks, MD, PhD

KEYWORDS

- Coagulation • Hemorrhage • Thrombocytopenia
- Thrombosis • Transfusion

Hemostasis results from the interplay among the vessel wall, the platelets, and the soluble coagulation factors.[1] Coagulation is initiated when von Willebrand factor is activated by substances such as exposed collagen in a blood vessel wall. Activated von Willebrand factor serves to recruit and activate platelets to the area of injury. In addition to serving as a physical barrier to blood loss from the vessel, platelets provide the phospholipid scaffold for activating the soluble coagulation cascade. The soluble factors include various proteolytic enzymes, including the vitamin K–dependent factors II, VII, IX, and X; the cofactors V and VIII; and the structural protein fibrinogen. Because the proteases involved in coagulation are potent, several different regulatory mechanisms exist to prevent excessive clot formation. These mechanisms include tissue factor pathway inhibitor, activated protein C, and antithrombin (**Fig. 1**).[2]

Although various coagulation tests are available, much diagnostic information can be obtained from thoughtful review of tests that are routinely available: the complete blood count, peripheral blood smear, prothrombin time (PT), and activated partial thromboplastic time (PTT). Some additional tests that are useful in specific circumstances include functional fibrinogen and d-dimer assays, inhibitor screen (mixing study), and specific factor assays.[3] When abnormalities in the PT or PTT are detected, these additional laboratory studies may be guided by consideration of the appropriate differential diagnosis (**Table 1**).

CAUSES OF THROMBOCYTOPENIA

Low platelet counts are commonly encountered in the ICU setting and may be associated with diverse conditions (**Box 1**). Determining whether or not a potentially life-threatening cause of thrombocytopenia is present is absolutely essential. A platelet count of 35,000/μL may require emergent intervention, or may require nothing more than observation. Such a low platelet count resulting from thrombotic thrombocytopenic purpura (TTP) or heparin-induced thrombocytopenia (HIT, see later discussion) may result in severe morbidity or mortality if immediate intervention is not undertaken. Alternatively, if a similarly low platelet count is the result of immune thrombocytopenic purpura, the risk for adverse consequences without immediate intervention is minimal.

Discussion of all the causes of thrombocytopenia is beyond the scope of this article; however, one general cause of thrombocytopenia is highly relevant in the ICU. Microangiopathic hemolytic anemia (MAHA) is manifest as fragmented red blood cells and thrombocytopenia. MAHA may be associated with various causes, including malignant hypertension and scleroderma renal crisis.[4] Malfunctioning prosthetic valves and prostheses with perivalvular leaks may present similarly, though the pathogenesis (a mechanical cause or turbulent blood flow) is different.[5] Other specific types of MAHA are determined by additional associated abnormalities.

TTP is manifest as thrombocytopenia and microangiopathic changes on blood smear, often, but not invariably, in association with fever, acute kidney injury, and neurologic abnormalities.[6] TTP is caused by deficiency in the ADAMTS13 protease that is involved in the regulation of von Willebrand multimer size. In its acquired form, TTP may be associated with the presence of an antibody inhibitor to ADAMSTS13. The most common presentation is of an otherwise healthy individual who suddenly, over the course of hours to days, becomes ill. Pregnancy, HIV infection, and certain

Section of Hematology, Department of Internal Medicine, Yale University School of Medicine, 333 Cedar Street, LCI 100, P.O. Box 208021, New Haven, CT 06520, USA
E-mail address: peter.marks@yale.edu

Clin Chest Med 30 (2009) 123–129
doi:10.1016/j.ccm.2008.11.003
0272-5231/08/$ – see front matter

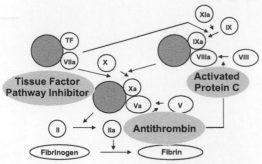

Fig.1. Coagulation is the result of the interplay among the vessel wall, the platelets, and the soluble coagulation factors. Coagulation is initiated in vivo through binding of factor VIIa to tissue factor (TF). Several of the soluble coagulation factors with enzymatic activity then form complexes with cofactors and are coordinated through calcium at phospholipid surfaces, ultimately leading to production of fibrin strands, the structural polymer that is critical in achieving effective hemostasis. The prothrombin time assesses the activity of factor VII and the common pathway factors (I, II, V, X), and the activated partial thromboplastin time assesses the activity of factors VIII, IX, XI and the common pathway. Abnormalities in factor XII, high-molecular-weight kininogen, and prekallikrein are also detected by the PTT, but these are not associated with bleeding. Light-gray shading represents the natural anticoagulant pathways, and darker gray shading represents phospholipid surfaces.

medications, such as clopidogrel, have also been associated with the development of TTP.[7] Rapid intervention with plasma exchange, or at the least, plasma administration, is indicated for this disorder, which otherwise can be rapidly fatal.

Hemolytic uremic syndrome (HUS) presents with many features in common with TTP, except that renal manifestations are more prominent, and fever and neurologic symptoms are not commonly observed.[8] HUS appears to result from vascular injury, and deficiencies in complement regulatory proteins have been identified in some cases.[9] Although some cases appear to be idiopathic in nature, many are associated with a prior diarrheal illness with Shiga toxin–producing bacteria, such as *Escherichia coli* H:0157. Other associations include treatment with medications such as the calcineurin inhibitors (cyclosporin A, tacrolimus) and mitomycin C, among others. The treatment of HUS in children is mainly supportive. However, plasma exchange is sometimes used in adults, although its efficacy has not been documented by well-controlled randomized trials.[10] A trial of this therapy may be warranted in adults who have severe or progressive HUS, although this is an area of controversy.

Disseminated intravascular coagulation (DIC) represents a consumptive coagulopathy that may develop in any number of settings, such as infection, malignancy, trauma, or amniotic fluid

Table 1
Differential diagnosis of coagulation disorders based on the prothrombin time/partial thromboplastin time

PT	PTT	Differential Diagnosis
Normal	Normal	von Willebrand disease Platelet function abnormality Factor XIII deficiency
Normal	Prolonged	Factor VIII, IX, XI, or XII deficiency Lupus anticoagulants Heparin/direct thrombin inhibitor treatment Spurious (improperly drawn or heparin contamination)
Prolonged	Normal	Factor VII deficiency Lupus anticoagulant Warfarin treatment Spurious (improperly drawn)
Prolonged	Prolonged	Factor II, V, X deficiency Abnormalities in fibrinogen Disseminated intravascular coagulation Lupus anticoagulant Excessive warfarin or heparin treatment Direct thrombin inhibitor treatment Spurious (improperly drawn or heparin contamination)

Box 1
Some of the more common causes of thrombocytopenia in the ICU setting
MAHA
DIC (due to infection, malignancy)
TTP
HUS
Malignant hypertension
Prosthetic valve malfunction
Immune-medicated thrombocytopenia
Idiopathic
Associated with rheumatologic disorders
Associated with lymphoproliferative disorders (ie, chronic lymphoid leukemia)
HIV-related
Hepatitis C-related
Medication-related (ie, penicillins, vancomycin, many others)
Drugs/toxins
Alcohol-induced marrow suppression
HIT
Intra-aortic balloon pump/intravascular device use
Hypersplenism

embolism.[11] In most cases, DIC presents with hemorrhage, although occasionally, thrombotic complications such as peripheral embolic phenomena may be observed. The pathogenesis in the different settings likely has in common the presence or release of phospholipid surfaces that serve to activate coagulation. Although a decreased platelet count, decreased fibrinogen, and elevated PT or PTT often accompany the microangiopathic change in DIC, in some cases only some of these abnormalities are present. The treatment of DIC consists of treatment of the underlying disorder in conjunction with replacement of coagulation factors, as appropriate.

In some cases when DIC is present, replacement may not be necessary. An example is the stable, nonbleeding patient who has an adequate platelet count and fibrinogen accompanied by modestly elevated PT or PTT. Patients who are bleeding, who have low fibrinogen levels (<80–100 mg/dL), or who require invasive procedures may require treatment. Fresh frozen plasma

(FFP) provides all the clotting factors, including fibrinogen. Repeated administration may be required because the efficacy of FFP is potentially limited by the half-life of the shortest-lived component, factor VII (4–6 hours). Cryoprecipitate mainly is a source of fibrinogen, factor VIII, and von Willebrand factor. Because other more purified concentrates exist for factor VIII and von Willebrand factor, its use is essentially restricted to the replacement of fibrinogen. The advantage of cryoprecipitate is that a 10-unit pool contains approximately the same amount of fibrinogen as 4 units of FFP in a volume of only about 50 to 100 mL of volume, which allows for rapid administration. Use of cryoprecipitate can be of great advantage in some circumstances. For example, in amniotic fluid embolism, often the blood is rapidly defibrinated, leading to bleeding accompanied by a marked rise in the PT and PTT. These two tests will be elevated when fibrinogen is depleted, even when the amount of the other soluble clotting factors is adequate.[12] Administration of cryoprecipitate may facilitate the rapid correction of a large portion of the coagulation defect. In some cases, the administration of platelets, FFP, and cryoprecipitate may be ineffective in DIC, and then consideration may be given to use of recombinant factor VIIa (see later discussion).

MANAGEMENT OF THROMBOCYTOPENIA

Thrombocytopenia may accompany the MAHAs. In addition, it may be an isolated finding, as in the case of marrow suppression due to sepsis, immune mediated thrombocytopenia, use of intra-aortic balloon pumps and other devices, and thrombocytopenia due to drugs commonly administered in the ICU setting (see **Box 1**).[13,14] Although determination of the definitive cause of thrombocytopenia may not be possible in the ICU setting, potential causes that would be a contraindication to platelet administration, such as TTP and HIT, should be eliminated from consideration based on clinical and laboratory evaluation.

Although no absolute threshold exists for platelet transfusion, the risk for complications such as intracranial hemorrhage increases as the count decreases, such that transfusion is reasonable even in the stable, nonbleeding patient when the platelet count declines below 10,000 to 20,000/μL.[15] Obviously, a lower threshold is required in patients who are bleeding or who require surgical procedures. In the absence of platelet dysfunction, line placement and most general surgical procedures can be performed safely with platelet count above the range of

30,000 to 50,000/µL. Neurosurgical procedures generally require a higher platelet count of 70,000 to 100,000/µL.

Patients may be refractory to platelet transfusion because of prior alloimmunization or increased consumption. Alternatively, platelet function may be impaired by the concomitant presence of uremia or by previously administered drugs. In such cases, use of desmopressin (DDAVP) or ε-aminocaproic acid may be considered. DDAVP may enhance the function of the existing platelets through improved signal transduction. It may be administered at a dose of 0.3 µg/kg every 12 to 24 hours for several doses, although care must be taken to watch for hypotension and hyponatremia.[16] ε-aminocaproic acid is an antifibrinolytic agent that has been associated with reduction or cessation in bleeding, particularly from mucosal sources, when thrombocytopenia is present.[17] Its use is contraindicated if DIC or upper urinary tract bleeding is present. Doses of ε-aminocaproic acid, 1 g every 6 hours by mouth or intravenously, are often effective in this setting. When uremia is present and continued bleeding is occurring despite more conservative measures, consideration may be given to the use of high-dose conjugated estrogens.[18]

MANAGEMENT OF AN ELEVATED PROTHROMBIN TIME/INTERNATIONAL NORMALIZED RATIO

An issue that often arises in the ICU is management of an elevated PT/international normalized ratio (INR). Two commonly encountered situations are the patient who presents with an elevated PT/INR in the setting of anticoagulation with vitamin K antagonists (ie, warfarin) and the patient who has an elevated PT/INR and requires an invasive diagnostic or therapeutic intervention.

Guidelines for the management of patients who have an elevated PT/INR have been published.[19] In the absence of bleeding or other complications, patients who have an INR less than 20 do not invariably require the emergent administration of FFP. Vitamin K should be administered at doses between 2 mg and 5 mg. In this regard, use of oral vitamin K is the preferred route for correction when urgent correction is not required (correction in about 24 hours). The slow intravenous route may be used when rapid correction is desirable (correction in 4–8 hours). Subcutaneous vitamin K is less reproducibly absorbed, particularly in the ICU setting.[20] Patients who are bleeding or who have high INR values do require the administration of FFP. In this case, the administration of 15 to 30 mL/kg of FFP will generally normalize the INR.[21] The FFP needs to be administered rapidly over the course of 1 to 2 hours, and repeated administration may be required, particularly if vitamin K is not also given. In the case of patients who cannot tolerate the volume of FFP required, prothrombin complex concentrate may be used to correct the INR.[22] Although available concentrates in the United States are not yet labeled for this indication, they facilitate correction of the INR in a rapid manner (10–15 minutes) with a small volume load (about 50 mL). Use of these agents may be preferable to the use of recombinant factor VIIa, which has also been used off-label for this purpose.[23]

The other issue often encountered in the ICU, correction of the PT/INR before invasive diagnostic procedures, is an area of some controversy. No definitive recommendations can be made. However, data suggest that in the absence of other hemostatic defects, most invasive procedures that do not involve the central nervous system can be performed safely at an INR less than 2, and certainly at an INR less than 1.5.[24,25] Unnecessary correction of the INR with FFP can be associated with a delay in required treatment and with transfusion-associated complications.

MANAGEMENT OF REFRACTORY HEMORRHAGE

Refractory hemorrhage may result from surgical or medical causes. Correction of surgical defects associated with blood loss is critical because even the most effective hemostatic agents cannot replace appropriately placed sutures when a vessel wall has a defect. In particular, refractory bleeding in a patient who has normal or only mildly abnormal coagulation parameters and a recent surgical history requires thorough evaluation for this possibility.

In some cases, no surgical cause will be found, or coagulation defects will be impossible to correct using conservative measures. In these cases, off-label use of recombinant factor VIIa may be entertained after a consideration of the potential benefits versus risks (thrombosis).[26] Optimally, documentation of an adequate platelet count ($\geq$30,000–50,000/µL) and fibrinogen level (>100 mg/dL) should be made before administration. Doses of 70 to 100 µg/kg have been used, and may be repeated if necessary. However, if hemostasis is not achieved after two to three doses, it is unlikely that this agent will be effective. As an alternative, or for patients who continue to bleed after the administration of recombinant factor VIIa, provided that DIC or upper urinary tract bleeding is not present, consideration may also be given to a trial of ε-aminocaproic acid, 1 g/hour by intravenous continuous infusion.

Sedation and Analgesia for the Mechanically Ventilated Patient

David R. Brush, MD, John P. Kress, MD*

KEYWORDS

- Analgesics • Opioid administration and dosage
- Conscious sedation methods
- Critical Illness • Humans
- Hypnotics and sedatives administration and dosage
- Intensive care units • Respiration • Artificial

Up to one third of ICU patients worldwide undergo mechanical ventilation.[1] These patients frequently require analgesics and sedatives—potent medications with clear benefits and significant side effects. Sedation and analgesic requirements can vary greatly among critically ill patients. This poses a challenge for clinicians hoping to maximize the benefits from controlled analgesia and sedation while attempting to minimize patient risk.

INDICATIONS FOR SEDATION AND ANALGESIA
Pain

Patients commonly experience pain while undergoing mechanical ventilation.[2,3] While pain from trauma, invasive operations, or procedures is often apparent, there are other sources of pain that may be underappreciated by clinicians such as routine nursing care, endotracheal tube suctioning, and prolonged immobility. Pain is associated with numerous adverse effects including increased endogenous catecholamine activity, sleep deprivation, anxiety and delirium.[4] Adequate treatment of pain may alleviate some of these adverse effects.[5] Although some discomfort may be alleviated by nonpharmacologic means such as patient positioning, minimizing invasive interventions, and prompt removal of unnecessary noxious stimuli, most patients will require opiates to adequately control their pain. Mechanically ventilated patients may be unable to communicate with care providers, and the physiologic variables of critically ill patients are often unreliable indicators of pain. Clinicians should direct their initial attention toward providing adequate analgesia when considering "sedation" in mechanically ventilated patients. Otherwise, agitated patients with pain may be given sedatives—an intervention with suboptimal results.

Anxiety

The intensive care unit can be a frightening place for patients. In addition to the anxiety caused by life-threatening illness, patients can often be isolated and in uncertain surroundings. Inadequately controlled pain, sleep deprivation, isolation, and the presence of invasive tubes and catheters are frequently listed as sources of stress and anxiety.[6,7] Although nonpharmacologic interventions such as comfortable positioning, verbal reassurance, and encouraging the presence of family and friends should be attempted, these interventions alone are often inadequate and medications must be employed.

Amnesia

Deep sedation is associated with memory impairment in mechanically ventilated patients.[8] Whereas amnesia is of clear benefit during surgical procedures and should be a mandatory goal when using neuromuscular blocking agents, there is growing evidence that critically ill patients may benefit from retaining an awareness of their

Section of Pulmonary and Critical Care Medicine, Department of Medicine, University of Chicago Medical Center, 5841 S. Maryland Avenue, MC 6076, Chicago, IL 60637, USA
* Corresponding author.
E-mail address: jkress@medicine.bsd.uchicago.edu (J.P. Kress).

Clin Chest Med 30 (2009) 131–141
doi:10.1016/j.ccm.2008.09.001

surroundings.[9,10] Some studies have shown that patients with a greater recall of adverse experiences may be likely to develop posttraumatic stress disorder (PTSD), leading some to suggest that deep sedation be routinely used to blunt patient awareness of the ICU experience.[11] More recently, investigators have demonstrated that patients who were most awake, or the most unresponsive, during mechanical ventilation had the lowest PTSD-like symptoms.[12] Given the increased morbidity associated with deep sedation, we recommend allowing patients to retain an awareness of their surroundings unless neuromuscular blocking agents are being used.

Decrease Oxygen Consumption

Sedatives can be used to decrease patient oxygen consumption. This reduction in oxygen consumption can be particularly important in patients suffering from acute lung injury or shock.

Facilitate Patient Care

Patients undergoing mechanical ventilation are sometimes dysynchronous with the ventilator. This may be more likely to occur with modern mechanical ventilation strategies such as low tidal volume or permissive hypercapnia. However, initial concerns that low tidal volume ventilation may lead to increased sedation requirements have not been substantiated.[13,14] Strategies involving high-frequency oscillatory ventilation and prone positioning may cause patients to require additional sedation. When ventilator dysynchrony is present, patients should be evaluated for sources of uncontrolled pain or discomfort. Despite adequate analgesia and ventilator-patient optimization, some patients require deeper sedation to meet the goals of care.

COMPLICATIONS ASSOCIATED WITH SEDATION AND ANALGESIA

The pharmacokinetic properties for short-term sedative and analgesic administration are not predictive of pharmacokinetics when the same drugs are used for long-term infusions in critically ill patients. Buildup of active drugs and metabolites, multicompartment tissue saturation, drug-drug interactions, and hepatic and renal dysfunction may result in unpredictable drug pharmacokinetics.[15] Administration of sedatives in the ICU by continuous infusion is associated with a higher risk for oversedation, particularly in the elderly or patients with hepatic dysfunction.[16] Kollef and colleagues[17] studied the outcomes of 240 mechanically ventilated patients who either received continuous sedation or received intermittent/no intravenous sedation. Continuous sedation was associated with prolonged mechanical ventilation, increased ICU and hospital length of stay, and increased rates of organ failure and re-intubation. Continuous sedation has also been shown to be an independent risk factor for developing ventilator-associated pneumonia.[18] Deep sedation may impair proper assessment of a patient's neurologic status, resulting in increased use of diagnostic procedures and imaging.[19] Long-term administration of sedatives and analgesic medications can also produce physical dependence, leading to withdrawal syndromes when these agents are discontinued.[20]

The role of sedation in the development of central nervous system dysfunction is receiving increased attention from investigators. Central nervous system dysfunction, measured as delirium, has been detected in 60% to 80% of patients undergoing mechanical ventilation.[21–23] ICU delirium is associated with greater hospital length of stay, and increased 6-month mortality.[24] Pandharipande and others[25] demonstrated that sedation with lorazepam is an independent risk factor for transitioning to delirium in ICU patients. This group also noted recently that newer agents such as dexmedetomidine had a lesser incidence of delirium than more conventional sedatives such as lorazepam. Investigators continue to evaluate which medications (or combinations of medications) can provide effective analgesia and sedation while minimizing unwanted side effects of drug accumulation and its associated risks.

INTRAVENOUS DRUGS FOR ANALGESIA AND SEDATION
Opioids

Opioids bind to receptors in the central nervous system and peripheral tissue. Mu-1 receptors mediate analgesia, while mu-2 receptor binding produces respiratory depression, nausea, vomiting, constipation, and euphoria. Kappa receptor activation causes sedation, miosis, and spinal analgesia. Whereas the primary effect of opioids is analgesia, they also may provide mild to moderate anxiolysis. Opioids have no reliable amnestic effect on patients.

Opioid administration is associated with dose-dependent, centrally mediated respiratory depression. Respiratory rate is depressed first, while tidal volume is initially preserved. Tidal volume is reduced with higher doses of opiates. The ventilatory response to hypoxia is eradicated and the CO_2 response curve is shifted to the right. Opioids are excellent drugs to help palliate coughing and the subjective sense of dyspnea. This pharmacologic property may be particularly important for many patients who are distressed during mechanical ventilation.

Opioids have little cardiovascular effect in euvolemic patients. The provision of opioids may decrease sympathetic tone, and thus may decrease heart rate and systemic vascular resistance. Additionally, opioids increase venous capacitance, thereby decreasing venous return. In hypovolemic patients with reduced cardiac output, this decrease in venous return, reduced sympathetic tone, and reduction in heart rate can result in significant hypotension.

Opioids decrease gastrointestinal motility and may induce ileus. Opioid-induced ileus is a common problem in critically ill patients. Treatment of this problem with stool softeners and/or laxatives is often ineffective. Methylnaltrexone bromide, a specific antagonist of peripheral mu-2 receptors in the gut, was recently approved by the Food and Drug Administration (FDA) for use in patients with late-stage advanced illnesses that are using opioids chronically. Thomas and colleagues[26] recently demonstrated that methylnaltrexone significantly restored bowel function in terminally ill patients on chronic opioid therapy, without adversely impacting analgesia. Currently, there is no literature evaluating this drug in ICU patients.

Morphine

Morphine is poorly lipid soluble, and thus has a relatively slow onset of action (5 to 10 minutes). For a typical single intravenous dose of 5 to 10 mg, the approximate half-life is 4 hours; however, with repeated dosing or continuous infusions, this half-life pharmacology is not applicable. Morphine is conjugated by the liver to metabolites that include morphine-6-glucuronide, a potent metabolite with 20 times the activity of morphine.[27] Both morphine and morphine-6-glucuronide are eliminated by the kidney, thus patients with renal dysfunction may suffer from prolonged drug effect. As such, morphine is a poor choice for patients with renal insufficiency.

Meperidine

Meperidine is more lipophilic than morphine and thus has a more rapid onset of action (3 to 5 minutes). However, meperidine's duration of action (1 to 4 hours) is shorter than morphine because of redistribution of the drug into peripheral tissues. Like morphine, meperidine is metabolized by the liver and is renally excreted. A metabolite of meperidine, normeperidine, is a potent central nervous system (CNS) stimulant that can precipitate seizures, especially in patients with renal

dysfunction.[28] Given the similar onset and half-life to morphine and the increased potential for CNS toxicity, meperidine should not be used routinely for analgesia in the ICU.[29]

Fentanyl

Fentanyl is highly lipid soluble with a rapid onset of action (1 minute) and rapidly redistributes into peripheral tissues, resulting in a short half-life (0.5 to 1 hour) after a single dose. Hepatic metabolism creates inactive metabolites that are renally excreted, making this drug a more attractive choice in patients with renal insufficiency. Continuous administration of fentanyl can result in altered pharmacokinetics, with build-up of drug into peripheral tissues that then reenters the plasma after drug discontinuation, causing a prolonged clinical effect.

Remifentanil

Remifentanil is a selective mu receptor agonist with unique pharmacokinetic properties. It is profoundly lipophilic, with an onset of action of about 1 minute. Unlike other opioids, it is rapidly metabolized by nonspecific blood and tissue esterases to a clinically inactive metabolite with a terminal half-life of approximately 10 to 20 minutes.[30] Remifentanil was first introduced as part of perioperative anesthesia, but its favorable pharmacokinetics have led to increased interest in its use as part of a sedative/analgesic regimen for nonsurgical mechanically ventilated patients. Because rapid metabolism leaves no residual opioid, clinicians should use care to anticipate the emergence of pain and discomfort following remifentanil discontinuation, and should consider using a more long-acting analgesic regimen to bridge patients through this period.

In a double-blind, randomized, controlled trial comparing remifentanil to fentanyl in postsurgical patients undergoing mechanical ventilation 12 to 72 hours, Muellejans and colleagues[31] demonstrated no significant difference in the time patients spent at an optimum level of sedation. Time to recovery from sedation was similar in both groups and both agents were well tolerated. Remifentanil is associated with a shorter time to extubation compared with sedation regimens using morphine.[32] Other studies have demonstrated that the pharmacokinetics of remifentanil are not significantly altered in ICU patients with renal dysfunction, even after continuous administration for up to 3 days.[33,34] Based on these initial studies, remifentanil shows exciting promise as a new analgesic for use in critically ill patients. However, more data are needed to guide clinicians on the use of this drug in ICU patients.

Benzodiazepines

Benzodiazepines are commonly used sedative agents in the ICU.[35–37] These drugs potentate gamma-aminobutyric acid (GABA) receptor complex–mediated inhibition of the CNS, leading to a dose-dependent effect that ranges from mild suppression of awareness to complete obtundation. Benzodiazepines are potent anxiolytic, anticonvulsant, and amnestic agents.[38] A paradoxical state of agitation, despite escalating doses, occasionally occurs, particularly in elderly patients. All benzodiazepines are lipophilic and are widely distributed throughout body tissues. With a single dose, the duration of action depends on the rate of redistribution to peripheral tissues, which terminates the clinical response. With longer infusions, the drug accumulates in peripheral tissues, and then is released back into the bloodstream after drug discontinuation, resulting in prolonged effect.

Benzodiazepine administration is associated with dose-dependent, centrally mediated respiratory depression. Although this depression is less pronounced than with opioid administration, there is a synergistic effect when the two drugs are combined. The pattern of respiratory depression is somewhat different than with opioids. Benzodiazepines depress tidal volume first, often with a compensatory increase in respiratory rate. The ventilatory response to hypoxia is eliminated at even low doses.

Similar to opioids, benzodiazepines have minimal cardiovascular effects in euvolemic patients. Hypotension may be seen in hypovolemic patients or in those with increased endogenous sympathetic activity.

Midazolam

Midazolam has a rapid onset of action (0.5 to 5 minutes) and a short duration of action after a single dose (2 hours). The drug undergoes oxidation through the cytochrome P450 pathway to form metabolites that are excreted in the urine. The primary metabolite, 1-hydroxymethylmidazolam, is a mild CNS depressant and may accumulate in patients with renal dysfunction.[39] Medications such as itraconazole, calcium channel blockers, and erythromycin may interfere with the cytochrome P450 enzyme and decrease midazolam metabolism. Hepatic dysfunction may also result in drug accumulation.

In critically ill patients undergoing continuous midazolam infusion, clinical recovery following drug discontinuation may take hours to days because of drug accumulation in peripheral tissues.[40] Elderly patients with decreased renal and hepatic function as well as obese patients with a greater volume of distribution are at greater risk for prolonged sedation.

Lorazepam

Intravenous lorazepam has an onset of action of approximately 5 minutes, with duration of action after a single dose of approximately 6 to 10 hours. Lorazepam is metabolized through hepatic glucuronidation to inactive metabolites that are renally excreted. High-dose infusion of lorazepam has been associated with severe metabolic acidosis from propylene glycol toxicity, a suspension agent used to enhance solubility in the intravenous solution.[41] Lorazepam administration has also been found to be an independent risk factor for the development of delirium in ICU patients.[25] In a study by Barr and colleagues,[42] midazolam outperformed lorazepam in areas of optimal sedation (Ramsey scale 3 to 4, 49% of the time with lorazepam, 69% for midazolam), depth of sedation (lorazepam patients were more likely to be deeply sedated), and time to emergence from sedation.

Propofol

Propofol (2, 6 diisopropylphenol) is a sterically hindered phenol that exhibits sedative and hypnotic effects.[43] Propofol acts on the GABA receptor, although at a different binding site than for benzodiazepines. Propofol is highly lipophillic and rapidly crosses the blood-brain barrier resulting in a rapid onset of action (1 to 5 minutes).[44] The duration of action is dose dependent but relatively short (2 to 8 minutes for a bolus injection). The depth of sedation increases in a dose-dependent fashion, and it rapidly redistributes into peripheral tissues resulting in a quick emergence from sedation when the drug is discontinued. Propofol is conjugated by the liver into inactive metabolites that are renally excreted, but unlike with benzodiazepines, the presence of hepatic or renal disease has little impact on its metabolism.[39] Elderly patients require a dosage reduction because of their decreased volume of distribution and decreased clearance of propofol. Like benzodiazepines, propofol exhibits dose-dependent sedation that may range from mild depression of responsiveness to obtundation. It has powerful anxiolytic and amnestic properties. Propofol has no analgesic effect, and patients may require higher doses of opioids compared with patients sedated with benzodiazepines.[45] Propofol may also be used as an effective anticonvulsant.[46]

Propofol causes profound respiratory depression and even apnea in some patients, and should be used only in patients with a secured airway or with personnel immediately available to intubate.

Similar to benzodiazepines, propofol decreases tidal volume with an associated increase in respiratory rate. Propofol administration can be associated with significant decreases in blood pressure, especially in hypovolemic patients. This is mainly because of increased venous capacitance and decreased venous return, although there may be some lesser effect stemming from myocardial depression. Long-term infusions of propofol may be associated with hypertriglyceridemia and subsequent pancreatitis, thus patients receiving propofol should have their serum triglyceride levels monitored.[47] Patients receiving long-term propofol infusion, those receiving parenteral lipids for nutrition, and patients with baseline hypertriglyceridemia are at greatest risk.

Propofol infusion syndrome (PRIS) is a rare, but potentially fatal, complication typically seen with infusion rates of more than 4 mg/kg/h for more than 48 hours.[48] Patients develop refractory bradycardia leading to asystole in the presence of metabolic acidosis, hyperkalemia, rhabdomyolysis, hyperlipidemia, or an enlarged fatty liver. Although the exact mechanism is unknown, current theories implicate impairment of mitochondrial respiratory chain function. Unexplained metabolic acidosis, elevations in serum lactate, creatinine kinase, or serum myoglobin may be early markers for the development of PRIS. Treatment consists of immediate discontinuation of propofol and correction of hemodynamic and metabolic abnormalities.

The pharmacokinetic properties of propofol offer significant advantages over other forms of hypnotic sedatives, such as benzodiazepines. Propofol has been demonstrated to be associated with a shorter duration of mechanical ventilation when compared with intermittent lorazepam in both retrospective studies and a recent randomized trial.[49,50] When combined with a strategy including daily interruption of sedation, propofol also provides a significant cost savings compared with intermittent lorazepam.[51] In a randomized trial by Barrientos-Vega and colleagues, long-term, continuous sedation with propofol and midazolam were equally effective at achieving goal sedation in patients undergoing mechanical ventilation, but propofol was associated with significantly shorter times from drug discontinuation to extubation.[52] This decreased time to extubation led to a cost savings in the propofol group, despite the higher drug cost of propofol compared with midazolam. Hall and colleagues[53] also demonstrated a decreased time to extubation after drug discontinuation of propofol compared with midazolam in their larger randomized multicenter trial.

Butyrophenones

Butyrophenones are sometimes provided for sedation in the ICU. These drugs appear to antagonize dopamine, especially in the basal ganglia, although the exact mechanism remains unclear. Drugs such as haloperidol induce a tranquil state, and patients often have a detached affect. Patients may even demonstrate a cataleptic, immobilized state. These drugs offer minimal analgesia, and have no amnestic or anticonvulsant properties. For patients with psychotic agitation resistant to other pharmacologic interventions, butyrophenones are sometimes required to maintain patient safety.

Butyrophenones do not have any significant respiratory effects. There may be some mild, synergistic respiratory depression when butyrophenones are used in combination with opioids. Butyrophenones may cause mild hypotension as a result of the effects of peripheral alpha-1 blockade.

Butyrophenones such as haloperidol are associated with QTc prolongation and, rarely, torsade de pointes.[54] Most reported cases in critically ill patients have occurred when patients were prescribed more than 50 mg/24 hours.[55] If the patient's baseline QTc interval is prolonged, if electrolyte disturbances are present, or they are receiving other drugs that may prolong the QTc interval, butyrophenones should be prescribed with caution.

Haloperidol

An intravenous dose of haloperidol will demonstrate an onset of effect within 2 to 5 minutes and will have a half-life of 2 hours. Doses of 1 to 10 mg are typically used initially, with titration depending on dose effect. In a retrospective cohort analysis of mechanically ventilated patients, Milbrandt and colleagues[56] detected a difference in hospital mortality between patients who received haloperidol within 2 days of initiation of mechanical ventilation when compared with patients who never received haloperidol (20.5% versus 36.1%; $P = .04$) even after adjusting for age, comorbidity, severity of illness, degree of organ dysfunction, and other potential cofounders. While intriguing, these findings must be interpreted with caution until confirmed by randomized, controlled trials.

Dexmedetomidine

Dexmedetomidine is a centrally acting alpha2-agonist approved for short-term use (<24 hrs) in patients receiving mechanical ventilation. It is an attractive drug for use in the ICU, given that it demonstrates sedative, analgesic, and anxiolytic properties without depressing respiratory drive.[57] Patients remain sedated if left undisturbed, but arouse easily with stimulation. Cardiovascular side effects include bradycardia and hypertension with initial bolus injection and hypotension with continuous infusion due to central sympatholysis.[39]

Most studies involving dexmedetomidine have been in postoperative patients, where it has been shown to decrease requirements for additional sedation and analgesic medications.[58] Currently, dexmedetomidine is FDA approved only for use up to 24 hours in mechanically ventilated patients, but a recent randomized trial comparing lorazepam to dexmedetomidine in critically ill, mechanically ventilated patients suggests that dexmedetomidine may be safely used for up to 120 hours.[59] Patients randomized to receive dexmedetomidine spent more days alive without delirium or coma (median days 7.0 versus 3.0, $P = .01$) and experienced a lower prevalence of coma (63% versus 92%; $P = .001$). Further long-term studies of dexmedetomidine are warranted before it can be routinely employed.

VOLATILE ANESTHETIC SEDATION

Volatile anesthetics such as isoflourane have been used for sedation in mechanically ventilated patients, but widespread use has been limited because of difficulty in administration. Compared with midazolam or propofol, isoflourane was found to have adequate sedative properties with predictable and quick awakening.[60,61] Recent technological advances such as the Anesthetic Conserving Device (AnaConDa, Hudson RCI, Uppsland Väsby, Sweden) can convert a standard ventilator to provide volatile sedation. Using this device, Sackey and colleagues[62] were able to provide prolonged isoflourane to ICU patients, with effective sedation and subsequent awakening times that were significantly shorter than seen with midazolam (time to follow verbal command 10 ± 8 versus 110 ± 132 minutes). In time, volatile sedation may become a viable alternative to routine intravenous sedation for mechanically ventilated patients.

ANALGOSEDATION VERSUS HYPNOTIC-BASED SEDATION

Traditional sedation practices focused primarily on hypnotic drugs such as benzodiazepines and propofol, with opioids added as needed to control pain. The introduction of shorter-acting opioids and dexmedetomidine has led to an increased interest in sedative strategies that focus primarily on analgesic medications, with hypnotic agents added on an as-needed basis. In a randomized, multicenter study by Breen and colleagues[63] of patients undergoing mechanical ventilation for up to 10 days, an analgesia-based sedation regimen using remifentanil reduced the duration of mechanical ventilation by 2 days compared with a midazolam-based sedation strategy where fentanyl or morphine was added as needed for analgesia. In neurosurgical and neurotrauma patients, analgesia-based sedation strategies using remifentanil plus propofol provided significantly faster and more predictable awakening for neurologic assessment compared with standard hypnotic-based regimens using propofol with fentanyl or morphine added for pain control.[64]

ASSESSING THE ADEQUACY OF SEDATION

Individual assessments of sedation adequacy can be hampered by lack of objectivity. The Society of Critical Care Medicine's Clinical Practice Guidelines for Sustained Use of Sedatives and Analgesics in the Critically Ill Adult recommend that a sedation goal or end point be established and regularly redefined for each patient using a validated sedation assessment scale, with documentation of regular assessment and response.[16]

There are several reliable instruments available to assess the adequacy of sedation. The Ramsay scale has been used for over 30 years in clinical investigations of sedation,[65] but has attracted criticism because of its lack of clear discrimination and lack of specific descriptors to differentiate between levels.[66] Other sedation scales such as the Sedation-Agitation Scale and the Richmond Agitation Sedation Scale (RASS) have been extensively tested for reliability and validity in critically ill patients.[67–69] The RASS has been validated to detect changes in sedation status over several days, to perform reliably in patients with altered levels of consciousness such as delirium, and to correlate with doses of sedatives and analgesic medications administered to critically ill patients. The Adaptation to the Intensive Care Unit Environment (ATICE) is a sedation scoring system that additionally rates patient agitation and ventilator synchrony.[70] It has demonstrated high internal consistency, inter-rater reliability across disciplines, and validity.

Limited data suggest that adoption of routine, structured assessments alone may substantially change patient outcomes, even without pairing assessments to a protocol dictating alteration in sedation administration. In a two-phase, prospective controlled study by Chanques and colleagues,[71] the implementation of a systematic evaluation of pain and agitation and using the Behavioral Pain Scale (BPS),[72] Numerical Rating

Scale (NRS),[73] and the Richmond Agitation Sedation Scale (RASS)[67] resulted in decreased incidence of pain and agitation in the intervention group (pain 63% versus 42% $P = .02$ and agitation 29% versus 12% $P = .02$). Compared with the control group, the patients in the intervention group experienced a decreased duration of mechanical ventilation (120 versus 65 hours, $P = .01$) and decreased nosocomial infection rate (17% versus 8%, $P < .05$). This study met with criticism because of the lack of independent observer scoring in the intervention group, which may have confounded sedation assessment because of lack of blinding. Nevertheless, it does lend support to the notion that a more objective methodology in sedation assessment may lead to improved outcomes.

Despite recommendations from the SCCM and other expert reviews[16,74–76] supporting the use of sedation scales and sedation algorithms, several studies suggest that this does not occur routinely in ICUs around the world. For example, a recent, large observational study in 44 French ICUs that had adopted sedation scales found only 43% patients on day 2 and 31% on day 6 had their level of sedation evaluated by a standardized assessment tool. Of the patients who were assessed, 57% on day 2 and 41% on day 6 were found to be deeply sedated.[77] In a recent cross-sectional survey of Canadian critical care physicians, only 49% of respondents used a sedation scoring system as part of routine patient assessment.[37]

PROTOCOLIZED SEDATION STRATEGIES

Patient-targeted sedation protocols provide a structured approach to the assessment of patient pain and distress, combined with an algorithm that directs drug escalation and de-escalation based on assessments. In a randomized, controlled trial of 321 patients receiving mechanical ventilation, Brook and colleagues[78] found that the use of protocol-directed sedation decreased the duration of mechanical ventilation, as well as hospital length of stay, compared with nonprotocol-directed sedation. In patients assigned to receive protocol-directed sedation, nurses were allowed to determine type of sedation used (sedatives, analgesics, or both), type of administration (intermittent or continuous), and dosages to target an "ideal level" of sedation (Ramsay score of 3: patient awake—responds to commands only). In contrast, patients in the nonprotocol-directed arm of the study had their sedation managed by treating physicians only. Nurses in this control group were allowed to communicate their observations and opinions to the treating

physicians, but were not allowed to make changes without a physician order. De Jonghe and colleagues[79] recently paired "Adaptation to the ICU Environment" (ATICE) assessments with a sedation protocol leading to a decreased time to arousal and decreased duration of mechanical ventilation. In addition to reducing duration of mechanical ventilation, nurse-implemented sedation protocols have also been shown to reduce the incidence of ventilator-associated pneumonia.[80] But even when protocols have been designed and put in place at an institution, they may not be optimally used. In a study by Marshall and others,[81] daily pharmacist-enforced intervention aimed at improving sedation guideline adherence resulted in further decreases in mechanical ventilation and ICU length of stay.

There have been some exceptions to the improvements seen with sedation protocols. In a study by Bucknall and colleagues,[82] protocol-directed sedation management did not change outcomes compared with usual local practice in an Australian ICU, where nurses are usually free to assess level of sedation, titrate sedative and analgesic medications, and stop sedation if the patient was deemed to be oversedated. Reasons for a lack of difference between the two groups may have been lack of blinding, and the significant increase in propofol prescribing in the control arm, which itself has been associated with decreased duration of mechanical ventilation.

DAILY INTERRUPTION OF SEDATION

Daily interruption of sedative infusion (DIS) allows a focused downward titration of sedative drugs over time, thus minimizing the tendency for drug accumulation to allow early patient awakening. Analgesic and sedative medications are interrupted once daily until the patient awakens to follow commands or exhibits distress that requires drug resumption. With drug interruption, the ICU team must be vigilant for the development of patient distress manifested by overt agitation, hemodynamic instability, or ventilator asynchrony. If excessive agitation is noted, providers should administer drugs as a bolus to de-escalate symptoms, and resume the sedatives and analgesics at half the previous doses. Further titration can then be performed to achieve the desired level of sedation. Alternatively, patients who awaken and are not agitated should have their sedatives restarted only *as needed*, thereby allowing them to spend some of their ICU time awake and interactive.

When mechanically ventilated patients undergoing DIS were compared with a control group where care was directed by the primary ICU team, the mean duration of mechanical ventilation was 4.9 days, compared with 7.3 days in the control group for whom drug infusions were only interrupted at the discretion of the ICU clinicians ($P = .004$)[19] **(Fig. 1)**. The median length of stay in the ICU was 6.4 days in the intervention group versus 9.9 days in the control group ($P = .02$), and patients in the DIS intervention spent more days awake and following commands (85.5% versus 9.0%, $P < .001$). Complications as a result of undersedation (eg, patient removal of endotracheal tube) were not different between groups.

This study met with criticism because of its single-center application and concerns for unrecognized patient harm such as psychologic distress, myocardial ischemia, and the risk of precipitating dangerous drug and alcohol withdrawal syndromes as a result of daily interruption of sedation.[83] Subsequent investigations into the long-term effects of DIS have shown no adverse psychologic outcomes, a reduction in PTSD symptoms after approximately 1 year, and a trend toward reductions in the incidence of PTSD.[10] In a subsequent cohort study of 74 mechanically ventilated patients undergoing DIS with coronary risk factors, sedative interruption was not associated with increased risk for ischemia

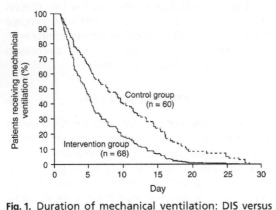

Fig. 1. Duration of mechanical ventilation: DIS versus control. Shown is a Kaplan-Meier analysis of the duration of mechanical ventilation, according to study group: an intervention group, in which sedative infusions were interrupted on a daily basis (DIS) until the patients were awake; and a control group, in which the infusions were interrupted only at the discretion of the clinicians in the intensive care unit. After adjustment for baseline variables (age, sex, weight, Acute Physiology and Chronic Health Evaluation II score, and type of respiratory failure), mechanical ventilation was discontinued earlier in the intervention group than in the control group (relative risk for extubation = 1.9, 95% CI 1.3 to 2.7; $P < .001$). (*From* Kress JP, Pohlman AS, O'Connor MF, Hall JB. Daily interruption of sedative infusions in critically ill patients undergoing mechanical ventilation. N Engl J Med 2000;342(20):1471–7; with permission. Copyright © 2000, Massachusetts Medical Society.)

determined by continuous three-lead Holter monitoring.[84] A recent trial by de Wit and colleagues[85] noted that a nursing-directed sedation protocol resulted in better outcomes than DIS. This study was hindered by early cessation. There was the suggestion that certain groups of patients, such as those with substance abuse histories, should have sedation strategies such as DIS undertaken with extreme caution. Further investigation into the safety of DIS in patients with alcohol and other drug use disorders is needed.

A recent multicenter, randomized trial assessed a protocol pairing spontaneous awakening trials (SATs), ie, daily interruption of sedatives, with spontaneous breathing trials (SBTs).[86] Patients in the intervention group (n = 168) underwent awakening with SAT before SBT, whereas patients in the control arm (n = 168) received patient-targeted sedation using a validated sedation scale and SBTs alone. Patients in the intervention group had more ventilator-free days during the 28-day study period (14.7 versus 11.6 days, $P = .02$), spent fewer days in the ICU (median time 9.1 days versus 12.9 days, $P = .01$), and were discharged from the hospital earlier (hospitalized 14.9 days versus 19.2 days, $P = .04$). There were more self-extubations in the intervention group compared with controls (16 patients versus 6 patients, $P = .03$), but the reintubation rates for both groups were similar. Last, patients in the intervention group were less likely to die than were patients in the control group (hazard ratio 0.68, 95% confidence interval [CI] 0.50 to 0.92,

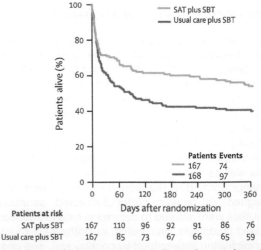

Fig. 2. Survival at 1 year. Events indicate the number of deaths in each group in the year after enrollment. (*From* Girard TD, Kress JP, Fuchs BD, et al. Efficacy and safety of a paired sedation and ventilator weaning protocol for mechanically ventilated patients in intensive care (Awakening and Breathing Controlled trial): a randomized controlled trial. Lancet 2008;371(9607):126–34; with permission.)

P = .01) (**Fig. 2**). For every seven patients treated with both SATs and SBTs, one life was saved (number needed to treat 7.4, 95% CI 4.2 to 35.5).

SUMMARY

Providing adequate sedation and analgesia to mechanically ventilated patients while avoiding the hazards of oversedation is challenging. Careful drug selection and frequent evaluation of the adequacy of sedation and analgesia can help minimize the risks of oversedation. Sedation scales, sedation protocols, and daily interruption of sedative can help minimize unwanted sedative effects, minimize the duration of mechanical ventilation, and may reduce ICU mortality. Further studies are warranted to determine how best to combine these tools as part of an overall sedation strategy, and new medications are being investigated that may also help minimize oversedation.

REFERENCES

1. Esteban A, Anzueto A, Frutos F, et al. Characteristics and outcomes in adult patients receiving mechanical ventilation: a 28-day international study. JAMA 2002;287(3):345–55.
2. Puntillo KA. Pain experiences of intensive care unit patients. Heart Lung 1990;19(5 Pt 1):526–33.
3. Turner JS, Briggs SJ, Springhorn HE, et al. Patient's recollection of intensive care unit experience. Crit Care Med 1990;18(9):966–8.
4. Epstein J, Breslow MJ. The stress response of critical illness. Crit Care Clin 1999;15(1):17–33.
5. Lewis KS, Whipple JK, Michael KA, et al. Effect of analgesic treatment on the physiologic consequences of acute pain. Am J Hosp Pharm 1994; 51(12):1539–54.
6. Biancofiore G, Bindi ML, Romanelli AM, et al. Stress-inducing factors in ICUs: what liver transplant recipients experience and what caregivers perceive. Liver Transpl 2005;11(8):967–72.
7. Novaes MA, Knobel E, Bork AM, et al. Stressors in ICU: perception of the patient, relatives and health care team. Intensive Care Med 2001;27(5):937.
8. Samuelson K, Lundberg D, Fridlund B. Memory in relation to depth of sedation in adult mechanically ventilated intensive care patients. Intensive Care Med 2006;32(5):660–7.
9. Jones C, Griffiths RD, Humphris G, et al. Memory, delusions, and the development of acute posttraumatic stress disorder-related symptoms after intensive care. Crit Care Med 2001;29(3):573–80.
10. Kress JP, Gehlbach B, Lacy M, et al. The long-term psychological effects of daily sedative interruption on critically ill patients. Am J Respir Crit Care Med 2003;168(12):1457–61.
11. Schelling G, Stoll C, Haller M, et al. Health-related quality of life and posttraumatic stress disorder in survivors of the acute respiratory distress syndrome. Crit Care Med 1998;26(4):651–9.
12. Weinert CR, Sprenkle M. Post-ICU consequences of patient wakefulness and sedative exposure during mechanical ventilation. Intensive Care Med 2008; 34(1):82–90.
13. Kahn JM, Andersson L, Karir V, et al. Low tidal volume ventilation does not increase sedation use in patients with acute lung injury. Crit Care Med 2005;33(4):903–4.
14. Cheng IW, Eisner MD, Thompson BT, et al. Acute effects of tidal volume strategy on hemodynamics, fluid balance, and sedation in acute lung injury. Crit Care Med 2005;33(1):239–40.
15. Spina SP, Ensom MH. Clinical pharmacokinetic monitoring of midazolam in critically ill patients. Pharmacology 2007;27(3):389–98.
16. Jacobi J, Fraser GL, Coursin DB, et al. Clinical practice guidelines for the sustained use of sedatives and analgesics in the critically ill adult. Crit Care Med 2002;30(1):119–41.
17. Kollef MH, Levy NT, Ahrens TS, et al. The use of continuous i.v. sedation is associated with prolongation of mechanical ventilation. Chest 1998;114(2):541–8.
18. Rello J, Diaz E, Roque M, et al. Risk factors for developing pneumonia within 48 hours of intubation. Am J Respir Crit Care Med 1999;159(6):1742–6.
19. Kress JP, Pohlman AS, O'Connor MF, et al. Daily interruption of sedative infusions in critically ill patients undergoing mechanical ventilation. N Engl J Med 2000;342(20):1471–7.
20. Cammarano WB, Pittet JF, Weitz S, et al. Acute withdrawal syndrome related to the administration of analgesic and sedative medications in adult intensive care unit patients. Crit Care Med 1998;26(4):676–84.
21. Ely EW, Inouye SK, Bernard GR, et al. Delirium in mechanically ventilated patients: validity and reliability of the confusion assessment method for the intensive care unit (CAM-ICU). JAMA 2001; 286(21):2703–10.
22. Ely EW, Margolin R, Francis J, et al. Evaluation of delirium in critically ill patients: validation of the Confusion Assessment Method for the Intensive Care Unit (CAM-ICU). Crit Care Med 2001;29(7):1370–9.
23. Lin SM, Liu CY, Wang CH, et al. The impact of delirium on the survival of mechanically ventilated patients. Crit Care Med 2004;32(11):2254–9.
24. Ely EW, Shintani A, Truman B, et al. Delirium as a predictor of mortality in mechanically ventilated patients in the intensive care unit. JAMA 2004;291(14): 1753–62.
25. Pandharipande P, Shintani A, Peterson J, et al. Lorazepam is an independent risk factor for transitioning to delirium in intensive care unit patients. Anesthesiology 2006;104(1):21–6.

26. Thomas J, Karver S, Cooney GA, et al. Methylnal-trexone for opioid-induced constipation in advanced illness. N Engl J Med 2008;358(22):2332–43.

27. Pasternak GW, Bodnar RJ, Clark JA, et al. Morphine-6-glucuronide, a potent mu agonist. Life Sci 1987; 41(26):2845–9.

28. Goetting M, Thirman M. Neurotoxicity of meperidine. Ann Emerg Med 1985;14(10):1007–9.

29. Gehlbach BK, Kress JP. Sedation in the intensive care unit. Curr Opin Crit Care 2002;8(4):290–8.

30. Westmoreland CL, Hoke JF, Sebel PS, et al. Pharmacokinetics of remifentanil (GI87084B) and its major metabolite (GR90291) in patients undergoing elective surgery. Anesthesiology 1993;79(5):893–903.

31. Muellejans B, Lopez A, Cross MH, et al. Remifentanyl versus fentanyl for analgesia based sedation to provide patient comfort in the intensive care unit: a randomized, double-blind controlled trial. Crit Care 2004;8(1):R1–11.

32. Dahaba AA, Grabner T, Rehak PH, et al. Remifentanil versus morphine analgesia and sedation for mechanically ventilated critically ill patients: a randomized double blind study. Anesthesiology 2004;101(3):640–6.

33. Pitsiu M, Wilmer A, Bodenham A, et al. Pharmacokinetics of remifentanil and its major metabolite, remifentanil acid, in ICU patients with renal impairment. Br J Anaesth 2004;92(4):493–503.

34. Breen D, Wilmer A, Bodenham A, et al. Offset of pharmacodynamic effects and safety of remifentanil in intensive care unit patients with various degrees of renal impairment. Crit Care 2004;8(1):R21–30.

35. Rhoney DH, Murry KR. National survey of the use of sedating drugs, neuromuscular blocking agents and reversal agents in the intensive care unit. J Intensive Care Med 2003;18(3):139–45.

36. Martin J, Franck M, Sigel S, et al. Changes in sedation management in German intensive care units between 2002 and 2006: a national follow-up survey. Crit Care 2007;11(6):R124.

37. Mehta S, Burry L, Fischer S, et al. Canadian survey of the use of sedatives, analgesics, and neuromuscular blocking agents in critically ill patients. Crit Care Med 2006;34(2):347–73.

38. George KA, Dundee JW. Relative amnesiac actions of diazepam, flunitrazepam and lorazepam in man. Br J Clin Pharmacol 1977;4(1):45–50.

39. Gommer D, Bakker J. Medications for analgesia and sedation in the intensive care unit: an overview. Crit Care 2008;12(Suppl 3):S4.

40. Byatt CM, Lewis LD, Dawling S, et al. Accumulation of midazolam after repeated dosage in patients receiving mechanical ventilation in an intensive care unit. BMJ 1984;289(6448):799–800.

41. Tayar J, Jabbour G, Saggi SJ. Severe hyperosmolar metabolic acidosis due to large dose of intravenous lorazepam. N Engl J Med 2002;346(16):1253–4.

42. Barr J, Zomorodi K, Bertaccini EJ, et al. A double-blind, randomized comparison of i.v. lorazepam versus midazolam for sedation of ICU patients via a pharmacologic model. Anesthesiology 2001; 95(2):324–33.

43. James R, Glen JB. Synthesis, biological evaluation and preliminary structure-activity considerations of a series of alkylphenols as intravenous anaesthetic agents. J Med Chem 1980;23(12):1350–7.

44. Mirenda J, Broyles G. Propofol as used for sedation in the ICU. Chest 1995;108(2):539–48.

45. Kress JP, O'Connor MF, Pohlman AS, et al. Sedation of critically ill patients during mechanical ventilation: a comparison of propofol and midazolam. Am J Respir Crit Care Med 1996;153(3):1012–8.

46. Marik PE, Varon J. The management of status epilepticus. Chest 2004;126(2):582–91.

47. Devlin JW, Lau AK, Tanios MA. Propofol-associated hypertriglyceridemia and pancreatitis in the intensive care unit: an analysis of frequency and risk factors. Pharmacotherapy 2005;25(10):1348–52.

48. Kam PC, Cardone D. Propofol infusion syndrome. Anaesthesia 2007;62(7):690–701.

49. Fong JJ, Kanji S, Dasta JF, et al. Propofol associated with a shorter duration of mechanical ventilation than scheduled intermittent lorazepam: a database analysis using Project IMPACT. Ann Pharmacother 2007; 41(12):1986–91.

50. Carson SS, Kress JP, Rodgers JE, et al. A randomized trial of intermittent lorazepam versus propofol with daily interruption in mechanically ventilated patients. Crit Care Med 2006;34(5):1326–32.

51. Cox CE, Reed SD, Govert JA, et al. Economic evaluation of propofol and lorazepam for critically ill patients undergoing mechanical ventilation. Crit Care Med 2008;36(3):706–14.

52. Barrientos-Vega R, Mar Sánchez-Soria M, Morales-García C, et al. Prolonged sedation of critically ill patients with midazolam or propofol: impact on weaning and costs. Crit Care Med 1997;25(1):33–40.

53. Hall RI, Sandham D, Cardinal P, et al. Propofol vs midazolam for ICU sedation: a Canadian multicenter randomized trial. Chest 2001;119(4):1151–9.

54. Glassman AH, Bigger JT Jr. Antipsychotic drugs: prolonged QTc interval, torsade de pointes, and sudden death. Am J Psychiatry 2001;158(11): 1774–82.

55. Lawrence KR, Nasraway SA. Conduction disturbances associated with administration of butyrophenone antipsychotics in the critically ill: a review of the literature. Pharmacotherapy 1997;17(3):531–7.

56. Milbrandt EB, Kersten A, Kong L, et al. Haloperidol use is associated with lower hospital mortality in mechanically ventilated patients. Crit Care Med 2005; 33(1):263–5.

57. Gerlach AT, Dasta JF. Dexmedetomidine: an updated review. Ann Pharmacother 2007;41(2):245–52.

58. Martin E, Ramsay G, Mantz J, et al. The role of alpha2-adrenoreceptor agonist dexmedetomidine in postsurgical sedation in the intensive care unit. J Intensive Care Med 2003;18(1):29–41.

59. Pandharipande PP, Pun BT, Herr DL, et al. Effect of sedation with dexmedetomidine vs lorazepam on acute brain dysfunction in mechanically ventilated patients: the MENDS randomized controlled trial. JAMA 2007;298(22):2644–53.

60. Kong KL, Willatts SM, Prys-Roberts C. Isoflurane compared with midazolam for sedation in the intensive care unit. BMJ 1989;298(6683):1277–80.

61. Millane TA, Bennett ED, Grounds RM. Isoflurane and propofol for long-term sedation in the intensive care unit. A crossover study. Anaesthesia 1992;47(9):768–74.

62. Sackey PV, Martling CR, Granath F, et al. Prolonged isoflurane sedation of intensive care unit patients with the Anesthetic Conserving Device. Crit Care Med 2004;32(11):2241–6.

63. Breen D, Karabinis A, Malbrain M, et al. Decreased duration of mechanical ventilation when comparing analgesia-based sedation using remifentanil with standard hypnotic based sedation for up to 10 days in intensive care unit patients: a randomized trial. Crit Care 2005;9(3):R200–10.

64. Karabinis A, Mandragos K, Stergiopoulos S, et al. Safety and efficacy of analgesia based sedation using remifentanil versus standard hypnotic based regimens in intensive care unit patients with brain injuries; a randomized, controlled trial [ISRCTN50308308]. Crit Care 2004;8(4):R268–80.

65. Ramsey MA, Savege TM, Simpson BR, et al. Controlled sedation with alphalaxone-alphadolone. BMJ 1974;2(5920):256–9.

66. Hansen-Flaschen J, Cowen J, Polomano RC. Beyond the Ramsay scale: need for a validated measure of sedating drug efficacy in the intensive care unit. Crit Care Med 1994;22(5):732–3.

67. Riker RR, Picard JT, Fraser GL. Prospective evaluation of the Sedation-Agitation Scale for adult critically ill patients. Crit Care Med 1999;27(7):1325–9.

68. Sessler CN, Gosnell MS, Grap MJ, et al. The Richmond Agitation-Sedation Scale: validity and reliability in adult intensive care unit patients. Am J Respir Crit Care Med 2002;166(10):1338–44.

69. Ely EW, Truman B, Shintani A, et al. Monitoring sedation status over time in ICU patients: reliability and validity of the Richmond Agitation Sedation scale (RASS). JAMA 2003;289(22):2983–91.

70. De Jonghe B, Cook D, Griffith L, et al. Adaptation to the Intensive Care Environment (ATICE): development and validation of a new sedation assessment instrument. Crit Care Med 2003;31(9):2344–54.

71. Chanques G, Jaber S, Barbotte E, et al. Impact of a systematic evaluation of pain and agitation in an intensive care unit. Crit Care Med 2006;34(6):1691–9.

72. Payen JF, Bru O, Bosson JL, et al. Assessing pain in critically ill sedated patients by using a behavioral pain scale. Crit Care Med 2001;29(12):2258–63.

73. Hamill-Ruth RJ, Marohn ML. Evaluation of pain in the critically ill patient. Crit Care Clin 1999;15(1):35–54, v–vi.

74. Sessler CN, Grap MJ, Brophy GM. Multidisciplinary management of sedation and analgesia in critical care. Semin Respir Crit Care Med 2001;22(2):211–25.

75. Riker RR, Fraser GL. Monitoring sedation, agitation, analgesia, neuromuscular blockade, and delirium in adult ICU patients. Semin Respir Crit Care Med 2001;22(2):189–98.

76. Kress JP, Hall JB. Sedation in the mechanically ventilated patient. Crit Care Med 2006;34(10):2541–6.

77. Payen JF, Chanques G, Mantz J, et al. Current practices in sedation and analgesia for mechanically ventilated critically ill patients: a prospective multicenter patient-based study. Anesthesiology 2007;106(4):687–95.

78. Brook AD, Ahrens TS, Schaiff R, et al. Effect of a nursing-implemented sedation protocol on the duration of mechanical ventilation. Crit Care Med 1999;27(12):2609–15.

79. De Jonghe B, Bastuji-Garin S, Fangio P, et al. Sedation algorithm in critically ill patients without acute brain injury. Crit Care Med 2005;33(1):120–7.

80. Quenot JP, Ladoire S, Devoucoux F, et al. Effect of a nurse implemented sedation protocol on the incidence of ventilator associated pneumonia. Crit Care Med 2007;35(9):2031–6.

81. Marshall J, Finn CA, Theodore AC. Impact of a clinical pharmacist-enforced intensive care unit sedation protocol on duration of mechanical ventilation and hospital stay. Crit Care Med 2008;36(2):626–8.

82. Bucknall TK, Manias E, Presneill JJ. A randomized trial of protocol-directed sedation management for mechanical ventialation in an Australian intensive care unit. Crit Care Med 2008;36(5):1444–50.

83. Hefner JE. A wake-up call in the intensive care unit. N Engl J Med 2000;342:1520–2.

84. Kress JP, Vinayak AG, Levitt J, et al. Daily sedative interruption in mechanically ventilated patients at risk for coronary artery disease. Crit Care Med 2007;35(2):365–71.

85. de Wit M, Gennings C, Jenvey WI, et al. Randomized trial comparing daily interruption of sedation and nursing-implemented sedation algorithm in medical intensive care unit patients. Crit Care 2008;12(3):R70.

86. Girard TD, Kress JP, Fuchs BD, et al. Efficacy and safety of a paired sedation and ventilator weaning protocol for mechanically ventilated patients in intensive care (awakening and breathing controlled trial): a randomized controlled trial. Lancet 2008;371(9607):126–34.

Short- and Long-Term Cognitive Outcomes in Intensive Care Unit Survivors

Ramona O. Hopkins, PhD[a,b,c,*], James C. Jackson, PsyD[d,e]

KEYWORDS

- Cognitive impairments
- Critical illness
- Critical care outcomes

Significant advances in critical care have led to improved survival rates among individuals admitted to intensive care units (ICUs). While some individuals—often younger and more robustly healthy individuals—leave the ICU and return to their normal lives with little difficulty, others are less fortunate. For the other survivors of critical illness, ICU hospitalization is a gateway to a life of new and emerging difficulties and limitations that are difficult to overestimate. Central nervous system or neurologic dysfunction is the least studied of the organ failures during critical illness. Current data suggest a high prevalence of neurologic disturbances in patients with critical illness admitted to medical or surgical (non-neurologic) ICUs. Medical technologic advances have improved central nervous system monitoring in critically ill patients, allowing physicians to diagnose quickly and reliably delirium, seizures, and encephalopathy. Furthermore, neuropsychologic tests provide reliable and valid assessment of long-term cognitive impairments. Neurologic dysfunction during critical illness can be severe and includes encephalopathy, cognitive, and psychiatric impairments. Chief among these problems are delirium and long-term cognitive impairment that are, in some respects, distinct and yet closely related. Recent investigations show that delirium is common during critical illness. Furthermore, long-term cognitive impairments may occur in well over half of all ICU survivors and are associated with poor functional outcomes.

DELIRIUM OR SHORT-TERM COGNITIVE OUTCOMES

Delirium is a neurobehavioral syndrome that occurs across health care settings, is associated with adverse outcomes, including death,[1,2] and is the most common manifestation of acute brain dysfunction during critical illness and among mechanically ventilated ICU cohorts.[2] Although many view delirium as transient, neuropathologic abnormalities are observed on brain imaging in delirious patients, including ventricular enlargement, and generalized and cortical and subcortical lesions.[3,4] A potentially toxic neuropsychiatric syndrome characterized by a fluctuating course and pronounced inattention, delirium is highly prevalent among hospitalized elderly, affecting between

a Psychology Department, Neuroscience Center, 1082 SWKT, Brigham Young University, Provo, UT, USA
b Pulmonary and Critical Care Division, Department of Medicine, LDS Hospital, 8th Avenue and C Street, Salt Lake City, UT, USA
c Pulmonary and Critical Care Medicine, Intermountain Medical Center, 5121 South Cottonwood Street, Murray, UT 84107, USA
d Division of Allergy/Pulmonary/Critical Care Medicine, Vanderbilt University School of Medicine, 6th Floor, Medical Center East #6109, Nashville, TN, USA
e Center for Health Services Research, Vanderbilt University School of Medicine, Nashville, TN, USA
* Corresponding author. Pulmonary and Critical Care Medicine, Intermountain Medical Center, 5121 South Cottonwood Street, Murray, UT 84107.
E-mail address: ramona.hopkins@imail.org (R.O. Hopkins).

Clin Chest Med 30 (2009) 143–153
doi:10.1016/j.ccm.2008.11.001

15% and 20% of hospitalized medical patients,[5] 25% to 65% of surgical patients,[6,7] and as many as 80% of patients in ICU settings.[8] While once considered benign, recent evidence has linked delirium with a variety of adverse outcomes, including prolonged hospitalization, poor surgical recovery, and increased morbidity and mortality.[9–12] Some researchers speculate that delirium may be a marker of subclinical dementia or cognitive impairment, which might not otherwise develop for years or decades. Indeed, data suggest that common pathogenic mechanisms might underlie development of cognitive impairments in delirium and dementia.[13]

Delirium is linked to adverse cognitive outcomes in a variety of patient populations, including critically ill patients. A recent review of nine studies summarized below found hospitalized patients with delirium had greater cognitive decline or developed dementia at follow-up.[14] For example, cognitive decline was twice as likely to occur in geriatric hip-fracture patients with delirium 2-years after surgery.[15,16] Hospitalized community-dwelling geriatric patients with delirium had cognitive decline at 6 months, and there was additional cognitive decline over the next 18 months.[17] Furthermore, hospitalized geriatric medical patients' Mini Mental State Examination (MMSE) scores were nearly five points lower in patients with delirium when compared with patients without delirium at 1-year follow-up after adjusting for premorbid function, comorbid diseases, and illness severity.[18] Older patients (age >84) who had an episode of delirium were significantly more likely to be diagnosed with dementia at 3-year follow-up, compared with patients without delirium.[19] One study found that over a 3-year period, in 60% of geriatric medical patients with delirium at hospital admission (evaluated for dementia at baseline) the incidence of dementia was 18.1% per year for patients with delirium compared with 5.6% per year for patients without delirium.[20] Koponen and colleagues[21] reported that one-third of patients who were delirious during psychiatric hospitalization evidenced cognitive deterioration. The above findings suggest that the presence of delirium may be one important factor that directly or indirectly contributes to the development of adverse long-term cognitive outcome.

Although delirium may be a sign of emerging cognitive impairment, it is clearly not the case that the cognitive decline experienced by large numbers of patients with delirium is solely or primarily related to pre-existing cognitive impairment. For example, Jackson and colleagues[22] excluded patients with probable early dementia and found nearly one-third of the ICU patients (all with delirium) had cognitive impairments at 6 months. Thus, delirium may be marker for development of cognitive impairments following critical illness and is not simply a marker of pre-existing subclinical or early dementia.

PREVALENCE OF COGNITIVE DYSFUNCTION

Cognitive impairment is generally long-lasting (observed as late as 6 years after ICU discharge) and is experienced among large numbers of ICU survivors. Among general medical ICU survivors, approximately one-third or more have long-term cognitive impairment.[22] It is difficult to determine the extent to which this impairment represents a new condition or reflects a worsening of an already existing impairment, as baseline data on cognitive functioning is generally unavailable in critically ill patients. However, the mean age of patients in the current studies of cognitive impairment in ICU survivors is 54 years, suggesting that exceedingly few of these patients could plausibly suffer from dementia. Similarly, it is difficult to make comparisons of prevalence across studies in light of discrepancies in the definitions of cognitive impairments employed, the neuropsychologic test batteries administered, and follow-up time points. To date, there have been 10 cohorts comprising approximately 450 patients in which cognitive impairment after critical illness have been studied.[23–33] The populations include six studies in acute respiratory distress syndrome (ARDS) patients,[23,25,26,29,31,32,34] one study in patients with respiratory failure,[34] two studies in medical ICU patients,[30,33] and one study in general ICU patients.[27] In one investigation, cognitive assessments were done via the telephone, which was validated in another cohort using in-person testing.[32] Follow-up times vary widely, with studies generally taking place within a year of hospital discharge,[35] but three studies assessed individuals beyond 1 year.[4,31,34] **Fig. 1** shows the prevalence of cognitive impairments in studies to date.

Data indicate cognitive impairments are strikingly widespread, as almost 80% of ICU survivors experience cognitive impairments early after hospital discharge, with the rate of cognitive impairments declining somewhat over time.[23–32,34] Among specific populations, notably patients with ARDS, the prevalence of cognitive impairments is particularly high as well as persistent, with 46% of patients at 1 year[23] and 25% of patients at 6 years[31] reporting ongoing difficulties. While highly prevalent, cognitive impairment demonstrated by ICU survivors is also often quite severe. For example, the aforementioned ARDS patients with cognitive sequelae all fell below the

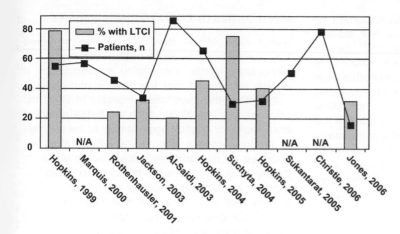

Fig. 1. Evidence from a total of 10 studies, totaling 450 patients, suggests that 25% to 78% of patients have long-term cognitive impairment following critical illness.

sixth percentile of the normal distribution of cognitive functioning, displaying marked neuropsychologic deficits in wide-ranging areas, including memory, executive functioning, attention, and mental processing abilities. Impairment does not impact all domains equally, and deficits in some areas rebound relatively more completely than others. With regard to global intellectual abilities, Hopkins and colleagues[34] showed that patients' estimated premorbid IQ was significantly higher than their measured IQ at hospital discharge, but improved to their premorbid level by 1-year follow-up. The finding that patients recovered over time with regard to IQ does not necessarily suggest a comparable recovery in all cognitive domains, as data from traumatic and anoxic brain injury literature suggests that some cognitive abilities are more likely to improve than others.

Even in ICU survivors without ARDS, cognitive impairment is widespread and similar cognitive functions are affected. Jackson and colleagues[22] studied 34 medical ICU survivors approximately 6 months after discharge and demonstrated that one-third of them had persistent cognitive impairment of at least moderate severity (using a very restrictive definition of two test scores two standard deviations below the mean or three test scores 1.5 standard deviations below the mean). While only 34 patients completed 6-month cognitive follow-up, 128 patients, all without pre-existing cognitive impairment assessed by the Informant Questionnaire of Cognitive Decline in the Elderly (IQCODE), were administered an initial MMSE at ICU discharge. The mean MMSE scores of those who did not participate in follow-up cognitive testing were below the impairment cut-off of 24 and were significantly lower than scores for those patients who completed follow-up, suggesting that those lost to follow-up likely had worse cognitive functioning than did the patients who completed

cognitive testing.[22] Furthermore, in a cohort of 32 critically ill medical patients with mechanical ventilation of greater than or equal to 5 days, 91% at hospital discharge and 41% at 6 months had cognitive impairments, primarily in attention, memory, mental processing speed, and executive function.[24]

While cognitive impairments experienced by ICU survivors occur across a range of cognitive domains, studies to date have typically evaluated these domains selectively. Some studies have focused on a broad range of cognitive abilities while others have focused on the assessment of a few specific abilities. In contrast to epidemiologic studies of traumatic brain injury and dementia, which routinely use exhaustive neuropsychologic testing batteries, the batteries employed with critically ill cohorts are relatively brief, as they are designed to accommodate the fatigue so common among ICU survivors. The impaired cognitive domains in ICU survivors may depend on the nature of the insults experienced during critical illness and its treatment, as well as the presence of pre-existing neurologic abnormalities, individual vulnerabilities such as older age, or comorbid disorders that might render specific domains more vulnerable to critical illness-induced brain injury. Information regarding the extent to which cognitive domains are differentially affected in ICU survivors is very preliminary, in part because studies to date have evaluated domains very unevenly. In general, impaired memory is the most frequently observed deficit, followed by executive function and attention deficits.[35] For example, a study that assessed executive function (eg, planning, organization, behavioral inhibition, decision making, and other functions) in medical and surgical ICU survivors found executive dysfunction occurred in 35% of the patients.[27] Few studies have predominately evaluated executive dysfunction, arguably one domain important to effective daily functioning. In the few studies designed to allow such comparisons,[27] perfor- mance on measures of executive functioning is poor relative to performance on tests of other cog- nitive abilities, suggesting that brain structures, regions, and systems under-girding executive functioning may be significantly implicated in the pathogenesis of ICU-related cognitive impairment. Investigations of executive dysfunction have been brief and incomplete, despite the apparent cen- trality of this problem to functional outcomes (see "Functional implications of cognitive impair- ments," below).

DURATION OF COGNITIVE IMPAIRMENTS

In general, it appears that the majority of ICU survivors experience marked improvement in cog- nitive functioning in the first 6 to 12 months after hospital discharge. However, despite demonstrat- ing a clear trajectory of improvement, many individuals continue to demonstrate persistent neuropsychologic difficulties over time, infre- quently returning to their pre-ICU baseline levels. For example, 70% of ARDS survivors had cogni- tive impairments at hospital discharge but only 45% had cognitive impairments at 1 year. There was little improvement in cognitive sequelae from 1 to 2 years.[34] A retrospective cohort study of 46 ARDS survivors found 25% had cognitive im- pairments 6 years following ICU treatment, only 21 patients returned to full-time employment, and all patients with cognitive impairments were disabled.[31] A second study in 30 ARDS survivors found impaired memory, attention, concentration, executive dysfunction, and motor impairments as- sessed one to greater than 6 years after hospital discharge (mean 6.2 years).[26] These studies suggest that the cognitive impairments in ARDS survivors are long-lasting and are likely perma- nent. It may be that the effects of ARDS on cogni- tive functioning may be accelerated among patients with specific sorts of vulnerabilities, such as the frail elderly. The effects of ARDS on cognitive function may be particularly striking in geriatric patients with pre-existing mild cognitive impairment or dementia, as ARDS-related neuro- logic insults may serve to heighten their cognitive decline and lead to what could be characterized as an "ICU-accelerated dementia." Such a pattern (eg, medical illness accelerating the trajectory of dementia) has been observed in other populations but has not been investigated in critically ill cohorts.[36,37]

MECHANISMS OF COGNITIVE IMPAIRMENTS

It was once believed that the brain was protected from most insults because of the existence of the blood-brain barrier and central autoregulation. It is now recognized that the brain is immunologi- cally active and therefore vulnerable to systemic inflammatory reactions, such as those resulting from sepsis or septic shock, similar to the findings in severe systemic illness. The inflammatory re- sponses are mediated by cytokines, nonantibody proteins that penetrate the blood-brain barrier di- rectly or indirectly to modulate and influence brain activity and potentially alter neurotransmitter re- lease.[38] Studies have shown that increased levels of biologic markers of inflammation, including in- terleukin-6 and tumor necrosis factor-α predict the development of cognitive impairments among older patients without acute illness.[39,40] However, there is probably not a single uniform cause of cognitive impairments but rather a number of more or less significant factors that interact dy- namically with premorbid and genetic variables, resulting in adverse outcomes. Other implicated mechanisms of brain injury include hypoxemia,[23] hyperglycemia,[41] delirium,[14] hypotension,[25] and the use of sedatives or analgesics.[42] The mecha- nisms of neurologic dysfunction are likely multifac- torial in nature and should be the subject of future research studies.

FUNCTIONAL IMPLICATIONS OF COGNITIVE IMPAIRMENTS

While knowledge regarding cognitive morbidity following critical illness is increasing, few studies have assessed the impact of cognitive impair- ments on patients' functional outcomes. The func- tional effects of cognitive impairments may be far reaching, including permanent disability or inability to return to work. Cognitive impairments can ren- der individuals unable to perform basic activities of daily living (ADLs), such as feeding, dressing, and bathing. Declines in instrumental activities of daily living (IADLs), which involve higher order functional abilities such as preparing meals and managing money, also occur especially in individ- uals with more severe cognitive deficits. **Table 1** describes several widely used questionnaires used to assess IADLs.

In a study of 2-year outcomes in ARDS survi- vors, nearly one-third of ARDS survivors were un- employed or had permanently left the workforce 2 years after hospital discharge.[34] In survivors of critical illness, 50% were unable to return to work, primarily because of the effects of cognitive impairment 6 years after ICU treatment.[31]

Table 1
Instrumental activities of daily living questionnaires

Test: IADL Questionnaires	Reference	Description	Administration Time	Number of Items	Cut-off Score	Comment
Older Americans Resource and Services Activities of Daily Living	Fillenbaum & Smyer, 1984[78]	Popular measure that assesses functional capacity in geriatric patients	10 minutes	7	?	**Pro:** Widely used in research and has strong psychometric properties **Con:** Relatively long and lacks clinical utility
Functional Activities Questionnaire	Pfeffer et al, 1982[79]	Informant based measure of high-order functional abilities	5 minutes	10	Score greater than 9 suggests the presence of dementia	**Pro:** Effective at distinguishing between dementia and normal aging **Con:** Scores are based on the perceptions of an informant and could be inaccurate
Lawton's IADL	Lawton, 1969[80]	Widely used measure of IADLs validated for use in elderly populations	5 minutes	8	Positive scores on four items—telephone use, transportation, medication management, and handling finances—correlate with diagnosis of dementia	**Pro:** Validated for use in elderly populations **Con:** Research on using Lawton's IADL as a dementia screening tool is equivocal.

Relatively little is known about the specific impact of cognitive impairments, secondary to critical illness, on important daily activities such as balancing a checkbook, following written directions, and complying with complex medication regimes, among other tasks. Research in other populations suggests that even mild cognitive impairments can lead to significant deficits in the completion of IADLs, such as driving and money management.[43,44] For example, in individuals with dementia and significant cognitive impairments, the cognitive impairments lead to changes in the ability to perform ADLs.[45]

As stated above, executive dysfunction is common in ICU survivors. Among many non-ICU medical, geriatric, and psychiatric populations, the functional correlates of executive dysfunction have been widely studied, with evidence documenting often robust associations between executive dysfunction, quality of life, and functional decrements.[46–50] Such findings are logically consistent in light of the fact that, at their most elemental level, higher order activities of daily living require capacities in areas such as planning, organization, and the generation of flexible and efficient strategies, all of which are limited by executive dysfunction.

Executive dysfunction in otherwise healthy elderly individuals is a harbinger of decreasing personal independence and is a risk factor for needing formal health care.[51,52] **Box 1** shows the adverse outcomes associated with executive dysfunction. Executive dysfunction contributes to an inability to effectively solve everyday problems[51] and effectively manage financial tasks, and predicts financial mismanagement better than overall cognitive impairment.[53,54] Executive dysfunction explains over 50% of the variance in the ability to provide informed consent and is a robust predictor of poor medication adherence, even in the absence of complex medication regimes.[55–57] Furthermore, executive dysfunction is related to the inability to successfully use certain medical devices, such as inhalers.[58] Executive dysfunction has consistently been identified as the most reliable neuropsychologic indicator of poor employment outcome after traumatic brain injury, and is associated with reduced occupational attainment and an inability to engage in complex workplace tasks.[59] In psychiatric and specific chronically ill populations, executive dysfunction is associated with problematic work behaviors as well as unemployment.[60,61]

Several studies have explored functional status in ICU survivors. In the largest study conducted to date (with a sample of 444 elderly survivors of critical illness), Vazquez Mata and colleagues[62]

Box 1
Adverse outcomes associated with executive dysfunction

Independent living/functioning deficits
- Decreased independence
- Greater levels of care
- Financial mismanagement

Poor health-care management
- Poor medication adherence
- Resistance to care
- Inability to use medical devices

Employment difficulties
- Unemployment
- Under-employment
- Poor work behavior

Impaired social functioning
- Interpersonal conflict
- Social maladjustment

Reduced quality of life

---

found the greatest decrease after ICU in functional abilities in medication management, mobility and dependence, work, and fine motor control. In an investigation of 240 elderly ICU survivors, Udekwu and colleagues[63] had a significant decrease in average functional levels at follow-up, although few patients were judged to be completely dependent. A recent investigation of 75 elderly (>70 years) patients found significant reduction in the ability to perform ADLs in all domains except for feeding.[64] These patients were assessed at a mean of 557 days after ICU discharge and had likely recovered from any transient decrements related to ICU-related physical debilitation. Among middle-aged trauma ICU survivors, Jackson and colleagues[65] found that nearly one in four (22%) trauma ICU survivors were impaired in instrumental activities of daily living (as measured by the Functional Activities Questionnaire), with particular problems in areas such as employment, managing financial or business affairs, and traveling or making travel arrangements. Additional research of functional decrements after critical illness and the degree to which they are related to the effects of cognitive impairment is needed to understand the full impact of these impairments on patients' lives. The study of functional decrements after critical illness and the degree to which they are related to the effects of cognitive impairment is a key component of a thorough research agenda.

ASSESSMENT OF PRE-ILLNESS COGNITIVE FUNCTION

Perhaps the one of the most methodologically challenging issue in the study of cognitive outcomes in ICU survivors is the assessment of premorbid neuropsychologic functioning.[66] As critically ill patients typically experience an acute onset of illness, it is rarely possible to evaluate them before hospitalization. Therefore, methods of estimating pre-illness cognitive functioning must be employed, especially because many patients have multiple comorbid chronic medical disorders. Assessment methods vary widely but generally rely on the use of information derived from surrogate evaluations. A number of brief surrogate-based screening tools designed to evaluate the presence or absence of cognitive impairment have been developed. These tools—originally designed for use with geriatric cohorts—have been widely used with medical populations including critically ill patients. The most prominent instruments in this category include the IQCODE and the AD-8.[67,68] The IQCODE short form (IQCODE-SF) consists of a total of 16 questions pertaining to the degree of change occurring over a 3-year period in cognitive and functional abilities of various kinds.[69] The AD-8 consists of eight similar questions, and it has the advantage of being validated with both surrogates and individual patients.

Another way to assess pre-illness cognitive function is through structured clinical interviews, which are often employed in the evaluation of patients with mild cognitive impairment, Alzheimer's disease (AD), and related dementias. These structured clinical interviews—notably, the Clinical Dementia Rating Scale (CDR)—are considered in many quarters to be gold standard diagnostic tools. The CDR was designed to be administered to both a patient and their surrogate, with a rating derived from information gleaned from both parties. However, the CDR can be employed using only the surrogate assessment form. While there are inherent limitations associated with this approach, it offers a degree of comprehensiveness that other surrogate evaluation tools lack, as well as the ability to rate patients according to cognitive impairment stages: CDR scores range from 0 (normal) to 3 (severe dementia).

Few instruments exist to assess pre-existing cognitive functioning in individual neuropsychologic domains, although recent efforts have been made to develop domain-specific clinical interviews. One of the most widely used in this regard is the Behavior Rating Inventory of Executive Function—Adult Version (BRIEF-A),[70] a standardized self-report measure that captures the views of adults and their surrogates of executive functioning in nine areas (inhibit, shift, emotional control, self-monitor, initiate, working memory, plan/organize, task monitor, and organization of materials). Recent evidence suggests that executive functioning is among the most common cognitive abilities to be effected as a result of critical illness. As such, it may be particularly important to identify the degree to which executive abilities are normal or abnormal at the time of hospital enrollment.

COGNITIVE REHABILITATION AND FOLLOW-UP CLINICS

ICU survivors not only demonstrate high rates of cognitive impairment as measured by neuropsychologic testing, but they also subjectively report the presence of diminished cognitive abilities, as well as persistent difficulties with memory, concentration, and planning and organizing. Cognitive impairments appear to be under-recognized by both ICU and rehabilitation providers. In non-ICU clinical settings, physicians fail to recognize (or assess) cognitive impairment in 35% to 90% of patients.[71] Cognitive impairments are rarely evaluated in critically ill patients and may be overlooked in one of every two cases.[72] This may be partly because the manifestations of cognitive impairment are often subtle and because patients may experience cognitive impairment in select domains, even if they are alert, oriented, and generally cognitively intact. Thus, few patients are referred for cognitive rehabilitation. A recent study found that 42% of ARDS survivors underwent rehabilitation therapy, but most were not evaluated for cognitive impairments and only 12% were identified as having cognitive impairments by the clinical rehabilitation team.[34]

Rehabilitation studies show that exercise regimes and psychologic interventions improve recovery as well as quality of life after a variety of medical conditions, including cardiac disease[73,74] and chronic and obstructive pulmonary disease.[75] Jones and colleagues[76] assessed the effectiveness of a rehabilitation program following critical illness to aid physical and psychologic recovery. Survivors were randomized to control and intervention, with the intervention group receiving a 6-week self-help rehabilitation manual. The intervention group had improved physical function and a trend to lower depression, compared with controls. Thus, rehabilitation with something as simple as a self-help manual was effective in aiding physical recovery and reducing depression in critically ill survivors.[76] To the authors' knowledge, there are no studies that have assessed the effectiveness of cognitive rehabilitation among medical ICU survivors.

Unfortunately, referrals for cognitive rehabilitation are rarely dealt with in any systematic way. In the current model of care-provision, patients often return to health care providers unrelated to those that provided life-saving treatment, with continuity of care only rarely maintained. Thus, primary care providers and sub-specialists that ICU survivors see upon their return home may lack the necessary context required to fully understand the array of new (or worsening) cognitive and emotional complaints expressed. In those situations, in which local physicians are concerned enough to make referrals, such referrals are hindered by the lack of availability of geriatric specialists, neuropsychologists, and others, particularly in rural or outlying areas. Together, these factors conspire to help ensure that individuals with brain injuries or significant emotional distress frequently fail to receive the treatment and interventions they need.

Increased identification of cognitive impairment in ICU survivors may benefit patients by increasing referrals to rehabilitation specialists, neuropsychologists, speech and language therapists, and other health care providers who can provide interventions, such as cognitive remediation. Against this backdrop, the need for the development of clinics designed to address the unique problems experienced by patients following critical illness is clear (such clinics are increasingly common fixtures on the health care landscape in parts of Europe,[77] but remain virtually nonexistent in North America). One principle purpose of such clinics should be to assess the nature and severity of the cognitive and emotional difficulties that are virtually ubiquitous among ICU survivors. This is beneficial for all parties, including and primarily for the patient, as it provides a valuable source of support and an opportunity to gain a deeper understanding of their condition, and to begin to develop realistic expectations about the probable natural history of their cognitive impairment or emotional distress.

SUMMARY

The significant and sometimes permanent effects of critical illness on cognitive functioning are increasingly recognized, so that a virtual consensus now exists among the intensive care community regarding the importance of this issue. Since the presence of cognitive impairment among medical ICU survivors was first systematically identified a decade or so ago, much progress has been made to study and better characterize this phenomenon. In the intervening years, we have learned that cognitive impairment is highly prevalent and functionally disruptive, and that it occurs in wide-ranging domains. Key questions remain unanswered with regard to vital questions, such as determining causes, risk factors, and mechanisms, as well as the degree to which brain injuries associated with critical illness are amenable to rehabilitation. Little remains known about the effects of critical illness on elderly ICU cohorts and on the neurologic functioning of individuals with pre-existing impairment versus those who are normal. Few data exist regarding the development of strategies designed to prevent the emergence of neuropsychologic deficits following critical illness. While great progress has been made and is ongoing, a pressing need exists for additional investigation of cognitive impairment following critical illness that will seek to untangle the many pertinent questions related to this condition, and which will ultimately offer help and hope to the thousands of survivors affected by this condition.

REFERENCES

1. Meagher DJ. Delirium: optimising management. Br Med J 2001;322(7279):144–9.
2. Pandharipande PP, Pun BT, Herr DL, et al. Effect of sedation with dexmedetomidine vs lorazepam on acute brain dysfunction in mechanically ventilated patients: the MENDS randomized controlled trial. JAMA 2007;298(22):2644–53.
3. Koponen H, Hurri L, Stenback U, et al. Computed tomography findings in delirium. J Nerv Ment Dis 1989;177(4):226–31.
4. Suchyta MR, Jephson A, Hopkins RO. Brain MR and CT findings associated with critical illness. Proc Am Thorac Soc 2005;2(1):A46.
5. Lipowski ZJ. Delirium in the elderly patient. N Engl J Med 1989;320(9):578–82.
6. Galanakis P, Bickel H, Gradinger R, et al. Acute confusional state in the elderly following hip surgery: Incidence, risk factors and complications. Int J Geriatr Psychiatry 2001;16(4):349–55.
7. O'Keefe ST, Chonchubhair AN. Postoperative delirium in the elderly. Br J Anaesth 1994;73:673–87.
8. Ely EW, Inouye SK, Bernard GR, et al. Delirium in mechanically ventilated patients: validity and reliability of the confusion assessment method for the intensive care unit (CAM-ICU). JAMA 2001; 286(21):2703–10.
9. Ely EW, Shintani A, Truman B, et al. Delirium as a predictor of mortality in mechanically ventilated patients in the intensive care unit. JAMA 2004;291(14):1753–62.
10. Inouye SK, Rushing JT, Foreman MD, et al. Does delirium contribute to poor hospital outcomes?

A three-site epidemiologic study. J Gen Intern Med 1998;13(4):234–42.

11. Second International Study of Infarct Survival. Randomised trial of intravenous streptokinase, oral aspirin, both, or neither among 17,187 cases of suspected acute myocardial infarction: ISIS-2. Lancet 1988;2: 349–60.

12. Uldall KK, Ryan R, Berghuis JP, et al. Association between delirium and death in AIDS patients. Aids Patient Care STDS 2000;14(2):95–100.

13. Eikelenboom P, Hoogendijk WJ. Do delirium and Alzheimer's dementia share specific pathogenetic mechanisms? Dement Geriatr Cogn Disord 1999; 10(5):319–24.

14. Jackson JC, Gordon SM, Hart RP, et al. The association between delirium and cognitive decline: a review of the empirical literature. Neuropsychol Rev 2004;14(2):87–98.

15. Dolan MM, Hawkes WG, Zimmerman SI, et al. Delirium on hospital admission in aged hip fracture patients: prediction of mortality and 2-year functional outcomes. J Gerontol A Biol Sci Med Sci 2001; 55A(9):M527–34.

16. Lawton MP, Brody EM. Assessment of older people: self-maintaining and instrumental activities of daily living. Gerontologist 1969;9(3):179–86.

17. Francis J, Kapoor WN. Prognosis after hospital discharge of older medical patients with delirium. J Am Geriatr Soc 1992;40(6):601–6.

18. McCusker J, Cole M, Dendukuri N, et al. Delirium in older medical inpatients and subsequent cognitive and functional status: a prospective study. Can Med Assoc J 2001;165(5):575.

19. Rahkonen T, Eloniemi-Sulkava U, Halonen P, et al. Delirium in the non-demented oldest old in the general population: risk factors and prognosis. Int J Geriatr Psychiatry 2001;16(4):415–21.

20. Rockwood K, Cosway S, Carver D, et al. The risk of dementia and death after delirium. Age Ageing 1999;28(6):551–6.

21. Koponen H, Stenback U, Mattila E, et al. Delirium among elderly persons admitted to a psychiatric hospital: clinical course during the acute stage and one-year follow-up. Acta Psychiatr Scand 1989;79(6):579–85.

22. Jackson JC, Hart RP, Gordon SM, et al. Six-month neuropsychological outcome of medical intensive care unit patients. Crit Care Med 2003;31(4): 1226–34.

23. Hopkins RO, Weaver LK, Pope D, et al. Neuropsychological sequelae and impaired health status in survivors of severe acute respiratory distress syndrome. Am J Respir Crit Care Med 1999;160(1):50–6.

24. Hopkins RO, Jackson JC, Wallace CJ. Neurocognitive impairments in ICU patients with prolonged mechanical ventilation. International Neuropsychological Society Meeting, St. Louis, MI, 2005.

25. Hopkins RO, Weaver LK, Chan KJ, et al. Quality of life, emotional, and cognitive function following acute respiratory distress syndrome. J Int Neuropsychol Soc 2004;10(7):1005–17.

26. Suchyta MR, Hopkins RO, White J, et al. The incidence of cognitive dysfunction after ARDS. Am J Respir Crit Care Med 2004;169(7):A18.

27. Sukantarat KT, Burgess PW, Williamson RC, et al. Prolonged cognitive dysfunction in survivors of critical illness. Anaesthesia 2005;60(9):847–53.

28. Marquis K, Curtis J, Caldwell E, et al. Neuropsychological sequelae in survivors of ARDS compared with critically ill control patients. Am J Respir Crit Care Med 2000;161:A383.

29. Al-Saidi F, McAndrews MP, Cheung AM, et al. Neuropsychological sequelae in ARDS survivors. Am J Respir Crit Care Med 2003;167(7):A737.

30. Jackson JC, Gordon SM, Burger C, et al. Acute respiratory distress syndrome and long-term cognitive impairment: A case study. Arch Clin Neuropsychol 2003;18(7):688.

31. Rothenhäusler HB, Ehrentraut S, Stoll C, et al. The relationship between cognitive performance and employment and health status in long-term survivors of the acute respiratory distress syndrome: Results of an exploratory study. Gen Hosp Psychiatry 2001;23(2):90–6.

32. Christie JD, Biester RC, Taichman DB, et al. Formation and validation of a telephone battery to assess cognitive function in acute respiratory distress syndrome survivors. J Crit Care 2006; 21(2):125–32.

33. Jones C, Griffiths RD, Slater T, et al. Significant cognitive dysfunction in non-delirious patients identified during and persisting following critical illness. Intensive Care Med 2006;32(6):923–6.

34. Hopkins RO, Weaver LK, Collingridge D, et al. Two-year cognitive, emotional, and quality-of-life outcomes in acute respiratory distress syndrome. Am J Respir Crit Care Med 2005;171(4):340–7.

35. Hopkins RO, Jackson JC. Long-term neurocognitive function after critical illness. Chest 2006; 130(3):869–78.

36. Lee TA, Wolozin B, Weiss KB, et al. Assessment of the emergence of Alzheimer's disease following coronary artery bypass graft surgery or percutaneous transluminal coronary angioplasty. J Alzheimers Dis 2005;7(4):319–24.

37. Lyketsos CG, Lopez O, Jones B, et al. Prevalence of neuropsychiatric symptoms in dementia and mild cognitive impairment: Results from the cardiovascular health study. JAMA 2002;288(12):1475–83.

38. Marshall JC. Inflammation, coagulopathy, and the pathogenesis of multiple organ dysfunction syndrome. Crit Care Med 2001;29(7 Suppl):S99–106.

39. Teunissen CE, van Boxtel MP, Bosma H, et al. Inflammation markers in relation to cognition in a healthy

aging population. J Neuroimmunol 2003;134(1–2): 142–50.

40. Yaffe K, Lindquist K, Penninx BW, et al. Inflammatory markers and cognition in well-functioning African-American and white elders. Neurology 2003;61(1): 76–80.

41. Hopkins RO, Suchyta MR, Jephson A, et al. Hyperglycemia and neurocognitive outcome in ARDS survivors. Proc Am Thorac Soc 2005;2(1):A36.

42. Starr JL, Whalley LJ. Drug induced dementia. Drug Saf 1994;11:310–7.

43. Griffith HR, Belue K, Sicola A, et al. Impaired financial abilities in mild cognitive impairment: a direct assessment approach. Neurology 2003;60:449–57.

44. Nygard L. Instrumental activities of daily living: a stepping stone towards Alzheimer's disease diagnosis in subjects with mild cognitive impairment? Acta Neurol Scand 2003;179:542–6.

45. Wadley VG, Crowe M, Marsiske M, et al. Changes in everyday function in individuals with psychometrically defined mild cognitive impairment in the advanced cognitive training for independent and vital elderly study. J Am Geriatr Soc 2007;55(8):1192–8.

46. Boyle PA, Cohen RA, Paul R, et al. Cognitive and motor impairments predict functional declines in patients with vascular dementia. Int J Geriatr Psychiatry 2002;17(2):164–9.

47. Boyle PA, Malloy PF, Salloway S, et al. Executive dysfunction and apathy predict functional impairment in Alzheimer disease. Am J Geriatr Psychiatry 2003;11(2):214–21.

48. Boyle PA, Paul RH, Moser DJ, et al. Executive impairments predict functional declines in vascular dementia. Clin Neuropsychol 2004;18(1):75–82.

49. Cahn-Weiner DA, Boyle PA, Malloy PF. Tests of executive function predict instrumental activities of daily living in community-dwelling older individuals. Appl Neuropsychol 2002;9(3):187–91.

50. Royall DR, Cabello M, Polk MJ. Executive dyscontrol: an important factor affecting the level of care received by older retirees. J Am Geriatr Soc 1998; 46(12):1519–24.

51. Burton CL, Strauss E, Hultsch DF, et al. Cognitive functioning and everyday problem solving in older adults. Clin Neuropsychol 2006;20(3):432–52.

52. Royall DR, Chiodo LK, Polk MJ. Correlates of disability among elderly retirees with "subclinical" cognitive impairment. J Gerontol A Biol Sci Med Sci 2007;55: M541–6.

53. Spinella M, Yang B, Lester D. Prefrontal system dysfunction and credit card debt. Int J Neurosci 2004; 114(10):1323–32.

54. Van Wielingen LE, Tuokko HA, Cramer K, et al. Awareness of financial skills in dementia. Aging Ment Health 2004;8(4):374–80.

55. Heaton RK, Marcotte TD, Mindt MR, et al. The impact of HIV-associated neuropsychological impairment on everyday functioning. J Int Neuropsychol Soc 2004;10(3):317–21.

56. Hinkin CH, Castellon SA, Durvasula RS, et al. Medication adherence among HIV+ adults: effects of cognitive dysfunction and regimen complexity. Neurology 2002;59(12):1944–50.

57. Insel K, Morrow D, Brewer B, et al. Executive function, working memory, and medication adherence among older adults. J Gerontol B Psychol Sci Soc Sci 2006;61(2):P102–7.

58. Allen SC, Jain M, Ragab S, et al. Acquisition and short-term retention of inhaler techniques require intact executive function in elderly subjects. Age Ageing 2003;32(3):299–302.

59. Biederman J, Petty C, Fried R, et al. Impact of psychometrically defined deficits of executive functioning in adults with attention deficit hyperactivity disorder. Am J Psychiatry 2006;163(10): 1730–8.

60. Evans JD, Bond GR, Meyer PS, et al. Cognitive and clinical predictors of success in vocational rehabilitation in schizophrenia. Schizophr Res 2004; 70(2–3):331–42.

61. McGurk SR, Mueser KT. Cognitive and clinical predictors of work outcomes in clients with schizophrenia receiving supported employment services: 4-year follow-up. Adm Policy Ment Health 2006; 33(5):598–606.

62. Vazquez Mata G, Rivera Fernandez R, Gonzalez Carmona A, et al. Factors related to quality of life 12 months after discharge from an intensive care unit. Crit Care Med 1992;20(9):1257–62.

63. Udekwu P, Gurkin B, Oller D, et al. Quality of life and functional level in elderly patients surviving surgical intensive care. J Am Coll Surg 2001; 193(3):245–9.

64. Montuclard L, Garrouste-Orgeas M, Timsit JF, et al. Outcome, functional autonomy, and quality of life of elderly patients with a long-term intensive care unit stay. Crit Care Med 2000;28(10): 3389–95.

65. Jackson JC, Obremskey W, Bauer R, et al. Long-term cognitive, emotional, and functional outcomes in trauma intensive care unit survivors without intracranial hemorrhage. J Trauma 2007; 62(1):80–8.

66. Jackson JC, Gordon SM, Ely EW, et al. Research issues in the evaluation of cognitive impairment in intensive care unit survivors. Intensive Care Med 2004;30(11):2009–16.

67. Galvin JE, Roe CM, Xiong C, et al. Validity and reliability of the AD8 informant interview in dementia. Neurology 2006;67(11):1942–8.

68. Jorm A, Scott R, Cullen J, et al. Performance of the informant questionnaire on cognitive decline in the elderly (IQCODE) as a screening test for dementia. Psychol Med 1991;21(3):785–90.

69. Jorm A, Jacomb P. The informant questionnaire on cognitive decline in the elderly (IQCODE): socio-demographic correlates, reliability, validity and some norms. Psychol Med 1989;19(4):1015–22.

70. Rabin LA, Roth RM, Isquith PK, et al. Self- and informant reports of executive function on the BRIEF-A in MCI and older adults with cognitive complaints. Arch Clin Neuropsychol 2006;21(7):721–32.

71. Callahan CM, Hendrie HC, Tierney WM. Documentation and evaluation of cognitive impairment in elderly primary care patients. Ann Intern Med 1995;122(6):422–9.

72. Wilkes MM, Navickis RJ. Patient survival after human albumin administration. A meta-analysis of randomized, controlled trials. Ann Intern Med 2001;135(3):149–64.

73. van Dixhoorn J, Duivenvoorden HJ, Staal HA, et al. Physical training and relaxation therapy in cardiac rehabilitation assessed through a composite criterion for training outcome. Am Heart J 1989;118(3):545–52.

74. Shephard RJ, Franklin B. Changes in the quality of life: A major goal of cardiac rehabilitation. J Cardiopulm Rehabil 2001;21(4):189–200.

75. Ries AL, Kaplan RM, Limberg TM, et al. Effects of pulmonary rehabilitation on physiologic and psychosocial outcomes in patients with chronic obstructive pulmonary disease. Ann Intern Med 1995;122(11):823–32.

76. Jones C, Skirrow P, Griffiths RD, et al. Rehabilitation after critical illness: A randomized, controlled trial. Crit Care Med 2003;31(10):2456–61.

77. Griffiths RD, Jones C. Seven lessons from 20 years of follow-up of intensive care unit survivors. Curr Opin Crit Care 2007;13(5):508–13.

78. Fillenbaum GG, Smyer MA. The development, validity and reliability of the OARS multidimensional functional assessment questionnaire. J Gerontol 1981;36(4):428–34.

79. Pfefer RI, Kurosaki TT Jr, Harrah CH, et al. Measurement of functional activities in older adults in the community 1982;37(3):323–9.

80. Brody MP, Jones EM. Assessment of older people: self-maintaining and instrumental activities of daily living. Gerontologist 1969;9(3):179–86.

Critical Care Outcomes in the Hematologic Transplant Recipient

John R. McArdle, MD

KEYWORDS

- Bone marrow transplantation • Stem cell transplantation
- Critical illness • Respiratory failure
- Multiorgan system failure • Mechanical ventilation

Bone marrow and peripheral blood stem cell transplantation provide the possibility of cure for a variety of hematologic malignancies and select nonmalignant diseases with otherwise poor prognoses. An estimated 50,000 to 60,000 such transplants were performed worldwide in 2006. An overwhelming majority of these transplants were performed because of hematologic malignancies, with a small minority of procedures performed because of nonmalignant conditions.[1] While such transplantations frequently prove life saving, substantial morbidity and mortality accompany the administration of this therapy, frequently resulting in serious complications for the recipient. Critical illness may result from a host of different complications, including toxicities related to the conditioning regimen or immunosuppressants, infection, graft-versus-host disease (GVHD), or recurrence of the underlying malignancy.[2] Intensive care unit (ICU) admission is necessary to manage such complications in a substantial number of these patients, with a wide variation in this number across series from under 10% to greater than 50%.[3–14]

Initial reports examining ICU outcome in recipients of bone marrow transplantation (BMT) or stem cell transplantation (SCT) suggest poor prognosis for short- and long-term survival.[6,15–17] Over the ensuing years, there have been significant changes in the management of patients prior to and during BMT. The use of peripheral blood as the source of stem cells has resulted in shorter duration of neutropenia. Prophylactic antimicrobial therapy has rendered many of the most worrisome infectious complications less common.[2] Evolving management strategies for GVHD may result in shorter duration of skin and mucosal breakdown. In certain populations, the pretransplant conditioning regimen is reduced, potentially diminishing the degree of regimen-related organ dysfunction. Since the initial reports on ICU outcome for hematologic transplant recipients, and concomitant with changes in the practice of transplantation, significant changes have come about in the management of such common ICU diagnoses, like severe sepsis and acute respiratory distress syndrome.

The evolution of the fields of transplantation science and ICU management may each be changing the landscape for what can be expected in the ICU care of hematologic transplant recipients. At the same time, a clear understanding of prognostic features predicting poor outcome may be of use to avoid undue discomfort for the patient and loved ones and appropriate allocation of ICU resources. This article describes the current understanding of ICU treatment and outcome of BMT and SCT patients suffering from critical illness.

CAUSES OF CRITICAL ILLNESS POST–BONE MARROW TRANSPLANTATION

Complications arising from BMT or SCT may make an impact on a variety of organs, with the spectrum of illnesses varying during different stages of the transplantation process. The conditioning

Section of Pulmonary and Critical Care Medicine, Department of Medicine, Yale University School of Medicine, 333 Cedar Street, P.O. Box 208057, New Haven, CT 06073, USA
E-mail address: john.mcardle@yale.edu

Clin Chest Med 30 (2009) 155–167
doi:10.1016/j.ccm.2008.10.002
0272-5231/08/$ – see front matter © 2009 Elsevier Inc. All rights reserved.

chestmed.theclinics.com

phase refers to the pretransplant period, during which patients receive chemotherapy, with or without total body irradiation,[2] for the purpose of cytoreduction of malignant cells and suppression or ablation of the patient's marrow. This is followed by return of hematopoietic stem cells, which may be harvested from bone marrow, peripheral blood, or umbilical cord. The third stage is engraftment, or return of a neutrophil count greater than 0.5×10^9/L and platelet count greater than 20×10^9/L without transfusion support for 3 consecutive days.[2] The time lapse between infusion of stem cells and engraftment is greater for bone marrow–derived stem cells than for peripheral blood–derived stem cells (median 21 days for BMT vs 14 days for peripheral blood–derived SCT),[18] leading to a longer duration of neutropenia and its associated infectious complications. While neutrophil counts may return to normal during the engraftment period, there remain abnormalities in lymphocyte number and function and immunoglobulin levels for months posttransplant.[2]

Posttransplant complications often mirror the status of the patient's immune reconstitution, with the first phase lasting for roughly the first 30 days posttransplant, during which complications related to acute toxicity of the conditioning regimen and prolonged neutropenia dominate. The second phase marks ongoing deficiencies in cell-mediated and humoral immunity, and persists out to roughly 100 days posttransplant. After day 100, immunity is more completely reconstituted, and the spectrum of complications is more likely to be related to GVHD, chronic toxicities of the conditioning or immunosuppressive regimens, or disease relapse.[19] Several of the more common disease processes leading to critical illness are outlined in **Table 1**.

PATIENT OUTCOMES AND FACTORS INFLUENCING OUTCOMES IN ADULT PATIENTS

The perception of futility as it relates to critical care in the hematologic transplant population stems from the observed patient outcomes in early series of BMT patients with critical illness. Crawford and colleagues[6] reported that among BMT patients requiring mechanical ventilation for respiratory failure, only 3% survived for 6 months beyond ICU admission. Paz and colleagues[12] reported similar results in their retrospective cohort of 36 patients requiring ICU admission post-BMT. The overall mortality in their cohort was 77.4%. However, among patients requiring mechanical ventilation, only 1 of 27 (2.7%) patients survived their ICU stay. There was no significant difference in outcome between those receiving an allogeneic as compared with an autologous transplant.[12] Likewise, a retrospective series of patients undergoing BMT from the Mayo Clinic demonstrated a mortality of 87% among patients who went to the ICU for reasons other than postsurgical recovery.[4] Of the patients requiring mechanical ventilation, mortality was 93%, and those with dysfunction of more than two organ systems demonstrated 100% mortality. Acute Physiology and Chronic Health Evaluation II (APACHE II) scoring were noted to underestimate the mortality in this cohort of patients.

Rubenfeld and Crawford[17] furthered our understanding of the factors associated with outcome in BMT recipients, performing a retrospective, nested case control study in which they evaluated the 53 survivors among their 865 mechanically ventilated BMT recipients between 1980 and 1992. They compared the survivors with 106 non-survivors matched for year of transplantation to identify variables associated with a poor outcome. In this cohort, they found that combinations of risk factors reflecting organ dysfunction were associated with increased mortality. The investigators defined acute lung injury as those patients requiring a fractional inspired oxygen content greater than 60% or positive end expiratory pressure greater than 5 cm H_2O after the first 24 hours of ventilation. Hepatic failure was defined as a serum bilirubin level greater than 4 mg/dL during the first 3 days of mechanical ventilation, and renal failure was defined as a serum creatinine level of greater than 2 mg/dL during this same time period. Vasopressor use was used as a surrogate for hemodynamic instability and was defined as any use of norepinephrine, epinephrine, phenylephrine, or dopamine at doses greater than 5 µg/kg/min for more than 4 hours in any 24-hour period. Among patients with acute lung injury and either (1) hepatic and renal failure or (2) the requirement for vasopressors for more than 4 hours, there were no survivors. The investigators concluded that this ability to predict futility within 4 days of the initiation of mechanical ventilation could be used to diminish the application of costly and invasive ICU procedures and therapies. An interesting sidebar in this series was the finding that the survival-to-discharge ratio in the cohort of BMT patients undergoing mechanical ventilation increased at the investigators' institution from 5% in the period from 1980 to 1987 to 16% from 1988 through the first half of 1992, though remained 0% in those with the above-mentioned combinations of risk factors. The loose definitions of hepatic and renal failure used in this study have been criticized as not truly indicative of acute organ failure, but the dramatic impact on mortality in this series lends credence to the idea that

Table 1
Common reasons for intensive care unit admission in hematologic transplant recipients

Reason for ICU Admission	Unique Features Related to Condition	Management Principles
Respiratory		
Pulmonary edema	Fluid loading, cardiotoxicity, and capillary leak related to conditioning therapy may lead to this condition, particularly in early posttransplant period	Diuresis; hemofiltration, if necessary; mechanical ventilation; prognosis favorable
Diffuse alveolar hemorrhage	Increasing bloody return, >20% hemosiderin-laden macrophages on bronchoalveolar lavage, total body irradiation, and intensive conditioning regimen are predispositions	Mechanical ventilation; correction of bleeding diathesis; high-dose steroids (controlled data lacking)
Infectious pneumonia	Bacterial and fungal pathogens most common during neutropenic phase; viruses and pneumocystis increase in frequency postengraftment	Prophylactic antifungal and antiviral therapy during most susceptible periods; empiric broad-spectrum therapy for prospective pathogens; bronchoalveolar lavage and adjunctive diagnostic techniques for viruses
Idiopathic pneumonia syndrome	Presence of widespread alveolar injury in absence of infectious agent; requires exclusion of infection with bronchoalveolar lavage	Corticosteroid and etanercept therapy may be helpful; high mortality
Shock		
Sepsis		Empiric broad-spectrum antibiotic therapy; fluid management/early goal-directed therapy
Hemorrhagic		Resuscitation and platelet and coagulation factor support; local management of bleeding source
Cardiogenic		Drainage of hemodynamically significant pericardial effusions; inotropic support; antiarrhythmic therapy as warranted
Neurologic complications		
Seizures related to busulfan calcineurin inhibitors	Pericardial effusions, rhythm disorders, or cardiac pump dysfunction	Antiseizure therapy
Intracranial hemorrhage	May benefit from phenytoin prophylaxis during therapy	Dose adjustment; consider alternative therapy; control hypertension
Iatrogenic multisystem diseases	Close monitoring of serum levels; dose adjustment of cyclosporine	Control of hypertension; correction of platelet and coagulation abnormalities; consideration of surgical evacuation if feasible
Veno-occlusive disease	Prophylactic ursodiol and heparin may reduce incidence; meticulous monitoring of fluid balance, bilirubin levels	Drug reversal; adjust dose of sedatives
GVHD	Frequent examination of skin; monitoring of liver function tests, gastrointestinal, and pulmonary symptoms with biopsy to guide diagnosis	Immunosuppression with corticosteroids, mycophenolic acid, monoclonal antibody therapy for immunomodulation; photopheresis may be beneficial

Adapted from Martin PL. To stop or not to stop: How much support should be provided to mechanically ventilated pediatric bone marrow and stem cell transplant patients? Respir Care Clin N Am 2006;12(3):403–9; with permission.

even relatively modest dysfunction of multiple organ systems is important prognostically.[17]

As had been suggested by the finding of improved survival among patients cared for in the latter years of Rubenfeld and Crawford's series, there has been a significant change in patient survival in series published in the past 10 years as compared with the prior decade (**Table 2**). Afessa and colleagues[3] published a retrospective cohort study of 112 SCT recipients requiring ICU care between April 1996 and December 2000. While they noted that organ failure, sepsis, the need for invasive mechanical ventilation, and use of vasopressors conferred higher mortality, significant minorities of such patients achieved 30-day survival (26% of those requiring invasive mechanical ventilation, 35% of those with multiorgan failure, and 19% of those requiring vasoactive medications). Among their entire cohort, the 30-day mortality was 52%, reflecting substantial gains as compared with prior series, including one published from the same institution. Similarly, Jackson and colleagues[9] published their experience over 6 years in 116 BMT patients requiring ICU care between 1988 and 1993, and found that 23% survived to hospital discharge, including 17% of those requiring mechanical ventilation. The need for mechanical ventilation, vasopressor use, and earlier year of transplantation were associated with worsened outcome.

To define whether outcomes differed after initial transplantation, Scales and colleagues[20] evaluated the outcome of critical care during hospitalizations that occurred subsequent to initial BMT. They evaluated subsequent ICU admission for 2653 patients receiving BMT between 1992 and March 2002. Of this cohort, 504 required subsequent ICU care, with an overall ICU mortality of 67%. Significantly higher mortality was associated with mechanical ventilation (87%), pulmonary artery catheterization (91%), and hemodialysis (94%).[20] The investigators found no difference in outcome related to autologous or allogeneic source or year of transplantation. No combination of factors was associated with 100% mortality.

Series predominantly retrospective in nature, such as these, run significant risk that bias may skew results. It is certainly conceivable that prior data may have led to more restrictive use of ICU beds or mechanical ventilation. This could certainly result in improvements in observed mortality when compared to results found in an earlier era. Several studies have suggested that traditional scoring systems, such as APACHE II, are less helpful among patients receiving BMT/SCT as compared with the general ICU population, tending to underestimate mortality.[4,9,21] The APACHE III scoring system, while not designed specifically for SCT patients, has been demonstrated to have improved performance characteristics, and likely reflects a more useful tool for predicting outcome in this population.[3] Several series have shown that recipients of allogeneic transplant and patients with severe GVHD fare worse during critical illness, and those receiving peripheral blood–derived SCT fare better than BMT recipients, although these results are not uniform across series.[3,22,23]

Umbilical cord blood has also served as a source of stem cells for patients requiring hematopoietic SCT given the poor availability of suitable donors for patients in need of SCT. Little data is available on the ICU outcomes of patients receiving umbilical cord blood SCT. Naeem and colleagues[10] published their experience with 44 adult patients and found that 57% required ICU transfer, most commonly in the first 90 days after transplantation, with mortality (72%) comparable to that observed in prior series of BMT and peripheral blood–derived SCT patients. ICU needs were noted to be more likely in patients receiving a myeloablative preparative regimen and less likely in those receiving a higher number of infused nucleated cells. The high use of ICU resources early in the posttransplant period may be related to the prolonged time to marrow recovery as compared with BMT or peripheral blood–derived SCT.

A careful review of the literature surrounding ICU outcomes of adult BMT/SCT recipients demonstrates that predicting mortality with 100% certainty remains quite difficult. Most series would suggest that the need for vasopressors, the need for mechanical ventilation, and the failure of multiple organs are associated with a particularly grim prognosis. Decisions regarding the utility of critical care in individual patients can be more difficult given the lack of prognostic certainty. The available literature can be helpful in defining groups particularly unlikely to survive, allowing more informed patient, family, and physician discussion of the appropriateness or desirability of critical care.

PATIENT OUTCOMES AND FACTORS INFLUENCING OUTCOMES IN PEDIATRIC PATIENTS

Early series describing ICU outcome among pediatric patients focused primarily on those BMT patients with respiratory failure. Todd and colleagues[24] presented their experience with 54 pediatric patients requiring mechanical ventilation after BMT. The overall mortality in this cohort was 89%, with 100% mortality noted in those with multiple organ system failure (MOSF) or leukemia as the

Table 2
Selected series of intensive care unit outcome in adult bone marrow transplant and stem cell transplant recipients

Investigators	Year Published	Number of Patients	Mortality	Factors Influencing Outcome
Torrecilla and colleagues[13]	1988	25	76%	Respiratory failure (83% mortality; if intubated >7 d, 100% mortality); ICU stay (if >10 d, 100% mortality)
Crawford and Peterson[6]	1992	348 (all mechanically ventilated)	79% ICU; 96% hospital; 97% 6 mo	Older age; active malignancy at time of transplant; HLA nonidentical transplant MOSF
Lloyd-Thomas and colleagues[16]	1988	60	22%	APACHE II >26 conferred 100% mortality; persistent malignancy, leukopenia, MOSF associated with mortality
Denardo and colleagues[15]	1989	50 patients with respiratory failure; 41 for nonsurgical reasons	95.2% mortality in nonsurgical population	Interstitial pneumonia associated with higher mortality
Afessa and colleagues[4]	1992	35	87% hospital mortality for nonsurgical patients	Mechanical ventilation (93% mortality); MOSF (100% mortality)
Paz and colleagues[12]	1993	36	77.4%	Mechanical ventilation (96.3% mortality)
Rubenfeld and Crawford[17]	1996	53 survivors, 106 nonsurvivors as controls among 865 mechanically ventilated patients	93.9%	Acute lung injury plus (1) vasopressors for >4 h or (2) hepatic and renal failure had 100% mortality
Jackson and colleagues[9]	1998	116	77%	Later year of transplant associated with improved outcome; APACHE II >45 conferred 100% mortality; increasing support (intubation, dialysis, vasopressors) associated with increased mortality
Price and colleagues[56]	1998	115	54%	Mechanical ventilation (18.8% survival); peripheral blood–derived SCT survival better than BMT survival (31% vs. 4%)
Huaringa and colleagues[21]	2000	60 (all mechanically ventilated)	82% ICU mortality; 95% 6-mo mortality	GVHD predicted worse outcome; onset of respiratory failure >30 d posttransplant and mechanical ventilation >14 d predicted worse outcome
Afessa and colleagues[3]	2003	112	33% ICU; 46% hospital; 52% 30 d	Allogeneic transplant, APACHE III score, invasive mechanical ventilation, vasopressors, sepsis, and organ failure associated with mortality
Kew and colleagues[57]	2006	38	62.2% ICU; 78.4% 12 mo	Vasopressor use associated with 95% mortality at 30 d and 100% at 12 mo

Abbreviation: MOSF, multiorgan system failure.

underlying diagnosis. Bojko and colleagues[25] documented the outcome of their 43 BMT patients with hypoxemic respiratory failure over a 7-year period, 1986 to 1993. Their mortality figure of 88.4% was strikingly similar to that found in the series by Todd and colleagues. Perhaps more ominously, only 1 of their 43 patients survived past 6 months with MOSF accounting for the vast majority of ICU deaths. Seventeen of the 43 patients developed respiratory failure in the first month post-BMT, with infection comprising the largest proportion of cases.

Nichols and colleagues[26] assessed factors contributing to the development of respiratory failure among pediatric BMT recipients. Thirty-nine of their 318 patients undergoing BMT between 1978 and 1988 required ICU admission. Factors predicting the development of respiratory failure included male gender, serum creatinine concentration greater than 1.5 mg/dL, and GVHD. Of those developing respiratory failure, 91% succumbed to their illness.[26]

Although the survival numbers differ between children and adults, the improvements in survival in adult BMT/SCT recipients over the past decade are similarly noted in the pediatric literature (**Table 3**). Kache and colleagues[27] presented their outcomes for 1992 to early 2004, during which time 183 patients received BMT at their institution, and 84 of them were admitted to the ICU. From 1992 to 1999, their ICU survival was 18%, compared with 59% from 2000 to early 2004. There was no difference in severity of illness noted prior to ICU transfer. During the latter time frame, 54% of survivors remained alive at 100 days posttransplant. The majority of both populations had received allogeneic transplants, and stem cell source was not noted to be associated with differences in ICU outcome.

Diaz de Heredia and colleagues[28] reported outcomes among their cohort of 176 patients undergoing BMT (92 allogeneic, 84 autologous) between 1991 and 1995. There were 31 ICU admissions during this time, with respiratory failure and septic shock accounting for two thirds of ICU admissions. Patients with allogeneic BMT were more likely to be admitted to the ICU as compared with those receiving autologous transplant (25.7% vs 10.8%), though there was no statistically significant differences in the outcome of ICU care by source of stem cell. The investigators found that grade III-IV GVHD was a risk factor for ICU admission and conferred greater risk of death. Among patients requiring mechanical ventilation (83% of ICU patients), ICU survival was 46.2%, substantially better than that seen in earlier series. The median number of failing organs among patients in this series was three, with the relative risk of death increasing 2.7-fold for each organ failure. The 3-year survival among this cohort was 29.7%, demonstrating the possibility of long-term benefits from ICU care.[28]

Similar results have been noted by Warwick and colleagues[14] (60% of mechanically ventilated patients successfully extubated), Jacobe and colleagues[29] (41.6% of mechanically ventilated patients discharged from the ICU), and Rossi and colleagues[30] (36% survival at 6 months). The survival among pediatric ICU patients appears favorable when compared with that seen in adult patients.

Bratton and colleagues[31] used a much larger database to assess outcomes of SCT patients from multiple institutions. They used the Kids Inpatient Database, which provides data on pediatric discharges from 2500 to 3500 community hospitals in the United States. The databases from 1997, 2000, and 2003 were evaluated to assess the outcome for patients undergoing SCT. Data were available from 22 states in 1997, from 27 states in 2000, and from 36 states in 2003. The investigators found that hospital mortality for pediatric SCT patients decreased to 6% in 2003 from 12% in 1997. Risk factors associated with death included allogeneic transplant without T cell depletion, umbilical cord blood SCT, mechanical ventilation, dialysis, and sepsis. Rates of GVHD, sepsis, and mechanical ventilation decreased significantly between 1997 and 2003.

Given the lack of uniform hopelessness seen in these cohorts, predicting outcome is perhaps of greater utility in the pediatric BMT/SCT population. Factors associated with poor survival are not uniform among patient cohorts, but include renal failure, GVHD, hepatic dysfunction, viral infection, respiratory failure, cord blood as source of stem cells, and MOSF. Schneider and colleagues[32] evaluated therapeutic interventions and the performance of prognostic scoring systems among their population of SCT recipients. They evaluated the Pediatric Risk of Mortality (PRISM) score, Therapeutic Intervention Score (TISS), and the Prehospital Therapeutic Intervention Score (p-TISS) in an effort to see whether survival could be predicted based on pre-ICU and ICU interventions or a traditional severity of illness assessment. The investigators found that patients who died in the ICU received more intensive therapy prior to ICU transfer as compared with those who survived, as assessed by p-TISS, as well as more intensive treatment in the ICU as reflected by TISS. The PRISM did not effectively discriminate between survivors and nonsurvivors. The addition of three clinical and laboratory features to

Table 3
Selected series of intensive care unit outcome in pediatric bone marrow transplant and stem cell transplant recipients

Investigators	Year Published	Number of Patients	Mortality	Factors Influencing Outcome
Todd and colleagues[24]	1994	54 (all intubated)	89%	All patients with leukemia or MOSF died
Bojko and colleagues[25]	1995	43 (acute hypoxemic respiratory failure)	88%	
Warwick and colleagues[14]	1998	196 (all intubated)	60% ICU; 86% 2 y	Acute GVHD and HLA-mismatched transplant predicted need for mechanical ventilation
Rossi and colleagues[30]	1999	39 (all intubated)	56% ICU; 64% 6 mo	MOSF predicted increased mortality
Diaz de Heredia and colleagues[28]	1999	31	53.8% ICU; 70.3% 3 y	Allogeneic recipients more likely to need ICU care; lung disease and mechanical ventilation associated with worse survival
Keenan and colleagues[58]	2000	121 (all intubated)	84% 30 d	Respiratory failure and pulmonary infection associated with mortality; impairment of more than one organ system at day 7 conferred 98% mortality
Schneider and colleagues[32]	2000	28	50% ICU	21% of patients lived at least 110 wk
Lamas and colleagues[59]	2003	44	70.4%	Male gender, grade III-IV GVHD, severe hemorrhagic cystitis, failure of >2 organs associated with mortality
Jacobe and colleagues[29]	2003	40	43.9% ICU; 64% 30 d	Respiratory failure with pulmonary infection had 100% mortality; ventilated population had 12.9% survival at 6 mo
Hagen and colleagues[8]	2003	86 (all intubated)	BMT: 53% ICU, 68% hospital, 79% 2 y; umbilical cord blood: 63% ICU, 75% hospital, 81% 2 y	Respiratory failure, sepsis, hepatic failure, and cord blood transplant associated with mortality
Tomaske and colleagues[34]	2003	26	57.7%; 66.9% 6 mo	O-PRISM score >10, sustained renal failure, and failed negative fluid balance predicted death
Cheuk and colleagues[5]	2004	19	46% ICU	Macroscopic hemorrhage and mechanical ventilation indicated increased mortality
González-Vicent and colleagues[7]	2005	36	53% ICU; 75.8% 3 y	O-PRISM score >10 associated with mortality
Kache and colleagues[27]	2006	81	82% transplant years 1992–1999; 41% transplant years 2000–2004	Malignancy as reason for transplant, dialysis, ratio of Pao_2 to fraction of inspired oxygen <300 associated with mortality

Abbreviation: O-PRISM, Oncological Pediatric Risk of Mortality.

the PRISM score (macroscopic bleeding, GVHD, and elevated C-reactive protein) allowed more accurate prediction of outcome in this cohort, and was designated as the Oncological Pediatric Risk of Mortality (O-PRISM) (Table 4).[32] Using this score in a prospective fashion, the same group demonstrated that an O-PRISM score of 10 or more was associated with increased risk of death or complications across multiple time points, as early as day 0 post-BMT.[33] O-PRISM has also been recognized in cohorts outside those described by Schneider and colleagues as predicting increased mortality, though a cutoff number beyond which care is hopeless has not been identified.[7,34] The early discrimination between those with a high likelihood of a complicated course may be useful to select those who might benefit from more aggressive therapeutic strategies earlier in their hospital course.

Table 4
Calculation of the pediatric risk of mortality and oncological pediatric risk of mortality scores

Variable	Measure For Infants	For Children	Score
Systolic blood pressure (mm Hg)	130–160 or 55–65	150–200 or 66–75	2
	>160 or 40–54	>200 or 50–64	6
	<40	<50	7
Diastolic blood Pressure (mm Hg)	>110	>110	4
Heart rate (beats/min)	>160 or <90	>150 or <80	4
Respiratory rate (breath/min)	61–90	51–70	1
	>90	>70	5
For all ages			
Ratio of Pao_2 to fraction of inspired oxygen	200–300		2
	<200		3
$Paco_2$ (mm Hg)	51–65		1
	>65		5
Bicarbonate (mmol/L)	<16 or >32		3
Glasgow Coma Scale	<8		6
Pupillary reactions	Unequal or dilated		4
	Fixed and dilated		10
Ratio of prothrombin time to partial thromboplastin time	>1.5 × control		2
Total bilurubin (>1 mo, mg/dL)	>3.5		6
Potassium (mmol/L)	3.0–3.5 or 6.5–7.5		1
	<3.0 or 7.5		5
Calcium (mmol/L)	1.7–2.0 or 3.0–3.7		2
	<1.7 or >3.7		6
Glucose (mg/dL)	40–60 or 250–400		4
	<40 or >400		8
Additional parameters included in the O-PRISM score			
Macroscopic bleeding	Yes		4
GVHD	Grade 2		2
	Grade >2		4
C reactive protein (mg/dL)	>10		4

From Schneider DT, Lemburg P, Sprock I, et al. Introduction of the Oncological Pediatric Risk of Mortality score (O-PRISM) for ICU support following stem cell transplantation in children. Bone Marrow Transplant 2000;25(10):1079–86; with permission.

POTENTIAL REASONS FOR IMPROVED INTENSIVE CARE UNIT OUTCOMES
Intensive Care Unit Related

Over the past decade, during which many of the gains in ICU mortality for BMT/SCT patients have been realized, there have been significant changes in the care of the critically ill. Several landmark trials have led to changes in the standard of care for patients admitted to the ICU. While most of these trials excluded BMT/SCT recipients, the changes the trials brought about may have contributed to the improvements noted in ICU outcome among SCT patients.

Rivers and colleagues[35] published a landmark trial in 2001 demonstrating that early goal-directed therapy (EGDT), a predefined approach to resuscitation and resuscitative endpoints in the early hours of sepsis, resulted in a significant survival benefit when compared with standard therapy (46.5% mortality vs 30.5%). The group randomized to EGDT had less organ dysfunction within 6 hours of institution of this treatment strategy, as measured by the Multiorgan Dysfunction Score. EGDT, or similar treatment, has become the standard of care in many ICUs. While the impact of EGDT on patients in the setting of BMT/SCT is not known, sepsis remains a common reason for ICU admission in this population, organ dysfunction is associated with increased risk of death, and any benefits this approach does accrue could positively impact a significant proportion of this population. The treatment of sepsis has also seen the advent of new pharmacologic therapy. Activated protein C was demonstrated in a multicenter, double-blind, randomized, placebo-controlled trial to result in significant mortality benefit in patients with severe sepsis (30.8% mortality for placebo group vs 24.7% mortality for the activated protein C group).[36] Patients with BMT were not included in this trial, and the anticoagulant properties of activated protein C render its use inappropriate for patients with severe thrombocytopenia or active hemorrhage. Even so, activated protein C it may provide a beneficial therapeutic option for select BMT patients with severe sepsis.

The treatment of acute respiratory distress syndrome has also undergone significant change in the last decade. A large multicenter trial evaluating the effects of low (6 mL/kg ideal body weight) vs high (12 mL/kg) tidal volume ventilation in patients with acute respiratory distress syndrome resulted in a significant mortality benefit favoring the group randomized to low tidal volumes (31.0% vs 39.8%).[37] Additionally, those randomized to low tidal volume had more days off the ventilator and more days without failure of nonpulmonary organs,

underscoring the favorable impact of this lung protective approach on the development of MOSF.[37] These benefits were seen in broad patient subgroups with acute respiratory distress syndrome, altering the way mechanical ventilation is delivered in many ICUs caring for BMT patients. Minimizing ventilator-induced lung injury may play an important role in the improved outcomes seen by various investigators in mechanically ventilated BMT patients.

Control of hyperglycemia often seen in the critically ill may also lead to decreased ICU-related complications. An intensive insulin regimen, employed in a randomized controlled fashion to compare tight glycemic control with insulin only when glucose levels rose to more than 215 mg/dL in a medical ICU population, resulted in a decrease in the development of newly acquired acute kidney injury, shortened time to ventilator weaning, and decreased ICU and hospital length of stay.[38] Among patients requiring ICU care for 3 or more days, there was a significant reduction in hospital mortality (52.5% vs 43.0%) in the group randomized to tight glycemic control (goal glucose 80–110 mg/dL). Among the subgroup with hematologic or oncologic disease (97 patients), there was a nonsignificant trend toward improved mortality in those receiving tight glycemic control. Insulin infusion protocols have become commonplace in ICUs and may underlie some of the improvements noted in ICU mortality in hematologic transplant recipients.

The use of noninvasive positive-pressure ventilation (NIPPV) has been evaluated in patients with immunocompromise and the development of acute respiratory failure in the setting of fever and pulmonary infiltrates. Fifty-two patients were randomized to intermittent NIPPV or treatment with supplemental oxygen.[39] Among this cohort, 58% had the diagnosis of hematologic cancer and neutropenia, with 33% of the total cohort having undergone BMT. The group randomized to intermittent NIPPV was less likely to require endotracheal intubation (46% vs 77%), and was less likely to die in the ICU (38% vs 69%) or hospital (50% vs 81%). The avoidance of intubation and invasive mechanical ventilation resulted in fewer cases of pneumonia and sinusitis in the group randomized to NIPPV.[39] These findings would support a strategy seeking to avoid intubation by the earlier application of NIPPV, which resulted in improved oxygenation over both the immediate and longer term in this study.

Transplant Related

Conditioning regimens prior to transplant are a course of significant organ injury, which may predispose patients to critical illness. Total body irradiation, employed in conjunction with chemotherapy, is frequently used as part of a myeloablative conditioning regimen. Total body irradiation is associated with increased risk for prolonged neutropenia as well as pulmonary toxicity, both of which may lead to complications requiring critical care. Nonmyeloablative regimens, now frequently used in leukemic patients undergoing allogeneic SCT, allows for lower regimen-related toxicity and a "graft-versus-tumor" effect, which can serve to decrease the risk of relapse of the underlying malignancy.[40]

Prophylactic regimens against infections likely also contribute to improved ICU outcome through the decrease in the overall burden of infection in the BMT population. The use of ciprofloxacin has been demonstrated to decrease the frequency of gram-negative infections when employed as prophylaxis beginning during the conditioning regimen and continuing to resolution of severe neutropenia.[41]

Measures to control the development of invasive fungal infections include environmental controls, such as air filtering in bone marrow transplant units and high efficiency particulate air filters in patient rooms.[42] The minimization of neutropenia with colony stimulating factors or nonmyeloablative regimens may also serve to decrease the risk of such infections. A number of different antifungal medications have been evaluated for their impact on the development of invasive fungal infections. Such medications include fluconazole, itraconazole, posaconazole, micafungin, and amphotericin B. While a number of meta-analyses have demonstrated a decreased rate of invasive fungal infections related to the use of antifungal prophylaxis, the impact on all-cause mortality has not been well established nor has the optimal agent been identified.[43–46] However, regimens containing itraconazole, posaconazole, and perhaps micafungin are associated with fewer aspergillus infections than is a fluconazole-based regimen.[47–49]

The use of acyclovir has been demonstrated to decrease the risk of reactivation of herpes simplex virus and varicella zoster virus in seropositive transplant recipients.[50,51] The optimal method of prophylaxis against cytomegalovirus disease remains uncertain. Other treatments tried include the use of prophylaxis, to prevent reactivation of disease, or the use of pre-emptive therapy only after the detection of viral antigen shedding, to avoid medication-induced toxicity. These may serve to decrease the occurrence of clinically significant end-organ disease.[52,53]

Hepatic veno-occlusive disease, marked by endothelial dysfunction and progressive vascular occlusion leading to organ dysfunction, has been associated with high mortality rates in patients undergoing BMT.[11] Improved response rates in both children and adults with hepatic veno-occlusive disease have been achieved with defibrotide, a polydeoxyribonucleotide with anticoagulant properties. Richardson and colleagues[54] demonstrated complete resolution in 36% of 88 adult and pediatric patients with veno-occlusive disease, with 35% survival at 100 days. Corbacioglu and colleagues[55] found a complete response rate of 76% in 45 pediatric SCT patients. These results represent significant gains compared with the traditionally poor survival rates with this disorder.

SUMMARY

Hematologic SCT provides hope for cure for patients with otherwise fatal malignancy or inherited metabolic disturbances. Profound immunosuppression and visceral organ toxicity related to the conditioning regimen, among other factors, confer a substantial risk for the development of critical illness among this patient population.

While the development of critical illness is associated with higher mortality in this population, the available literature suggests that survival of patients who develop critical illness among both adult and pediatric populations is increasing. The development of MOSF and respiratory failure continues to identify a subgroup of patients with a poor prognosis. Our understanding of this patient population is still evolving. The available literature is largely retrospective in nature, with most series reported from single centers. Gaps in effective prognostic scoring systems remain, and assessment of ICU treatment approaches in critically ill SCT patients in a prospective fashion are still lacking. However, a nihilistic view of the utility of critical care in the hematologic transplant recipient appears not to be warranted, and continued close collaboration among intensivists, hematologists, and oncologists may well lead to further gains in this area.

REFERENCES

1. Center for International Blood and Marrow Transplant Research. Current use and outcome of hematopoietic stem cell transplantation 2007. Available at: http://www.cibmtr.org/SERVICES/observation_research/summary_slides/index.html.
2. Yen KT, Lee AS, Krowka MJ, et al. Pulmonary complications in bone marrow transplantation: a practical approach to diagnosis and treatment. Clin Chest Med 2004;25(1):189–201.

3. Afessa B, Tefferi A, Dunn WF, et al. Intensive care unit support and Acute Physiology and Chronic Health Evaluation III performance in hematopoietic stem cell transplant recipients. Crit Care Med 2003;31(6):1715–21.

4. Afessa B, Tefferi A, Hoagland HC, et al. Outcome of recipients of bone marrow transplants who require intensive-care unit support. Mayo Clin Proc 1992; 67(2):117–22.

5. Cheuk DK, Ha SY, Lee SL, et al. Prognostic factors in children requiring admission to an intensive care unit after hematopoietic stem cell transplant. Hematol Oncol 2004;22(1):1–9.

6. Crawford SW, Petersen FB. Long-term survival from respiratory failure after marrow transplantation for malignancy. Am Rev Respir Dis 1992;145(3):510–4.

7. Gonzalez-Vicent M, Marin C, Madero L, et al. Risk score for pediatric intensive care unit admission in children undergoing hematopoietic stem cell transplantation and analysis of predictive factors for survival. J Pediatr Hematol Oncol 2005;27(10):526–31.

8. Hagen SA, Craig DM, Martin PL, et al. Mechanically ventilated pediatric stem cell transplant recipients: effect of cord blood transplant and organ dysfunction on outcome. Pediatr Crit Care Med 2003;4(2): 206–13.

9. Jackson SR, Tweeddale MG, Barnett MJ, et al. Admission of bone marrow transplant recipients to the intensive care unit: outcome, survival and prognostic factors. Bone Marrow Transplant 1998;21(7): 697–704.

10. Naeem N, Eyzaguirre A, Kern JA, et al. Outcome of adult umbilical cord blood transplant patients admitted to a medical intensive care unit. Bone Marrow Transplant 2006;38(11):733–8.

11. Naeem N, Reed MD, Creger RJ, et al. Transfer of the hematopoietic stem cell transplant patient to the intensive care unit: does it really matter? Bone Marrow Transplant 2006;37(2):119–33.

12. Paz HL, Crilley P, Weinar M, et al. Outcome of patients requiring medical ICU admission following bone marrow transplantation. Chest 1993;104(2): 527–31.

13. Torrecilla C, Cortes JL, Chamorro C, et al. Prognostic assessment of the acute complications of bone marrow transplantation requiring intensive therapy. Intensive Care Med 1988;14(4):393–8.

14. Warwick AB, Mertens AC, Shu XO, et al. Outcomes following mechanical ventilation in children undergoing bone marrow transplantation. Bone Marrow Transplant 1998;22(8):787–94.

15. Denardo SJ, Oye RK, Bellamy PE. Efficacy of intensive care for bone marrow transplant patients with respiratory failure. Crit Care Med 1989;17(1):4–6.

16. Lloyd-Thomas AR, Wright I, Lister TA, et al. Prognosis of patients receiving intensive care for life-threatening medical complications of haematological

malignancy. Br Med J (Clin Res Ed) 1988; 296(6628):1025–9.

17. Rubenfeld GD, Crawford SW. Withdrawing life support from mechanically ventilated recipients of bone marrow transplants: a case for evidence-based guidelines. Ann Intern Med 1996;125(8): 625–33.

18. Allogeneic peripheral blood stem-cell compared with bone marrow transplantation in the management of hematologic malignancies: an individual patient data meta-analysis of nine randomized trials. J Clin Oncol 2005;23(22):5074–87.

19. Krowka MJ, Rosenow EC 3rd, Hoagland HC. Pulmonary complications of bone marrow transplantation. Chest 1985;87(2):237–46.

20. Scales DC, Thiruchelvam D, Kiss A, et al. Intensive care outcomes in bone marrow transplant recipients: a population-based cohort analysis. Crit Care 2008;12(3):R77.

21. Huaringa AJ, Leyva FJ, Giralt SA, et al. Outcome of bone marrow transplantation patients requiring mechanical ventilation. Crit Care Med 2000;28(4): 1014–7.

22. Afessa B, Tefferi A, Litzow MR, et al. Outcome of diffuse alveolar hemorrhage in hematopoietic stem cell transplant recipients. Am J Respir Crit Care Med 2002;166(10):1364–8.

23. Scott PH, Morgan TJ, Durrant S, et al. Survival following mechanical ventilation of recipients of bone marrow transplants and peripheral blood stem cell transplants. Anaesth Intensive Care 2002;30(3): 289–94.

24. Todd K, Wiley F, Landaw E, et al. Survival outcome among 54 intubated pediatric bone marrow transplant patients. Crit Care Med 1994;22(1):171–6.

25. Bojko T, Notterman DA, Greenwald BM, et al. Acute hypoxemic respiratory failure in children following bone marrow transplantation: an outcome and pathologic study. Crit Care Med 1995;23(4):755–9.

26. Nichols DG, Walker LK, Wingard JR, et al. Predictors of acute respiratory failure after bone marrow transplantation in children. Crit Care Med 1994;22(9): 1485–91.

27. Kache S, Weiss IK, Moore TB. Changing outcomes for children requiring intensive care following hematopoietic stem cell transplantation. Pediatr Transplant 2006;10(3):299–303.

28. Diaz de Heredia C, Moreno A, Olive T, et al. Role of the intensive care unit in children undergoing bone marrow transplantation with life-threatening complications. Bone Marrow Transplant 1999;24(2):163–8.

29. Jacobe SJ, Hassan A, Veys P, et al. Outcome of children requiring admission to an intensive care unit after bone marrow transplantation. Crit Care Med 2003;31(5):1299–305.

30. Rossi R, Shemie SD, Calderwood S. Prognosis of pediatric bone marrow transplant recipients

requiring mechanical ventilation. Crit Care Med 1999;27(6):1181–6.

31. Bratton SL, Van Duker H, Statler KD, et al. Lower hospital mortality and complications after pediatric hematopoietic stem cell transplantation. Crit Care Med 2008;36(3):923–7.

32. Schneider DT, Lemburg P, Sprock I, et al. Introduction of the Oncological Pediatric Risk of Mortality score (O-PRISM) for ICU support following stem cell transplantation in children. Bone Marrow Transplant 2000;25(10):1079–86.

33. Schneider DT, Cho J, Laws HJ, et al. Serial evaluation of the Oncological Pediatric Risk of Mortality (O-PRISM) score following allogeneic bone marrow transplantation in children. Bone Marrow Transplant 2002;29(5):383–9.

34. Tomaske M, Bosk A, Eyrich M, et al. Risks of mortality in children admitted to the paediatric intensive care unit after haematopoietic stem cell transplantation. Br J Haematol 2003;121(6):886–91.

35. Rivers E, Nguyen B, Havstad S, et al. Early goal-directed therapy in the treatment of severe sepsis and septic shock. N Engl J Med 2001;345(19):1368–77.

36. Bernard GR, Vincent JL, Laterre PF, et al. Efficacy and safety of recombinant human activated protein C for severe sepsis. N Engl J Med 2001;344(10):699–709.

37. Ventilation with lower tidal volumes as compared with traditional tidal volumes for acute lung injury and the acute respiratory distress syndrome. The Acute Respiratory Distress Syndrome Network. N Engl J Med 2000;342(18):1301–8.

38. Van den Berghe G, Wilmer A, Hermans G, et al. Intensive insulin therapy in the medical ICU. N Engl J Med 2006;354(5):449–61.

39. Hilbert G, Gruson D, Vargas F, et al. Noninvasive ventilation in immunosuppressed patients with pulmonary infiltrates, fever, and acute respiratory failure. N Engl J Med 2001;344(7):481–7.

40. Champlin R, Khouri I, Komblau S, et al. Reinventing bone marrow transplantation. Nonmyeloablative preparative regimens and induction of graft-vs-malignancy effect. Oncology (Williston Park) 1999;13(5):621–8 [discussion: 631, 635–8, 641].

41. Lew MA, Kehoe K, Ritz J, et al. Ciprofloxacin versus trimethoprim/sulfamethoxazole for prophylaxis of bacterial infections in bone marrow transplant recipients: a randomized, controlled trial. J Clin Oncol 1995;13(1):239–50.

42. Loo VG, Bertrand C, Dixon C, et al. Control of construction-associated nosocomial aspergillosis in an antiquated hematology unit. Infect Control Hosp Epidemiol 1996;17(6):360–4.

43. Bow EJ, Laverdiere M, Lussier N, et al. Antifungal prophylaxis for severely neutropenic chemotherapy recipients: a meta analysis of randomized-controlled clinical trials. Cancer 2002;94(12):3230–46.

44. Glasmacher A, Prentice A, Gorschluter M, et al. Itraconazole prevents invasive fungal infections in neutropenic patients treated for hematologic malignancies: evidence from a meta-analysis of 3,597 patients. J Clin Oncol 2003;21(24):4615–26.

45. Kanda Y, Yamamoto R, Chizuka A, et al. Prophylactic action of oral fluconazole against fungal infection in neutropenic patients. A meta-analysis of 16 randomized, controlled trials. Cancer 2000;89(7):1611–25.

46. Vardakas KZ, Michalopoulos A, Falagas ME. Fluconazole versus itraconazole for antifungal prophylaxis in neutropenic patients with haematological malignancies: a meta-analysis of randomised-controlled trials. Br J Haematol 2005;131(1):22–8.

47. Ullmann AJ, Lipton JH, Vesole DH, et al. Posaconazole or fluconazole for prophylaxis in severe graft-versus-host disease. N Engl J Med 2007;356(4):335–47.

48. van Burik JA, Ratanatharathorn V, Stepan DE, et al. Micafungin versus fluconazole for prophylaxis against invasive fungal infections during neutropenia in patients undergoing hematopoietic stem cell transplantation. Clin Infect Dis 2004;39(10):1407–16.

49. Winston DJ, Maziarz RT, Chandrasekar PH, et al. Intravenous and oral itraconazole versus intravenous and oral fluconazole for long-term antifungal prophylaxis in allogeneic hematopoietic stem-cell transplant recipients. A multicenter, randomized trial. Ann Intern Med 2003;138(9):705–13.

50. Erard V, Wald A, Corey L, et al. Use of long-term suppressive acyclovir after hematopoietic stem-cell transplantation: impact on herpes simplex virus (HSV) disease and drug-resistant HSV disease. J Infect Dis 2007;196(2):266–70.

51. Meyers JD. Chemoprophylaxis of viral infection in immunocompromised patients. Eur J Cancer Clin Oncol 1989;25(9):1369–74.

52. Winston DJ, Yeager AM, Chandrasekar PH, et al. Randomized comparison of oral valacyclovir and intravenous ganciclovir for prevention of cytomegalovirus disease after allogeneic bone marrow transplantation. Clin Infect Dis 2003;36(6):749–58.

53. Zaia JA, Gallez-Hawkins GM, Tegtmeier BR, et al. Late cytomegalovirus disease in marrow transplantation is predicted by virus load in plasma. J Infect Dis 1997;176(3):782–5.

54. Richardson PG, Murakami C, Jin Z, et al. Multi-institutional use of defibrotide in 88 patients after stem cell transplantation with severe veno-occlusive disease and multisystem organ failure: response without significant toxicity in a high-risk population and factors predictive of outcome. Blood 2002;100(13):4337–43.

55. Corbacioglu S, Greil J, Peters C, et al. Defibrotide in the treatment of children with veno-occlusive

disease (VOD): a retrospective multicentre study demonstrates therapeutic efficacy upon early intervention. Bone Marrow Transplant 2004;33(2): 189–95.

56. Price KJ, Thall PF, Kish SK, et al. Prognostic indicators for blood and marrow transplant patients admitted to an intensive care unit. Am J Respir Crit Care Med 1998;158(3):876–84.

57. Kew AK, Couban S, Patrick W, et al. Outcome of hematopoietic stem cell transplant recipients admitted to the intensive care unit. Biol Blood Marrow Transplant 2006;12(3):301–5.

58. Keenan HT, Bratton SL, Martin LD, et al. Outcome of children who require mechanical ventilatory support after bone marrow transplantation. Crit Care Med 2000;28(3):830–5.

59. Lamas A, Otheo E, Ros P, et al. Prognosis of child recipients of hematopoietic stem cell transplantation requiring intensive care. Intensive Care Med 2003; 29(1):91–6.

Measurement of Quality and Assurance of Safety in the Critically Ill

Peter J. Pronovost, MD, PhD[a,b,c,*], J. Bryan Sexton, PhD[a,c],
Julius Cuong Pham, MD, PhD[a,d],
Christine A. Goeschel, RN, MPA, MPS[a,e],
Bradford D. Winters, MD, PhD[f], Marlene R. Miller, MD, MSc[e,g,h]

KEYWORDS
- Patient safety • Quality of care
- Measurement • Outcomes • Measuring patient safety

The author (P.J.P.) recently testified before the Government Oversight Committee in the US Congress regarding patient safety. The hearing focused on US efforts to improve patient safety in general and catheter-related bloodstream infections in particular. During the back and forth of these hearings, the committee members kept asking how we knew if we were safer. Patients who had been harmed were particularly adamant. They wanted empiric valid evidence that the medical care patients receive today would be less likely to harm them. Although many efforts were discussed, there was little evidence that care had substantially improved over the past decade. After this hearing, Representative Waxman surveyed states about their efforts to prevent catheter-related bloodstream infections. Although all states said they were making efforts to prevent them, only eight had gathered data showing their infection rates. We believe patients and indeed everyone deserves a valid and empiric answer to the question posed about safety.

Almost a decade after *To Err is Human*[1] reported major patient safety problems, the global health care community is still floundering to definitively answer whether patients are safer. Despite continued rhetoric and work to improve safety, little attention has focused on rigorously evaluating patient safety.[2,3] While the Government Oversight Committee may be the most visible forum, the general public, Congress, and health care payers are also demanding safer care and proof that safety has improved. For example, the Centers for Medicare and Medicaid Services (CMS)

[a] Department of Anesthesiology and Critical Care Medicine, Johns Hopkins University, School of Medicine, 1909 Thames Street, 2nd Floor, Baltimore, MD 21231, USA
[b] Department of Surgery, Johns Hopkins University, School of Medicine, 720 Rutland Avenue, Ross 759, Baltimore, MD 21205, USA
[c] Department of Health Policy and Management, Johns Hopkins University, School of Medicine, 720 Rutland Avenue, Ross 759, Baltimore, MD 21205, USA
[d] Department of Emergency Medicine, Johns Hopkins University, School of Medicine, 615 N. Wolfe Street, Baltimore, MD 21205, USA
[e] Quality and Patient Safety Initiatives, Johns Hopkins University, School of Medicine, 1909 Thames Street, 2nd Floor, Baltimore, MD 21231, USA
[f] Department of Anesthesiology and Critical Care Medicine, The Johns Hopkins University, School of Medicine, 600 North Wolfe Street, Meyer 299B, Baltimore, MD 21287, USA
[g] Department of Pediatrics, Johns Hopkins University, School of Medicine, Johns Hopkins Children's Center, 600 North Wolfe Street, CMSC 1-141, Baltimore, MD 21287, USA
[h] National Association of Children's Hospitals and Related Institutions, 401 Wythe Street, Alexandria, VA 22314, USA
* Corresponding author. Department of Anesthesiology and Critical Care Medicine, Johns Hopkins University, School of Medicine, 1909 Thames Street, 2nd Floor, Baltimore, MD 21231.
E-mail address: ppronovo@jhmi.edu (P. Pronovost).

Clin Chest Med 30 (2009) 169–179
doi:10.1016/j.ccm.2008.09.004

(http://www.cms.hhs.gov) and other payers are starting to deny full payment when a patient suffers a preventable complication on their target list.[4]

While the push to measure safety outcomes is universal, the main barrier to accomplish this has been poor investment in the "basic science" of patient safety. This science would allow us to comprehend the causes of harm, design and pilot test interventions to reduce harm, and robustly evaluate their impact. Nevertheless, we continue to invest a dollar on basic and clinical research for every penny we allocate to ensure patients receive safe care.[5]

Unfortunately, the field of patient safety has often been slow to embrace the need for valid measurement. In this article, we describe some of the dilemmas in measuring patient safety, outline a conceptual model and present a framework for measuring safety, and offer future directions.

MEASUREMENT DILEMMAS

There are many challenges to measuring patient safety that have slowed our progress to make improvements. The dilemmas faced include deciding which measures will identify hazards and which will evaluate patient safety progress, how to balance between universal (generic) and specific measures of patient safety, how to efficiently collect data, how to manage data and data quality control, and how to find a balance between scientifically sound and feasible measures.

The methods used to identify hazards, such as error-reporting systems, are different from the methods used to evaluate progress toward improving patient safety. The first and prime challenge in measuring safety is clarifying which indicators identify hazards and which evaluate patient safety progress. Measures used to evaluate progress must produce reliable and validly measured rates. Most safety parameters are hard or impossible to capture as valid rates because events are uncommon (eg, serious medication errors) or rare (eg, retained foreign object); few events have standardized definitions; surveillance systems depend upon self-reporting; denominators (the populations at risk) are largely unknown or poorly defined; and the time period for exposure (patient day or device day) is unspecified. All of these reasons may introduce bias. Creating measurement systems that are relatively free of such bias would be intricate and expensive.

Despite these problematic issues, measures of patient safety are often inappropriately presented as valid rates. Many hospitals use their patient safety or incident reporting systems to monitor, trend, and benchmark error rates, then present these rates as indicators of safety. Although these reporting systems are invaluable to identify hazards, they cannot rigorously evaluate progress in improving safety. For instance, if a hospital's reported incidents per 1000 discharges decreased from 150 last year to 50 this year, is that hospital safer? The answer is obscure because only a small, nonrandom fraction of incidents are submitted to reporting systems.[1] Sometimes it is impossible to determine if the decrease in incident reports means that fewer errors occurred or that clinicians reported fewer. For example, when we investigated a threefold decrease in our rate of laboratory specimen errors, we found that the incidence dropped because the officer in charge of reporting errors had gone on vacation. Self-reported measures are useful to identify hazards but not to validly monitor progress.

Regardless of whether all incidents are reported, the ambiguity of what comprises a medical error makes inferences about safety problematic. Common quality measures, such as the "door-to-balloon time" for acute myocardial infarction, are relatively unambiguous.[6] Conversely, clinicians often disagree when an action is labeled as an error, and tend to be biased by the outcome and their involvement in the case.[7] Sometimes, clinicians remain unaware of their mistakes even after harm has occurred. Given the bias inherent in identifying and reporting incidents, it is unlikely that "rates" of errors obtained from reporting systems will accurately represent the true incidence of errors or harm.

Choosing the best denominator is another dilemma in the error-rate equation. In general, the denominator should quantify exposure to risk for the outcome of interest. For example, when a hospitalized patient experiences a narcotic overdose, is the appropriate denominator the patient or patient day, the prescribed or dispensed doses, all administered medication doses, or all administered narcotic doses? The results (rate of errors) will vary substantially depending on the denominator chosen. Without valid rates, methods to monitor health care reliability will not be informative. For example, you can improve reliability by changing the denominator from the patient to the drug dose without fundamentally changing patient safety.

Self-reporting may be valid for rare events when harm is clearly evident (low surveillance bias) and the definitions for the numerator and denominator are standardized. Examples include wrong-patient or wrong-site surgery. The National Quality Forum (NQF) assembled a list of "never events" (serious reportable events) that include these examples, which is a good place to begin addressing the current measurement conundrum (www. qualityforum.org). Still, highly visible events may also be underreported. Underreporting plus the relative rarity of these events will compromise their usefulness in measuring safety.

A second challenge is finding a balance between universal and specific measures. While a specific measure or narrow aspect of care (eg, hospital-acquired infections) will enable us to calculate a valid rate, we will need many indicators to achieve a more complete view of safety. Broader safety measures, such as "trigger tools that scan a patient's medical record to detect potential adverse events,"[8] will afford a panoramic view of potentially problematic areas, but we will lack explicit definitions for numerators and denominators. Also, denominators will vary depending on the trigger tool, whether standardized surveillance mechanisms are undefined, if interrater reliability is low, and if no differentiation is made between preventable and inevitable harm. For example, trigger tools can screen medical records for a low platelet count; however, this does not show whether an error or the patient's disease caused the low count. Bottom line, broad measures of safety should be used to screen for potential problems (eg, identify hazards) that warrant further investigation. They should not be used to evaluate progress toward improving patient safety.

A third challenge is how to efficiently capture data. Most quality measures are collected by manual chart review. This is feasible if an organization is collecting a small number of measures. As the number of measures increases, this collection method will quickly become expensive and unsustainable, particularly given the small financial margins at most hospitals. To illustrate, because CMS measures are generally collected manually, each new measure typically requires that a hospital hire one or more staff to collect the data. CMS has over 70 new measures in the pipeline that hospitals may have to collect.

Automatic data collection offers some hope. However, because most electronic medical records have limited amounts of structured data elements relative to quality measures, data mining (searching text for key words) will likely not provide accurate enough data for quality measurement. While such approaches are useful to identify hazards (much like error reports), they will not be valid enough to monitor progress in patient safety. Rather, clinicians will need to define data elements and include structured data fields in their electronic medical records.

One promising approach for automated data collection has been efforts to integrate the documentation from physicians, nurses, and other health care professionals. Each profession typically documents in silos and as a result, many data elements have been duplicative and often not standardized. We created an interdisciplinary team, defined the measures we wanted to get from the documentation system, wrote specifications for those measures, and then agreed on who and how the data elements would be documented. Some measures required physician documentation and some nurse documentation. The result, however, was a valid set of ICU safety measures. Such team-oriented approaches should be encouraged.

A fourth challenge is data quality control and data management. Far too often, hospitals are using quality performance data for marketing even though these locally developed measures and measurement methods are neither standardized nor consistently accurate and reliable. Although much of the data are used internally to improve a hospital's quality of care, measures are also publicly reported on Web sites and in brochures.[9] Unfortunately, these data are not part of any national reporting initiatives and we have no assurance of their accuracy. In an age when advertising is less about the caliber of a product and more about the sell, it is important that health care rise above the opaque marketing ploys used to sell sports drinks and energy bars. This behavior is at best misleading and at worst fraudulent. If consumers cannot trust the quality measures we report, they may lose faith in the quality and integrity of the health care profession.

Invalid quality-of-care measures that are publicly reported also pose substantial risks to patients, providers, and potentially to payers. Patients could choose a doctor or hospital based on misinformation and make bad decisions.[10,11] In addition, health care organizations may become overly confident about the quality of care they provide and cut back on improvement efforts, which will likely introduce preventable harm. Finally, payers may mistakenly reward or deny reimbursement, wrongly drop preferred providers, channel patients to low-quality providers, or make inaccurate inferences about the value (quality per cost) they are purchasing.[12–14] While internal health care quality improvement efforts that use invalid measures may misinform staff and senior leaders, they pose little risks to the public.[15] Clearly, our greatest concern is with rapidly growing measures that hospitals voluntarily develop and publicly report. While this enthusiasm is good and long overdue, there is little assurance that these publicly reported measures are free of unintentional biases, outright false-hoods, or are even accurate.

A fifth and final challenge is developing measures that are both scientifically sound (valid and reliable) and feasible given existing resources. To date, many measures are feasible but not scientifically sound. For example, measures of ventilator-associated pneumonia (VAP) obtained from administrative data are feasible to obtain, but correlate poorly with data collected from each medical record.[16] However, screening all ventilated patients with a bronchioalveolar lavage (one accepted definition for pneumonia) is scientifically sound, but not feasible (highly labor intensive and costly).

After addressing these challenges, it is still difficult to develop and implement effective patient safety measures. Measures must be important to a variety of stakeholders, scientifically sound, feasible, and usable.[17] Whereas consumers and employers believe outcome measures are important, clinicians prefer process measures given their concern over the validity of outcome measures. There is no shortage of important measures, but the above tension must be rectified. Based on our experience with measuring patient safety, we found it was efficacious and efficient to reduce the quantity but not the quality of data collected. When studying hospital-acquired infection rates for example, a National Institutes of Health (NIH)-funded randomized trial may collect many variables (eg, age, gender) to understand the context of the outcome. While interesting, such nonessential variables may not be feasible to collect in a patient safety project.

CONCEPTUAL MODEL FOR MEASURING SAFETY

For nearly a quarter century, health care organizations have used Donabedian's model to evaluate quality: specifically, *structure*, how care is organized, plus *process*, how care is delivered, which influence *outcomes*, the health care results achieved.[18] We have added context or culture to this model (**Fig. 1**).

There are tradeoffs with measuring each of these components. Perhaps not surprisingly for any measure, the resources required for the measurement, and the validity of the measure are often inversely related. Structural measures, such as ICU physician staffing, are often the least burdensome to measure but sometimes are not valid. For example, in ICUs that reported compliance with the Leapfrog Group's ICU physician staffing standard, patients were often not treated by an intensivist. This may be because the unit of analysis for structural measures is the ICU or hospital,

whereas care varies among patients and physicians.[19]

Process measures typically target the care patients received and are generally more valid. These measures can be collected while patients are in the hospital, require little risk adjustment (other than defining inclusion and exclusion criteria), and provide meaningful and generally unambiguous performance feedback to clinicians. Process measures also generally have face validity with clinicians: if the evidence demonstrates that a patient should get a therapy and the patient does not, physicians can use this feedback. One problem with process measures is poor correlation with outcomes.[20] This may be because the treatments that worked in the confines of a clinical study (efficacy) may not work in the uncontrolled real world (effectiveness). The process measured may be but one component of a larger process map (set of processes), and the effect of the measured process on the outcome overshadowed by the whole process. The process measured may also either not have correlated with the outcome (like smoking cessation to reduce mortality after acute myocardial infarction [AMI]), or it was not measured appropriately. For example, we measure smoking cessation education by auditing whether or not a checkbox affirming the education has been performed is checked off in the chart. This likely corresponds poorly with patient knowledge or behavior change.

The absence of strong scientific evidence linking processes to meaningful outcomes has limited the usefulness of process measures when studying patient safety. For example, although having surgeons sign their surgical sites seems like a sensible method to prevent wrong site surgeries, no scientific evidence links this process to the desired outcomes.

Outcome measures are what patients, clinicians, and health care payers are most concerned about. Unfortunately, outcomes are also the most difficult to measure. They require relatively sophisticated risk-adjustment methods, and substantial resources for patient follow-up after discharge (long-term outcomes are generally more informative than short-term).

Culture is a relatively new measure and increasingly recognized as important. Culture and communication shortcomings are the most frequently cited contributing factors for sentinel events reported to the Joint Commission (http://www.jointcommission.org). There are now valid tools to measure culture,[21,22] and culture is responsive to interventions.[23,24] Culture is assessed by surveying staff regarding their perceptions of safety and teamwork.

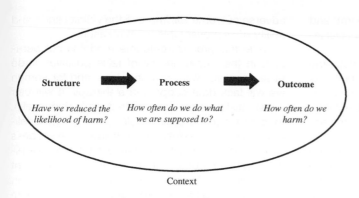

Fig. 1. A conceptual model for measuring safety that includes the three measurement types in Donabedian's model (structure, process, outcome) plus a fourth type of measure (context). Associated with each type of measure is the underlying question that will help us measure safety and evaluate if safety has improved. (*Data from* Donabedian A. Evaluating the quality of medical care. Milbank Mem Fund Q 1966;44:166–206.)

TYPES OF PATIENT SAFETY MEASURES

Using this conceptual model, we developed a framework for measuring patient safety that includes the following: how often do we harm (outcome measure), how often do we use evidence-based interventions (process measure), how do we know we learned from mistakes (structural measure), and have we created a safe culture (culture measure). We have used this framework at the Johns Hopkins Hospital and in more than 100 ICUs in Michigan.[23] We will discuss each measure in turn.

How Often Do We Harm?

The pubic is increasingly demanding that health care monitor outcomes, generally in the form of preventable harm rates. This is a difficult task. The first and foremost challenge in measuring safety outcomes is separating preventable from inevitable harm. In aviation, all fatal crashes are viewed as preventable. The implicit premise of preventable harm is that clinicians either did or failed to do something (the error) that caused harm, which could have been prevented if the error had not occurred. Although there are many similarities, health care is significantly different from aviation and other industries that handle high-risk situations. Despite receiving the best-known medical therapies, some patients will inevitably die or suffer complications.

To advance the science of evaluating whether we are safer, we must tackle the muddled issue of separating preventable from inevitable harm. To make this separation, we need valid measures of harm.[2] Valid measures will require a clear definition of the event (numerator), those at risk for the event (denominator), and a standardized surveillance system to identify events and those at risk for them.

There are three methods to estimate preventable harm. First, if the harm should be completely preventable (eg, wrong-site surgery), we can simply measure rates of harm. While there may be a small margin of error (some harm may truly not be preventable), the error will likely be insignificant. To determine with certainty that most harm is preventable, we will need demonstrated evidence from a valid study. Yet for most harm, the analysis will not be this simple. Most harm is preventable to some degree and researchers will have to develop methods to untangle preventability and inevitability.

If the harm is only practically preventable, we have two options to make this separation and estimate preventable harm. First, if the population of interest is clearly defined and valid risk-adjustment models exist, we can use risk adjustment to determine the observed and expected mortality.[20,25] This type of approach works well for very circumscribed diseases (eg, acute myocardial infarction) in which risk-adjustment models work well. Risk adjustment is less useful for diverse populations, such as overall hospital or ICU mortality.

The second option to make this separation when harm is practically preventable is to link the failure to use an evidence-based intervention (process) with the harm (outcome). Although implicit review may help us understand how communication errors contribute to harm, it will probably not be helpful for this option because clinician consensus regarding preventability is poor.[26]

An explicit review is a more precise method for option two and has been effective in previous research of errors.[27] It can reveal if a patient suffering an adverse outcome received the appropriate evidence-based therapy (process) and can more clearly demonstrate that an error did occur when diagnosing an adverse outcome as a preventable harm. Health care organizations could then monitor counts or rates of preventable harm, and payers could use these data to create financial incentives to minimize these events.

To demonstrate how this process-outcome model works, consider deep venous thrombosis (DVT) and pulmonary embolism (PE). These complications are commonly labeled as preventable, but the evidence for this generally presents relative rather than absolute risk reductions.[28] Relative risk alone does not provide information about the incidence rates needed to estimate the degree of preventability. Absolute risk reductions can give us this information. Also, because we lack standardized methods of surveillance, rates of DVT and PE will vary by how hard clinicians look for this complication. For example, instituting a new screening process for DVT increased this rate 10 fold at one academic institution.[29] Finally, some patients will develop these complications despite receiving the best-known therapy, which suggests that the adverse event is not completely preventable. Thus, to identify patients who suffer a preventable harm, we can detect patients who developed a DVT (the outcome and the denominator) and those who did not receive evidence-based prophylaxis or treatment (the process and the numerator).[28] This process-outcome model minimizes surveillance bias, which plagues many harm measures, when identifying patients with preventable harm. Therefore, only patients who suffered the outcome and did not receive the recommended interventions are diagnosed with a preventable harm.

A precondition of using this process-outcome model is that evidence-based therapies exist to prevent the harm. This is not always the case. To increase this evidence base and avoid deterring innovative efforts, hospitals should be encouraged to continue their efforts to prevent all adverse events. During this process, they develop new interventions to prevent harm and inevitably learn how often the harm is truly preventable. When this evidence is robust, it can be used to inform practice and policy. At this point, policy efforts could select events from this evidence for inclusion in pay-for-performance programs.[4] Among the best measures of harm that we have are central line–associated blood stream infections (CLABSI). However, the Centers for Disease Control and Prevention's definition for CLABSI was developed when the stakes were lower (eg, no public reporting or pay for performance) and uses a surveillance rather than a clinical definition, which emphasizes sensitivity over specificity (they contain many false positives). Thus, linking a process error (failure to use recommended therapies) with the

adverse outcome will improve the validity and reliability of all preventable harm measures.

While this process-outcome model is not perfect, in that some degree of false positives and false negatives will occur in events and for some we will lack data supporting a therapy, it will be substantially better than current error-ridden efforts to diagnose preventable harm. This model will help inform a safety research agenda. Also, because this model links evidence-based interventions with outcomes, it may help to meet the needs of clinicians who seek more specific measures of preventable harm, and consumers like Representative Waxman who want more information about preventable harm.

How Often Do Patients Receive Recommended Therapies?

Process measures monitor clinician activities and are among the most common measures available. Rates of administering beta blockers (AMI), elevating the head of bed (VAP), or providing smoking cessation education are examples of established process measures. As mentioned earlier, process measures are often informative, have high face validity to clinicians, require little risk adjustment, and are generally easier to collect.

The methods used to develop process measures have been previously described.[17,30] When evaluating whether process measures are scientifically sound, it is important to assess validity of a measure at two levels. The first level involves the patient safety domain. If the domain is an outcome measure, is it an important aspect of quality, and does either variation in practice among organizations or interventions that improve the outcome demonstrate it is largely preventable? If the domain is a process measure, is there evidence that the intervention will improve patient outcomes?[31]

The second level of validity must consider how that important domain of patient safety is measured. To minimize bias, efforts should use the measurement principles from clinical research. Clinical research studies typically have well-defined research protocols, explicit data collection tools, well-designed databases, clear quality control plans, and detailed analytic plans.[31] Also, quality improvement and patient safety studies should use a study design that is appropriate for the research question. Whereas randomized trials are often impractical, robust results can be achieved with other study designs.[15] Some examples are cluster randomized designs, a stepped wedge trial design,[32] or a quasiexperimental (time series) design–observational study with the intervention and control groups evaluated over time. If a pre-post design is used, it is particularly important to control for historical bias or performance changes over time.[33] If historical and other biases are not controlled for, investigators may make incorrect inferences. Moreover, although study design issues often address selection bias, they do not address measurement bias that is often significant in quality improvement efforts.[31] Regardless of the study design, robust data collection can minimize measurement error.

If process measures are valid and performance standardized, they can achieve profound improvements in quality of care and patient safety. An example is a set of five practices one of the authors (P.J.P.) and several other clinician-researchers at the Johns Hopkins Hospital culled out from the Centers for Disease Control and Prevention's 100-page practice guideline for preventing CLABSIs. These practices had the greatest impact on preventing infections, and when converted into behaviors had the lowest barriers to implement in daily use. These behaviors were organized on a checklist, and the form used by frontline clinicians to standardize the performance of these behaviors. This standardized process for inserting and monitoring removal of central lines was piloted in a surgical ICU at Hopkins in 1999 and nearly eliminated CLABSIs;[34] the same evidence-based process resulted in a large and sustained reduction in CLABSIs in 103 ICUs participating in the Michigan collaborative from March 2004 to September 2005.[35,36]

How Do We Know We Learned From Mistakes?

Identifying, learning from, and mitigating safety hazards are an important aspect of patient safety research and practice. Efforts to identify hazards involve analysis of the health care system at multiple levels (unit, department, and hospital) to determine where potential or known risks of patient harm can occur to try and prevent an adverse outcome.

Most patient safety research involves retrospective analysis of medical errors. On a unit or departmental (microscopic) level, this involves in-depth analysis of sentinel events. Analyses may be formal (eg, root cause analysis), or informal (eg, case review by a departmental safety or quality improvement committee). The purpose of an analysis is to identify the causes and contributing factors associated with an adverse medical event, then plan and implement strategies to prevent the event from recurring.

On an institutional or regional level (macroscopic), retrospective analysis of medical errors can occur through patient safety reporting systems (PSRS). These systems are advocated by the Institute of Medicine as an important mechanism for identifying hazards.[1] National or multi-institutional PSRS, such as the United Kingdom's National Reporting and Learning System, US Pharmacopeia's (Rockville, MD) MEDMARX system (http://www.usp.org/medmarx), and the Johns Hopkins University's Intensive Care Unit Safety Reporting System have emerged.[37–39] The collective objectives of these reporting systems are to detect events, disseminate information about medical errors, aid health care organizations in prioritizing safety efforts given their limited resources, and design and implement interventions to mitigate risks for harm.

But how do we know if these interventions have reduced a patient's risk of harm? We previously discussed the challenges in separating preventable from inevitable harm, and the inability to measure many as valid rates. Yet a method is needed to evaluate whether we mitigated the risk for future similar events.

In general, we can measure whether we reduced risk at three levels. First, we can evaluate the probability that the intervention was effective. This will involve an assessment to see if the intervention addressed the most important factors that increased risk, and an assessment to determine if the intervention can be implemented as intended.

Second, we can measure whether the intervention was actually implemented. For some interventions, this may mean assessing whether or not an effective policy or procedure was created. An example would be the creation of a policy to perform EKGs within 5 minutes of arrival to the Emergency Department for all patients with chest pain. For other interventions, an actual assessment of staff awareness of the new policy or procedure may be warranted. In this case, surveying staff to see who is aware of the EKG policy. Finally, an actual assessment of the intervention itself may be required. In our EKG example, an audit of time from patient arrival to EKG may be required. If the intervention being evaluated targets improved teamwork, direct observation to evaluate team behaviors will be required. The type of assessment chosen for an intervention will depend on the magnitude of the risk, the quality of data desired, and the resources available. Generally, the higher the quality of data desired, the greater the resources required to gather the data.

Third, we can evaluate whether staff perceive (after the intervention has been implemented) a reduction in risk for the event. This evaluation holds promise for being an important measure because it samples the perceptions and local wisdom of frontline clinicians. However, it also poses a number of methodological challenges. Staff perceptions of risk will likely vary depending on their knowledge of the event, their participation in the event, and their knowledge of the interventions resulting from the event. Research in this area will be particularly important and could be closely linked with assessments and improvements in safety culture.

Have We Created a Safe Culture?

After the *To Err is Human* report,[1] the National Quality Forum and the Joint Commission recommended "improving the culture of safety" as a strategy to improve safety. Implicit in that recommendation are four key questions about safety culture: what is it; how do you measure it; how do you use it; and how do you improve it?

What is safety culture?

Safety culture is a shared sense of norms, beliefs, attitudes, artifacts, and values, but the popular and practical lay definition is "the way we do things around here (in this clinical area)." *Culture* is typically connected with lengthy anthropological and ethnographic studies of one culture or group. In contrast, health care organizations need scientifically sound yet feasible methods to regularly assess safety culture. The demand for relatively low-cost and quick annual assessments of safety culture has resulted in *climate* questionnaires. *Climate* instruments measure a snapshot of the larger culture through multiple dimensions such as *safety climate* or *teamwork climate*.[21,40]

How do you measure safety culture?

Safety culture assessments evaluate staffs' attitudes toward patient safety. With 12 translations used in more than 2000 hospitals, the most thoroughly validated and widely used instrument to assess safety culture in health care to date is the Safety Attitudes Questionnaire (SAQ).[21,22,41–43]

Safety culture responds positively to interventions,[23,44,45] and extracts attitudes that are associated with length of stay and error rates.[24] The SAQ clusters caregiver assessments into six factor-analytically derived scales (domains): safety climate, perceptions of management, teamwork climate, job satisfaction, stress recognition, and working conditions.

We use a census approach to capture the consensus of caregivers in a given clinical area (annually). The criteria for participant inclusion are all clinical and nonclinical staff with a 50% or more commitment to one clinical area for at least 4 consecutive weeks before survey administration. Physicians who admit two or more patients per month (eg, ICU), or conduct five or more procedures per month (eg, cardiac catheterization laboratory) are also included. In addition, we require a 60% or higher response rate for an accurate interpretation of results at the clinical-area level; SAQ administrations average an 80% response rate annually.[46,47] We use the clinical area (unit) to group and interpret SAQ results because unit cultures within a hospital vary far more than cultures among hospitals.[46]

How do you use safety culture results?

To interpret results on a hospital or health system level, hospitals are represented by the percentage of units above the 60% threshold. Focusing on unit-level results helps hospitals recognize units that need resources or leadership support, and helps health systems identify hospitals that are struggling versus thriving. Either way, the focus of interpreting culture results is on the consensus view of caregivers who work in a particular clinical area.

How do you "improve" safety culture?

In our experience, culture is local and efforts to make improvements must occur at the clinical-area level. Extant understanding of how to improve safety culture is still evolving and maturing rapidly. We developed and use the comprehensive unit-based safety program (CUSP) to improve safety culture.[23,24] Briefly, CUSP assesses safety culture, involves staff in identifying and mitigating safety hazards and investigating defects;[48] assigns a senior hospital leader to support unit-level safety activities; and provides tools to improve communication, teamwork, and other areas that pose safety hazards.[24,48–51] Some other approaches to improving culture include operating room briefings;[52,53] executive walkrounds;[45,54] simulation; situation, background, assessment, and recommendation;[55] and culture debriefings.[56] Most of these tools are incorporated into the CUSP program. The processes we recommend for assessing safety culture[47] and feeding back results in an operationally relevant and engaging way[56] are critical to the successful integration of annual culture assessments into routine operations.

FUTURE DIRECTIONS

The public, government agencies, health care payers, and others will continue to rightly demand an answer to the question, Are we safer? There needs to be greater accountability from the health care community. However, this must be done with scientifically valid yet feasible measures that inform patients about health care purchasing decisions. To date, this has not been the case.

Future directions should include a larger number of valid measures, more effective and efficient means to collect data, and better integration of safety measures with broader measures of quality such as equity and efficiency. But we must select measures more wisely. Much of what is currently collected is of questionable validity and lacks face validity with the clinicians who use the data to improve care. If clinicians question a measure's validity, we have little hope of improving. Greater scientific and methodological input is needed to develop and pilot test measures.

In US health policy, the three significant issues are costs, quality (safety), and access to care. Most efforts try to address one of these issues alone. The result is like squeezing a balloon at one end and causing a bulge at the other end. Future efforts should simultaneously address all three of these issues.

Yet our efforts to make progress in the basic science of patient safety measurement and improvement must start by building scholarly capacity within our health care systems. We have learned from basic and clinical researchers that to accomplish this will require formal training (such as a public health degree), mentoring, and participating in a research project. There are very few people with formal training in patient safety and very few programs to train clinicians to become leaders in this field. Progress will require an investment that no doubt will reap substantial returns. Only then will we be able to improve the science of health care delivery and answer the critical question about whether we are safer with a resounding and valid yes.

ACKNOWLEDGMENTS

We acknowledge Christine G. Holzmueller, BLA, for her assistance with editing this article. Financial disclosures include contractual support for quality and safety projects through the Society of Cardiovascular Anesthesia Foundation, the Michigan Health and Hospital Association, and the World Alliance for Patient Safety.

REFERENCES

1. Institute of Medicine. To err is human: building a safer health system. Institute of Medicine Report. Washington DC: National Academies Press; 1999.
2. Pronovost PJ, Miller MR, Wachter RM. Tracking progress in patient safety: an elusive target. JAMA 2006;296(6):696–9.
3. Leape LL, Berwick DM. Five years after to err is human: what have we learned? JAMA 2005;293(19):2384–90.
4. Pronovost PJ, Goeschel CA, Wachter RM. The wisdom and justice of not paying for "preventable complications." JAMA 2008;299(18):2197–9.
5. Moses H 3rd, Dorsey ER, Matheson DH, et al. Financial anatomy of biomedical research. JAMA 2005;294(11):1333–42.
6. Bradley EH, Curry LA, Webster TR, et al. Achieving rapid door-to-balloon times: how top hospitals improve complex clinical systems. Circulation 2006;113(8):1079–85.
7. Caplan R, Posner K, Cheney F. Effects of outcome on physician judgments of appropriateness of care. JAMA 1991;265:1957–60.
8. Rozich J, Haraden C, Resar RK. Adverse drug event trigger tool: a practical methodology for measuring medication related harm. Qual Saf Health Care 2003;12:194–200.
9. Pronovost PJ, Miller M, Wachter RM. The GAAP in quality measurement and reporting. JAMA 2007;298(15):1800–2.
10. Hibbard JH, Stockard J, Tusler M. Hospital performance reports: impact on quality, market share, and reputation. Health Aff (Millwood) 2005;24(4):1150–60.
11. Hibbard J, Stockard J, Tusler M. Does publicizing hospital performance stimulate quality improvement efforts? Health Aff (Millwood) 2003;22(2):84–94.
12. Porter ME, Teisberg EO. How physicians can change the future of health care. JAMA 2007;297(10):1103–11.
13. Glickman SW, Ou FS, DeLong ER, et al. Pay for performance, quality of care, and outcomes in acute myocardial infarction. JAMA 2007;297(21):2373–80.
14. Shortell SM, Rundall TG, Hsu J. Improving patient care by linking evidence-based medicine and evidence-based management. JAMA 2007;298(6):673–6.
15. Auerbach AD, Landefeld CS, Shojania KG. The tension between needing to improve care and knowing how to do it. N Engl J Med 2007;357(6):608–13.
16. Klompas M, Platt R. Ventilator-associated pneumonia—the wrong quality measure for benchmarking. Ann Intern Med 2007;147(11):803–5.
17. McGlynn EA. Choosing and evaluating clinical performance measures. Jt Comm J Qual Improv 1998;24(9):470–9.
18. Donabedian A. Evaluating the quality of medical care. Mill Mem Fund Quar 1966;44:166–206.
19. Pronovost PJ, Thompson DA, Holzmueller CG, et al. The organization of intensive care unit physician services. Crit Care Med 2007;35(10):2256–61.
20. Bradley EH, Herrin J, Elbel B, et al. Hospital quality for acute myocardial infarction: correlation among

process measures and relationship with short-term mortality. JAMA 2006;296(1):72–8.

21. Colla J, Bracken A, Kinney L, et al. Measuring patient safety climate: a review of surveys. Qual Saf Health Care 2005;14:364–6.

22. Sexton JB, Helmreich RL, Neilands TB, et al. The safety attitudes questionnaire: psychometric properties benchmarking data, and emerging research. BMC Health Serv Res 2006;6(44).

23. Pronovost PJ, Berenholtz SM, Goeschel C, et al. Improving patient safety in intensive care units in Michigan. J Crit Care 2008;23(2):207–21.

24. Pronovost P, Weast B, Rosenstein B, et al. Implementing and validating a comprehensive unit-based safety program. J Patient Saf 2005;1(1):33–40.

25. Werner RM, Bradlow ET. Relationship between Medicare's hospital compare performance measures and mortality rates. JAMA 2006;296(22): 2694–702.

26. Lawthers A, McCarthy E, Davis R, et al. Identification of in-hospital complications from claims data. Is it valid? Med Care 2000;38(8):785–95.

27. Hofer TP, Kerr EA, Hayward RA. What is an error? Eff Clin Pract 2000;3(6):261–9.

28. Geerts WH, Bergqvist D, Pineo GF, et al. Prevention of venous thromboembolism: American College of Chest Physicians evidence-based clinical practice guidelines. [8th edition]. Chest 2008;133(6 Suppl): 381S–453S.

29. Haut ER, Noll K, Efron DT, et al. Can increased incidence of deep vein thrombosis (DVT) be used as a marker of quality of care in the absence of standardized screening? The potential effect of surveillance bias on reported DVT rates after trauma. J Trauma 2007;63(5):1132–5 [discussion: 1135–7].

30. Berenholtz SM, Pronovost PJ, Ngo K, et al. Developing quality measures for sepsis care in the ICU. Jt Comm J Qual Patient Saf 2007;33(9): 559–68.

31. Pronovost PJ, Berenholtz SM, Needham DM. A framework for healthcare organizations to develop and evaluate a safety scorecard. JAMA 2007; 298(17):2063–5.

32. Brown CA, Lilford RJ. The stepped wedge trial design: a systematic review. BMC Med Res Methodol 2006;6:54.

33. Wachter RM, Pronovost PJ. The 100,000 lives campaign: a scientific and policy review. Jt Comm J Qual Patient Saf 2006;32(11):621–7.

34. Berenholtz SM, Pronovost PJ, Lipsett PA, et al. Eliminating catheter-related bloodstream infections in the intensive care unit. Crit Care Med 2004;32(10): 2014–20.

35. Pronovost P, Needham D, Berenholtz S, et al. An intervention to decrease catheter-related bloodstream infections in the ICU. N Engl J Med 2006;355(26): 2725–32.

36. Gawande A. The checklist. Annals of Medicine. The New Yorker 2007;1–8.

37. Pronovost PJ, Thompson DA, Holzmueller CG, et al. Toward learning from patient safety reporting systems. J Crit Care 2006;21(4):305–15.

38. Holzmueller CG, Pronovost PJ, Dickman F, et al. Creating the web-based intensive care unit safety reporting system. J Am Med Inform Assoc 2005; 12(2):130–9.

39. Chuo J, Lambert G, Hicks RW. Intralipid medication errors in the neonatal intensive care unit. Jt Comm J Qual Patient Saf 2007;33(2):104–11.

40. Singla AK, Kitch BT, Weissman JS, et al. Assessing patient safety culture: a review and synthesis of the measurement tools. J Patient Saf 2006;2(3):105–15.

41. Makary MA, Sexton JB, Freischlag JA, et al. Patient safety in surgery. Ann Surg 2006;243(5):628–32.

42. Sexton JB, Makary MA, Tersigni AR, et al. Teamwork in the operating room: frontline perspectives among hospitals and operating room personnel. Anesthesiology 2006;105(5):877–84.

43. Sexton JB, Holzmueller CG, Pronovost PJ, et al. Variation in caregiver perceptions of teamwork climate in labor and delivery units. J Perinatol 2006;26(8): 463–70.

44. Pronovost PJ, Berenholtz SM, Goeschel CA, et al. Creating high reliability in healthcare organizations. Health Serv Res 2006;41(4):1599–617.

45. Frankel A, Grillo SP, Pittman M, et al. Revealing and resolving patient safety defects: the impact of leadership walkrounds on safey climate. Health Serv Res July 2008, Epub ahead of print.

46. Rose JS, Thomas CS, Tersigni A, et al. A leadership framework for culture change in health care. Jt Comm J Qual Patient Saf 2006;32(9):433–42.

47. Pronovost PJ, Sexton JB. Assessing safety culture: guidelines and recommendations. Qual Saf Health Care 2005;14:231–3.

48. Pronovost PJ, Holzmueller CG, Martinez E, et al. A practical tool to learn from defects in patient care. Jt Comm J Qual Saf 2006;32(2):102–8.

49. Pronovost P, Berenholtz S, Dorman T, et al. Improving communication in the ICU using daily goals. J Crit Care 2003;18(2):71–5.

50. Pronovost PJ, Weast B, Bishop K, et al. Senior executive adopt-a-work unit: a model for safety improvement. Jt Comm J Qual Saf 2004;30(2):59–68.

51. Thompson DA, Holzmueller CG, Cafeo CL, et al. A morning briefing: setting the stage for a clinically and operationally good day. Jt Comm J Qual Patient Saf 2005;31(8):476–9.

52. Makary MA, Holzmueller CG, Thompson DA, et al. Operating room briefings: working on the same page. Jt Comm J Qual Saf 2006;32(6):351–5.

53. Makary MA, Mukherjee A, Sexton JB, et al. Operating room briefings and wrong site surgery. J Am Coll Surg 2007;204(2):236–43.

54. Thomas EJ, Sexton JB, Neilands TB, et al. The effect of executive walk rounds on nurse safety climate attitudes: a randomized trial of clinical units. BMC Health Serv Res 2005;5(1):28.

55. Haig KM, Sutton S, Whittington J. SBAR: a shared mental model for improving communication between clinicians. Jt Comm J Qual Patient Saf 2006;32(3):167–75.

56. Sexton JB, Paine LA, Manfuso J, et al. A check-up for safety culture in "my patient care area."Jt Comm J Qual Patient Saf 2007;33(11):699–703.

End-of-Life Decision Making in the ICU

Mark D. Siegel, MD

KEYWORDS

- Death • Decision making • Ethics • Triage • Futility
- Bereavement • End-of-life care

Twenty percent of deaths in the United States follow admission to an ICU,[1] often in association with decisions to forego life support.[2] In recent years, end-of-life decision making has become a key feature of critical care practice.[3–7]

Unfortunately, numerous shortcomings afflict end-of-life care in the ICU. Patients unlikely to benefit are admitted frequently, leading to needless suffering and wasted resources.[8,9] Inadequate treatment of pain and dyspnea are common.[10,11] Patients' relatives frequently develop psychiatric morbidity, which may be partly related to conflict with physicians and stress connected with end-of-life decisions.[4,12–18]

End-of-life care varies dramatically among physicians, hospitals, and countries, and this variability fuels concern that factors besides a patient's illness and preferences drive treatment. In one study, clinicians shown identical hypothetic cases suggested widely different treatments, ranging from aggressive care to palliation.[19] Other studies have shown widely varying rates of decisions to forego life support, use of "do not resuscitate" (DNR) orders, and willingness to treat patients who are permanently unconscious or terminally ill.[2,8,20,21] The reasons for this variability are unknown but probably include differences in practice style, access to care, and local cultural and religious traditions.[6,8,22–25]

ICU management clearly improves survival for appropriately targeted patients.[26,27] To some degree, end-of-life decisions determine if patients live or die.[28–30] Careful decision making is essential to ensure that care provided is consistent with patients' wishes.[31–33] Given their expertise, intensivists are well positioned to provide outstanding end-of-life care and promote family satisfaction.[34,35] The remainder of this article is devoted to building a framework on which to guide end-of-life decision making in the ICU.

AN APPROACH TO END-OF-LIFE DECISION MAKING

The goal of end-of-life decision making is to meet patients' wishes and needs by choosing appropriate treatments. In Western society, these choices occur within an ethical framework dominated by key precepts: respect for patient autonomy, the physician's duty toward beneficence and nonmaleficence, and an obligation to ensure just distribution of resources.[36]

These precepts sometimes pose internal conflicts. For example, patients may refuse treatment or request care physicians believe nonbeneficial. Alternatively, desired care may be unavailable, for example, if a shortage exists in ICU beds. Respect for autonomy generally allows patients to refuse recommended care, although most agree this it does not require that physicians offer nonstandard interventions or care they believe harmful.

End-of-life choices fall into two broad categories, those that are constrained and those that are unconstrained. Unconstrained choices imply the opportunity to choose among multiple treatment options. In contrast, constraint occurs when options are limited, either because treatments are unavailable or because they cannot work. Specifically, under some circumstances, rationing and triage may be necessary when resources are limited. In other circumstances, medical futility may constrain treatment. In practice, most end-of-life choices are unconstrained,

Section of Pulmonary and Critical Care Medicine, Department of Medicine, Yale University School of Medicine, 333 Cedar Street, LCI 105, P.O. Box 208057, New Haven, CT 06520-8057, USA
E-mail address: mark.siegel@yale.edu

Clin Chest Med 30 (2009) 181–194
doi:10.1016/j.ccm.2008.11.002
0272-5231/08/$ – see front matter © 2009 Elsevier Inc. All rights reserved.

but constrained choices impose ethical and practical considerations that must be addressed.

RATIONING AND TRIAGE

Rationing is defined as "the allocation of health care resources in the face of limited availability."[37] Triage refers to a specific system or plan to prioritize individual patients based on their underlying conditions (**Box 1**).[38] Rationing and triage are uncommon in American ICUs, where it is unusual to refuse admission, even to patients who have end-stage illness.[21,39,40] Limitations have long affected care in countries with fewer resources.[41] The need to triage will likely become more common in the United States with growing concern about pandemics, bioterrorism, and the expanding population of critically ill patients.[27,37,41–44]

At first glance, the need to restrict services may strike some physicians as ethically troublesome.

However, when resources are limited, rationing cannot be avoided and physicians are obligated to maximize benefit to the population and distribute services fairly.[37] Policies must be designed to identify those patients most likely to benefit from the ICU, recognizing that triage has the potential to place patients refused admission at risk for worse outcomes.[27,37,41,45,46]

Protocols using objective parameters can help guide decision making. Several models are available,[43,44,47] as are reviews and position pieces that highlight essential principles.[27,37,45,46,48] Institutions should prepare for shortages in advance and ensure that triage protocols are appropriately vetted, understood by affected clinicians, and ready to be implemented when needed.[48] Good clinical practice should be promoted to minimize the need to triage. Examples include adhering to standard admission and discharge criteria; addressing end-of-life issues; expediting bed flow; expanding the capacity of acute care floors to manage seriously ill patients; and following practices that decrease length of stay, such as avoiding excess sedation and weaning in a timely manner.[49] To avoid conflict of interest, triage physicians should be distinct from those providing patient care.

Objective, transparent principles of prioritization must be implemented that encompass two factors: the need for ICU care and the likelihood of benefit (**Box 2**). Patients requiring interventions typically limited to the ICU, such as mechanical ventilation through an endotracheal tube, should generally take priority over patients admitted for monitoring only. Similarly, patients most likely to survive and resume a functional life should take priority over those unlikely to achieve an acceptable outcome. Examples of patients unlikely to benefit include those uninterested in aggressive care and those who have rapidly fatal illness,

---

Box 1
Key triage principles

- Triage is required when need (eg, for ICU beds) exceeds supply.
- The goal of triage is to provide the greatest good to a target population.
- Objective criteria are used to assign priority to one patient over another.
- Policies must be fair, transparent, and objective.
- Institutions should minimize the need to triage by

  Expanding ICU bed capacity if possible

  Improving their ability to care for patients outside the ICU

  Encouraging efficient patient throughput

  Promoting practices that decrease ICU length of stay

  Addressing end-of-life issues

- Appropriate ICU bed use should be promoted before crises occur.
- Triage policy must be understood by all stakeholders.
- Triage responsibility must be separated from patient care responsibility.
- Oversight by experts in bioethics, legal affairs, and hospital administration must be provided for.
- One must remember that triage does not condone abandonment

Data from Refs.[27,37,44–46,48]

Box 2
An example of a triage scoring system

Level I: Requires ICU-only interventions/high likelihood of benefit

Level II: No ICU-only interventions needed/high likelihood of benefit

Level III: Requires ICU-only interventions/low likelihood of benefit

Level IV: No ICU-only interventions needed/low likelihood of benefit

Level V: Does not meet standard ICU admission criteria

Adapted from Yale-New Haven Hospital ICU Triage Policy. March 5, 2008.

advanced, irreversible cognitive impairment, or progressive multiple organ failure. Objective measures, such as severity of illness scores, clearly identified "ICU-only" interventions, and expert input should promote appropriate triage.

Even if denied ICU admission, critically ill patients merit treatment to the extent that resources are available. When implementing triage, institutions should consider whether prioritization should apply only within or also between individual ICUs (eg, to consider if a medical ICU patient should displace a patient who has lesser need from a surgical ICU). Similarly, policies should address whether candidates should be limited to those already within the institution or should include those hospitalized elsewhere (eg, those seeking transfer for specialty services). Finally, oversight and support should be provided by ethics committees, legal experts, and hospital administrators, to ensure that triage is implemented ethically, legally, and effectively.

FUTILITY

Few issues inspire more passion than medical futility.[50-58] The definition of futility is hotly debated. However, any reasonable definition should recognize a condition as futile if no effective treatment exists. Futile care is inherently unethical, incurring cost and possible suffering without benefit.[59] Identifying futility has critical implications for decision making. Many physicians and professional societies agree that physicians should not provide futile care, even if requested,[53,55,60] although some dissent.[56] Identifying futility may relieve physicians, patients, and families from difficult decisions when it is recognized that the outcome cannot be altered.

Disputes over the definition of futility make it difficult to determine its frequency. In a European study, 73% of ICUs frequently admitted patients without hope of survival.[8] In a study from California, 4.8% of Medicare beneficiaries received "potentially ineffective care," defined as expensive hospital care given shortly before death.[61]

Unfortunately, many physicians define futility loosely in practice.[62] Quantitative and qualitative criteria have been promoted.[50,53,60,63,64] A commonly cited quantitative definition denotes futility when treatments fail despite 100 attempts.[53] Some object to using quantitative criteria if success remains possible, even if exceedingly unlikely.[50] Others have suggested restricting futility designations to conditions meeting narrow physiologic criteria, such as recalcitrant hypotension or hypoxemia.[64] In contrast, others support broader use, including states of permanent unconsciousness

or inability to overcome dependence on intensive care.[53,60] The more narrow the definition, the less commonly futility will be identified.

Citing futility as a rationale to limit care raises numerous concerns. For example, not all patients agree that futility should entitle physicians to withhold offers of mechanical ventilation.[65] In addition, it is difficult for physicians and nurses to identify futile cases reliably.[66] Several investigators have tried to identify clinical factors in specific populations that precluded survival,[67] but survival estimates can become obsolete quickly as practice evolves and outcomes improve.[68,69]

Rigid notions of futility can create self-fulfilling prophecies.[70] Clearly, concerns about causing needless suffering must be balanced with the imperative to seek better outcomes in our sickest patients.[71] Many reasonable ethical concerns have been raised regarding the use of the futility rationale to justify decision making.[56] In practice, it is difficult to cite in all but the most obvious cases. For these reasons, it is usually best to approach end-of-life decision making using the methods used in nonfutile, unconstrained, situations.

UNCONSTRAINED DECISION MAKING

Most end-of-life decisions are unconstrained by resource limitations or futility, and are restricted only by patient preference and practice standards. In North America (and, increasingly, elsewhere), respect for patient autonomy dominates decision making, empowering patients to choose among treatment options. In other places, paternalism often dominates, with physicians choosing treatments they think best for the patient, although this practice is becoming less frequent.[23]

Respect for autonomy parallels the principles of informed decision making. To make decisions, patients must understand their conditions and receive enough information to weigh the risks and benefits of treatment options. Physicians may, and often should, provide recommendations, although patients have the final say.

In the ICU, cognitive impairment due to factors such as delirium, sedation, and dementia prevent most patients from making decisions.[72-75] Cognitive impairment can be subtle[76] and mandates a thorough assessment to confirm decision-making capacity. In practice, most end-of-life decisions depend on surrogate decision makers, usually family members[3,77-79] except under unusual circumstances when none are available.[80]

Surrogate Decision Making

Surrogates face special challenges, particularly because patients' wishes are often unknown.

A hierarchy for surrogate decision making has been described.[3,78] First, surrogates should report the patient's specific preferences if known. Second, if this is not possible, surrogates should attempt substituted judgment, relying on available evidence to express what they believe the patient would choose if able. Finally, if preferences are completely unknown, surrogates should choose the treatment they believe to be in the patient's best interest.

Surrogate decision making requires flexibility.[78] Many patients would prefer their relatives to exercise discretion or make decisions for them rather than limit themselves to being spokespeople.[81] Families from certain cultures may not recognize traditional Western views of autonomy.[82–84] For example, some families may not be able to or want to consider patients' interests as distinct from their own.[82,83] Some families may not want to engage in decision making.[84] It is reasonable to take a flexible approach to surrogate decision making as long as the patient's wishes are not compromised.

Advance Directives

Physicians and families often do not know patients' end-of-life preferences.[31,85,86] To encourage accurate decision making, physicians should discuss preferences with patients preemptively, while they can still speak for themselves.[87] Advance directives (ADs) have been proposed as a way to ensure patients' wishes are respected if they become incapacitated. The most common ADs instruct physicians to forego life-sustaining treatment if patients become terminally ill or permanently unconsciousness.[88]

Unfortunately, few patients have ADs and little evidence exists that they aid decision making.[89,90] As written, they generally apply to limited, specific circumstances, such as permanent unconsciousness and terminal illness. They often are unhelpful if incapacitation is temporary, the illness is not terminal, or the interventions in question are not specifically addressed.[91,92] ADs do not improve surrogates' abilities to represent patients' preferences accurately.[93] Patients frequently misunderstand their own ADs, which may also fail to reflect their wishes.[89]

Discussing preferences in advance can be helpful.[92] Prior discussions can diminish the family's burden when asked to make decisions.[17] Outpatient discussions offer opportunities to consider treatment options, including hospice, should life-threatening illness develop. Patients who have advanced cancer who have end-of-life discussions appear to have a better quality of life before death and their family members experience fewer bereavement-related psychiatric disorders.[94] Unfortunately, outpatient discussions occur inconsistently, even among patients who would benefit.[94]

Special Challenges Facing Surrogate Decision Makers

Surrogate decision makers face enormous pressure.[79] Many family members, especially spouses, experience anxiety, depression, and features of posttraumatic stress disorder.[12–14,95] Participation in end-of-life decisions may contribute to psychiatric morbidity, although further work is needed to confirm this finding and to identify the mechanisms involved.[13]

Decision making is especially difficult when patients' preferences are unknown. In general, preferences are not consistently related to factors such as age, underlying illness, prognosis, presence of ADs, or quality of life.[96–98] Physicians and family members often cannot predict preferences, although certain factors, such as level of surrogate and patient education and prior end-of-life discussions may improve accuracy.[31,85,86,97–100]

Wishes expressed as outpatients may be unstable over time.[101–104] Factors associated with instability include a long time between interviews, changes in health status and quality of life, not having children, absence of a living will, and previous desire for aggressive care.[101–104] To some degree, changes in treatment preferences are understandable. Willingness to accept treatment may change if a patient's condition or the likelihood of successful treatment evolves.[105] Similarly, as illness progresses and quality of life deteriorates, some patients may be more willing to accept lower functional outcomes.[106] Alternatively, they may be less willing to pursue highly burdensome therapies or risk severe disability.[107]

Certain common observations are worth noting. A strong will to live will cause many patients to endure ICU care, even when prognosis is poor.[108] Most survivors would return to the ICU even if the benefit was only 1 month of survival.[97] In contrast, many outpatients who have chronic illness report little interest in aggressive therapy if the likely outcome is poor; many, but not all, would view survival with a poor quality of life or major functional or cognitive impairment as a fate worse than death.[96,109]

FAMILY MEETINGS

Family meetings precede most end-of-life decisions in North America. Well-conducted meetings promote appropriate decisions and family satisfaction and well-being.[3,4,77,110,111] Meetings should occur shortly after ICU admission and not wait until decisions are urgent.[4,112] As with any medical procedure, successful meetings include several components, including a clear description of the medical facts, a discussion of goals and treatment options, and decision making (**Box 3**).[3,4,77,111,113,114] Meetings should be held in a private, quiet place to minimize interruptions and should include all important members of the team, including attending physicians, medical trainees, nurses, social workers, and chaplains if possible. Caregivers should meet beforehand to achieve consensus regarding prognosis and treatment options.[77]

Discussing Prognosis

Physicians leading meetings should review the patient's course with the family, including ongoing and previous treatments attempted. Prognostic estimates are essential. Although precision may be difficult,[106] decision making requires some prognostic quantification. Prognosis may vary depending on the outcome considered, whether it be survival, return of cognitive function, or quality of life.[77] Severity of illness scores may help identify patients unlikely to survive,[59,115] although population-based scores are often misleading when applied to individual cases.

A poor prognosis alone is unlikely to dictate treatment. Many families will support aggressive treatment as long as an acceptable outcome is possible. With appropriate support, families should be able to balance hope with realistic expectations.[3,116] Patients can receive palliative care even as life-saving efforts continue; they are not mutually exclusive.[117] One should not worry that an honest discussion regarding prognosis will destroy hope or cause psychologic harm; rather, honest discussions appear to improve end-of-life care for both patients and families.[94]

Making Decisions

Agreement regarding treatment goals sets the stage for specific decisions.[118] A clear identification of goals followed by an assessment of whether they can be achieved should help families and caregivers choose appropriate treatments.[51] Goals can be grouped into three categories. On one end of the spectrum, the goal may be to cure or ameliorate the patient's illness using all available therapies, without imposing limitations. On the other end, the goal may be to emphasize symptom management, sometimes to the point of providing "comfort measures only." A midrange

goal would be to attempt disease treatment while limiting those interventions and treatments considered overly burdensome. As distinct from treatments, goals should include outcomes expressed in nonmedical terms, such as a wish to return home, avoid disability, or be free of pain.

Once goals are established, decisions regarding specific interventions should follow logically.[118] For example, if the decision is made to treat without limitations, it generally follows that all necessary interventions will be provided, including cardiopulmonary resuscitation (CPR) or mechanical ventilation. In contrast, if comfort is to be emphasized, these interventions would make little sense. A more nuanced discussion may be necessary if the decision is to provide limited treatment. Plans should be internally logical, recognizing that individual treatment decisions are not inherently independent. For example, it would be inappropriate to provide CPR to a patient who arrests after foregoing intubation for respiratory failure.

The implications of decisions made must be fully understood by clinicians and surrogates. By itself, a decision to make a patient DNR implies only that resuscitation would be withheld after cardiac arrest. DNR orders have no bearing on other decisions, and fully aggressive management may be provided otherwise.[119] The distinction between therapies deemed heroic or not is arbitrary. Although it is common to draw certain "lines in the sand," such as withholding vasopressors for shock, the rationale for imposing certain limitations and not others can be illogical.[120] It is much more important to weigh the benefits and burdens of individual therapies to determine if they are consistent with the established treatment goals.

Pitfalls can result from mistaken assumptions. For example, patients who have metastatic cancer or dementia can vary widely in prognosis and functional status. ICU care may be appropriate for some but not others. Similarly, the fact that a patient has an AD or wants to be DNR says little about overall preferences. Finally, just because families and physicians agree does not ensure appropriate decision making. All decisions require careful deliberation to maximize the likelihood that they are appropriate.

Families should not be pressured to make decisions,[15] and they should never simply be asked "what they want done."[63] It is the physician's responsibility to determine if treatment preferences are achievable and to offer recommendations.[63,114] Most families prefer to share decision making with physicians and should be allowed to do so.[3,77,121–123]

Explicit language can reinforce the concept of surrogacy. For example, family members may be

---

Box 3
Key components of successful family meetings

- Meet early in the hospitalization, before decision making is urgent.
- Prepare in advance.

  Find an appropriate, private location.

  Enlist all team members, including attending physicians, trainees, nurses, social workers, chaplains, and translators (if necessary).

  Achieve team consensus regarding prognosis and treatment options.

- Introduce everyone present.

  Sit in a circle if possible.

  Clarify everyone's roles or relationship to the patient.

  Explain the purpose of the meeting.

- Explain key concepts:

  The purpose of the meeting

  Surrogate decision making

  Shared decision making

- Clearly describe the patient's condition.

  Explain the disease process.

  Discuss what the patient is experiencing.

  Discuss ongoing and previous treatments attempted.

  Discuss prognosis.

- Allow time for questions, comments, and clarification.

- Discuss goals and treatment options.

  Focus on general goals, using lay language.

  Try to determine what the patient would want if possible.

  Consider the risks, benefits, and implications of specific treatment options.

    Focus on treatments designed to meet established goals.

    Explain why certain options are not available, if necessary.

  Determine the degree of shared decision making required.

    Provide recommendations as appropriate.

    Allow time for questions and deliberation.

  Make explicit treatment decisions.

    Ensure that decisions are consistent with treatment goals.

    Ensure the treatment plan is internally logical and consistent.

Ensure consensus and comprehension.

- Wrap up.

  Provide explicit, empathic statements of support for the family.

  Ensure ongoing care for patient, including

    Full efforts to meet the established goals

    Management of symptoms as necessary

  Provide opportunities for follow-up meetings if needed.

A flexible approach is necessary to meet the needs of individual patients and families.

Data from Refs.[3,4,77,111,118,122]

---

asked what they believe the patient would say if present.[4] Many families prefer to function as a group. It is important to strive for consensus among all present to avoid burdening any individual with sole decision-making responsibility.[4,79]

Families should be given sufficient time to speak and ask questions.[111,124] Physicians should listen carefully, recognizing that concerns expressed may be subtle.[77,111,113] Empathic statements foster family satisfaction.[125] Finally, conferences should conclude with positive statements ensuring support for the patient and family, and, if the decision is made to forego life support, assurance that the patient will not suffer.[126]

OBSTACLES TO SUCCESSFUL FAMILY MEETINGS

Several factors pose challenges to reaching consensus with families. Real or perceived conflict between families and physicians is common.[17,18] Physicians may be confounded by what they perceive to be a family's illogical thinking,[63] which should be taken as a sign that important issues need to be addressed. Inadequate or delayed communication is a common problem, contributing to misconceptions about prognosis and treatment options.[112,127] Insufficient physician time to meet with families may also contribute.[5] Insurmountable disagreements should be rare, however, and conflict should dissipate when communication improves, misunderstandings are corrected, and emotional and spiritual needs are met (**Box 4**).[4,63,77,110,111,113]

Significant shortcomings plague many family meetings. Many are led by unsupervised trainees.[128] Discussions of prognosis, particularly likelihood of survival, occur inconsistently.[128–130] Physicians often miss opportunities to share

Box 4
Avoiding conflict and barriers to consensus

- Form supportive relationships with families.

  Meet early.

  Meet frequently.

  Ensure open visitation.

  Invite participation on rounds.

- Focus on overriding goals rather than narrow issues (such as code status).

- Allow families to express feelings and concerns.

- Be mindful of language and cultural barriers.

  Use professional translators.

  Avoid sloppy language and jargon.

  Consider cultural context and family's background and past experiences.

  Explore common informal statements by family.

    "We're hoping for a miracle."

    "We want everything done."

- Be aware of religious and spiritual concerns.

  Avoid assumptions about preferences.

  Enlist chaplain support.

- Address potential knowledge deficits:

  Nature of illness

  Risks and benefits of specific interventions

  Awareness of treatment options

  Assumptions about ADs and implications of DNR orders

- Ensure senior physician involvement.

- Do not place undue pressure on families to make decisions.

  Avoid placing the burden on individual family members.

  Place decisions in perspective (generally it's not "if" but "how" death occurs).

  Share in decision making as requested.

- Do not rush families.

  Allow them time to consider new findings and recommendations.

  Allow time for treatment trials.

  Schedule follow-up meetings.

- Recognize stress and the potential for psychiatric morbidity in families.

  Be empathic.

  Be patient.

Enlist support of social workers and mental health professionals.

Data from Refs.[4,5,12–14,63,77,82,83,110–113,128,134]

essential information or give emotional support.[113] In one study, only a few meetings included efforts to confirm that families understood the decisions made.[121]

Misdirected focus can impose obstacles to consensus. No reason exists to ask families if they wish futile or unavailable therapy. Similarly, excessive time spent considering narrow issues such as "code status" (which addresses only how to respond to a cardiac arrest) might be better spent considering overriding goals such as whether to emphasize aggressive treatment or comfort.

The burden felt to make decisions may delay consensus. In addition to sharing in decision making, physicians may help families by placing decision making in appropriate perspective. Although some end-of-life decisions can influence outcome,[28–30,70,131] the patient's underlying illness almost certainly plays a bigger role in most cases. Fear that they are responsible for "pulling the plug" can make decision making difficult for some families and set the stage for subsequent misgivings. When prognosis is poor, it may be helpful to acknowledge that decisions are more likely to influence how, not whether, a patient dies.

Physicians may overestimate what families understand.[123,127,132,133] Insufficient information may prevent families from making informed choices or trusting what physicians say. In one French study, half of families reported inadequate communication with physicians.[134] In an American study, many families were not given enough information to make informed decisions regarding tracheotomy.[127] Physicians may fail to distinguish between permanent and temporary conditions (eg, those related to cognitive impairment).[135] Lacking understanding, many families may overestimate the likelihood of success of CPR,[133] whereas accurate information may lead fewer to choose it.[136] Similarly, some families may be concerned that a decision to choose intubation and mechanical ventilation commits patients to long-term life support, not recognizing that withdrawal of support is an option if treatments fail or preferences change.[2]

Specific interventions should be described in an unbiased manner, addressing the risks and benefits in sufficient, but not overwhelming, detail.

Families may not understand why physicians have concluded that a prognosis is poor or why recommendations are being made to limit life support. When patients are doing poorly, it may be especially helpful to recount the efforts made so families understand that deterioration has occurred despite treatment attempts.

Language may impose a significant barrier to communication.[83,137–139] A growing number of residents of the United States are not comfortable with English.[140] Inasmuch as possible, it is essential to use professional interpreters;[82,139,141] family members and untrained hospital staff are not appropriate substitutes. Certain English terms do not translate easily. Allowing interpreters flexibility may be preferable to translating verbatim.[139,141] Interpreters may be particularly useful as "cultural brokers," helping physicians to better understand the issues in the context of the family's cultural background.[139,141]

Although qualified interpreters play a crucial role, translated conferences pose potential difficulties. Interpreters may inadvertently alter language and the information may be conveyed in ways that could influence decisions.[137] In addition, families may receive less information and emotional support during translated conferences.[142] When impasse arises, it may be helpful to consider if key information is being "lost in translation."[138]

Even when everyone is speaking English, it is critical to ensure they are "speaking the same language." Family members may misconstrue terms such as "DNR," "CPR," and "intubation" if not carefully defined. Imprecise phrases such as "poor prognosis" or "unlikely to work" are prone to misinterpretation; more precise terms may help prevent misunderstanding.[77] Families may misinterpret intent when jargon such as "withdrawal of care" is used, as opposed to "withdrawal of life-sustaining treatment."[3] Attempts to soften language, for example with euphemisms such as "letting nature take its course," may soften the blow when bad news is given, but may risk misunderstanding. Physicians may also misinterpret terms used by families, such as requests to "do everything,"[63] which mean little if not explored and defined. Similarly, expressions of hope do not inherently imply that families are unrealistic.

In addition to language barriers, cultural differences may impose pitfalls.[78,82,138,139,141–144] Families from many regions of the world may find the concept of patient autonomy alien.[78,82,83] Some may consider it their responsibility to make decisions for their relatives, as opposed to trying to represent their preferences.[83] Certain Western norms, such as truth telling, may be seen as cruel and some may be concerned that even talking about death may make it more likely.[83] Some African Americans may view suffering as an obstacle to overcome rather than a rationale for palliative care, and some may be more willing than families from other backgrounds to accept life in a severely impaired state.[143] Finally, negative experiences in other settings, for example in refugee camps or under conditions of racial discrimination, may make it difficult for families to trust physicians. While recognizing the existence of certain cultural traditions, it is also critical to avoid making assumptions about attitudes and wishes, which must be deliberately explored.

Physicians should be sensitive to religious and spiritual concerns. The relationship among religion, spirituality, and decision making is complex and not entirely predictable. Many families harbor non-Western beliefs regarding the cause of illness or the role God plays in outcomes.[144] It is important not to assume that religious beliefs or belief in miracles preclude any particular treatment option. For example, hope for a miracle does not necessarily imply that physicians should offer nonstandard therapy or withhold recommendations to emphasize palliation or referral to hospice.[145]

Many families report significant burdens placed on them when treatment decisions are made. According to families, helpful physician and nursing behaviors include timely communication, clarification of the family's role, facilitating family consensus, and accommodating grief; in contrast, unhelpful behaviors include postponing end-of-life discussions, placing the decision-making burden on one person, withdrawing from the family, and defining death as a failure.[16] Often, the burden of decision making may be lessened if physicians take a more active role.[122,146]

IF CONFLICT PERSISTS

One of the greatest challenges facing intensivists is how best to address impasses created when families request potentially futile or inappropriate treatments. Although it is widely held that physicians are not obligated to provide futile care,[53,55,60] it is rarely necessary to forego therapy over a family's wishes.[118] Conflict usually dissipates in response to empathic, comprehensive communication and patience.[147]

Impasses involving psychologic, spiritual, and social issues may require mediation and support from psychologists or psychiatrists, chaplains, or social workers. Some families may be more comfortable talking with nursing staff. Undue pressure should not be placed on families to make decisions.[15] A lack of trust may explain why some families fail to accept physicians' recommendations.[58] Families may need extra time to form working relationships with physicians they barely know.[79] Many families simply need more time to grapple with and accept new findings. Treatment trials may help them come to terms with recommendations they initially resist.[54,148]

How to proceed when impasse persists remains an unsettled controversy. Some ethicists argue that physicians should defer to the wishes of families in these rare circumstances,[56] although this is a minority view.[53,55,60] If the decision is made to override a family's wishes, due process must be followed to ensure that the patient's and family's rights are respected.[149,150] Due process may include obtaining second opinions, providing opportunities to transfer care, and requesting oversight by an ethics committee. Institutional policies should ensure that decisions are fair and rational and eliminate the possibility that physicians would exert undue influence on patients and families.[151]

The American Medical Association has recommended a process-based approach to decision making under these circumstances,[149] although it is not clear that this approach would be legally supported in all jurisdictions.[54] To date, one state, Texas, has devised legislation to ensure due process when unilateral decisions are made.[150] It must be emphasized, however, that unilateral decision making should only occur as a last resort.

SUMMARY

A large proportion of deaths, particularly in the developed world, follows admission to an ICU. For intensivists, managing death in the critically ill has become a key professional skill. Intensivists must be thoroughly familiar with the ethical framework that guides end-of-life decision making. Moreover, they must become skilled in the nuanced practice of working closely with family members serving as surrogate decision makers. A combination of rational thinking, empathy, and patience will almost always foster effective decision making and exceptional end-of-life care.

REFERENCES

1. Angus DC, Barnato AE, Linde-Zwirble WT, et al. Use of intensive care at the end of life in the United States: an epidemiologic study. Crit Care Med 2004;32:638–43.

2. Prendergast TJ, Claessens MT, Luce JM. A national survey of end-of-life care for critically ill patients. Am J Respir Crit Care Med 1998;158:1163–7.

3. Truog RD, Campbell ML, Curtis JR, et al. Recommendations for end-of-life care in the intensive care unit: a consensus statement by the American College [corrected] of Critical Care Medicine. [erratum appears in Crit Care Med. 2008 May;36(5):1699]. Crit Care Med 2008;36:953–63.

4. Davidson JE, Powers K, Hedayat KM, et al. Clinical practice guidelines for support of the family in the patient-centered intensive care unit: American College of Critical Care Medicine Task Force 2004–2005. Crit Care Med 2007;35:605–22.

5. Nelson JE, Angus DC, Weissfeld LA, et al. End-of-life care for the critically ill: a national intensive care unit survey. Crit Care Med 2006;34:2547–53.

6. Cook D, Rocker G, Marshall J, et al. Withdrawal of mechanical ventilation in anticipation of death in the intensive care unit. N Engl J Med 2003;349:1123–32.

7. Prendergast TJ, Puntillo KA. Withdrawal of life support: intensive caring at the end of life. JAMA 2002;288:2732–40.

8. Vincent JL. Forgoing life support in western European intensive care units: the results of an ethical questionnaire. Crit Care Med 1999;27:1626–33.

9. Hamel MB, Phillips R, Teno J, et al. Cost effectiveness of aggressive care for patients with nontraumatic coma. Crit Care Med 2002;30:1191–6.

10. Mularski RA, Heine CE, Osborne ML, et al. Quality of dying in the ICU: ratings by family members. Chest 2005;128:280–7.

11. Levy CR, Ely EW, Payne K, et al. Quality of dying and death in two medical ICUs: perceptions of family and clinicians. Chest 2005;127:1775–83.

12. Pochard F, Darmon M, Fassier T, et al. Symptoms of anxiety and depression in family members of intensive care unit patients before discharge or death. A prospective multicenter study. J Crit Care 2005;20:90–6.

13. Azoulay E, Pochard F, Kentish-Barnes N, et al. Risk of post-traumatic stress symptoms in family members of intensive care unit patients. Am J Respir Crit Care Med 2005;171:987–94.

14. Pochard F, Azoulay E, Chevret S, et al. Symptoms of anxiety and depression in family members of intensive care unit patients: ethical hypothesis regarding decision-making capacity. Crit Care Med 2001;29:1893–7.

15. Luce JM, White DB. The pressure to withhold or withdraw life-sustaining therapy from critically ill patients in the United States. Am J Respir Crit Care Med 2007;175:1104–8.

16. Tilden VP, Tolle SW, Garland MJ, et al. Decisions about life-sustaining treatment: impact of physicians' behaviors on the family. Arch Intern Med 1995;155:633–8.

17. Abbott KH, Sago JG, Breen CM, et al. Families looking back: one year after discussion of withdrawal or withholding of life-sustaining support. Crit Care Med 2001;29:197–201.

18. Breen CM, Abernethy AP, Abbott KH, et al. Conflict associated with decisions to limit life-sustaining treatment in intensive care units. J Gen Intern Med 2001;16:283–9.

19. Cook DJ, Guyatt GH, Jaeschke R, et al. Determinants in Canadian health care workers of the decision to withdraw life support from the critically ill. Canadian Critical Care Trials Group. JAMA 1995; 273:703–8.

20. Yaguchi A, Truog RD, Curtis JR, et al. International differences in end-of-life attitudes in the intensive care unit: results of a survey. Arch Intern Med 2005;165:1970–5.

21. Anonymous. Attitudes of critical care medicine professionals concerning distribution of intensive care resources. The Society of Critical Care Medicine Ethics Committee. Crit Care Med 1994;22: 358–62.

22. Luce JM, Lemaire F. Two transatlantic viewpoints on an ethical quandary. Am J Respir Crit Care Med 2001;163:818–21.

23. Pochard F, Azoulay E, Chevret S, et al. French intensivists do not apply American recommendations regarding decisions to forgo life-sustaining therapy. Crit Care Med 2001;29:1887–92.

24. Ferrand E, Robert R, Ingrand P, et al. Withholding and withdrawal of life support in intensive-care units in France: a prospective survey. Lancet 2001;357:9–14.

25. Sprung CL, Maia P, Bulow HH, et al. The importance of religious affiliation and culture on end-of-life decisions in European intensive care units. Intensive Care Med 2007;33:1732–9.

26. Sprung CL, Geber D, Eidelman LA, et al. Evaluation of triage decisions for intensive care admission. Crit Care Med 1999;27:1073–9.

27. Sinuff T, Kahnamoui K, Cook DJ, et al. Rationing critical care beds: a systematic review. Crit Care Med 2004;32:1588–97.

28. Azoulay E, Pochard F, Garrouste-Orgeas M, et al. Decisions to forgo life-sustaining therapy in ICU patients independently predict hospital death. Intensive Care Med 2003;29:1895–901.

29. Azoulay E, Adrie C, De Lassence A, et al. Determinants of postintensive care unit mortality: a prospective multicenter study. Crit Care Med 2003;31:428–32.

30. Chen Y-Y, Connors AF Jr, Garland A. Effect of decisions to withhold life support on prolonged survival. Chest 2008;133:1312–8.

31. Anonymous. A controlled trial to improve care for seriously ill hospitalized patients. The Study to Understand Prognoses and Preferences for Outcomes and Risks of Treatments (SUPPORT). The SUPPORT principal investigators. [erratum appears in JAMA 1996 Apr 24;275(16):1232]. JAMA 1995;274:1591–8.

32. Cosgriff JA, Pisani M, Bradley EH, et al. The association between treatment preferences and trajectories of care at the end-of-life. J Gen Intern Med 2007;22:1566–71.

33. Asch DA, Hansen-Flaschen J, Lanken PN. Decisions to limit or continue life-sustaining treatment by critical care physicians in the United States: conflicts between physicians' practices and patients' wishes. Am J Respir Crit Care Med 1995;151:288–92.

34. Clarke EB, Curtis JR, Luce JM, et al. Quality indicators for end-of-life care in the intensive care unit. Crit Care Med 2003;31:2255–62.

35. Gries CJ, Curtis JR, Wall RJ, et al. Family member satisfaction with end-of-life decision making in the ICU. Chest 2008;133:704–12.

36. Carrese JA, Sugarman J. The inescapable relevance of bioethics for the practicing clinician. Chest 2006;130:1864–72.

37. Truog RD, Brock DW, Cook DJ, et al. Rationing in the intensive care unit. Crit Care Med 2006;34: 958–63.

38. Iserson KV, Moskop JC. Triage in medicine, part I: concept, history, and types. Ann Emerg Med 2007;49:275–81.

39. Walter KL, Siegler M, Hall JB. How decisions are made to admit patients to medical intensive care units (MICUs): a survey of MICU directors at academic medical centers across the United States. Crit Care Med 2008;36:414–20.

40. Ward NS, Teno JM, Curtis JR, et al. Perceptions of cost constraints, resource limitations, and rationing in United States intensive care units: results of a national survey. Crit Care Med 2008;36:471–6.

41. Simchen E, Sprung CL, Galai N, et al. Survival of critically ill patients hospitalized in and out of intensive care units under paucity of intensive care unit beds. Crit Care Med 2004;32:1654–61.

42. Powell T, Christ KC, Birkhead GS. Allocation of ventilators in a public health disaster. Disaster Med Public Health Prep 2008;2:20–6.

43. Talmor D, Jones AE, Rubinson L, et al. Simple triage scoring system predicting death and the need for critical care resources for use during epidemics. Crit Care Med 2007;35:1251–6.

44. Christian MD, Hawryluck L, Wax RS, et al. Development of a triage protocol for critical care during an influenza pandemic. CMAJ 2006;175:1377–81.

45. Anonymous. Consensus statement on the triage of critically ill patients. Society of Critical Care Medicine Ethics Committee. JAMA 1994;271:1200–3.

46. Anonymous. Guidelines for intensive care unit admission, discharge, and triage. Task Force of the American College of Critical Care Medicine,

Society of Critical Care Medicine. Crit Care Med 1999;27:633–8.

47. Daly K, Beale R, Chang RW. Reduction in mortality after inappropriate early discharge from intensive care unit: logistic regression triage model. BMJ 2001;322:1274–6.

48. Rubinson L, Nuzzo JB, Talmor DS, et al. Augmentation of hospital critical care capacity after bioterrorist attacks or epidemics: recommendations of the Working Group on Emergency Mass Critical Care. Crit Care Med 2005;33:2393–403.

49. Girard TD, Kress JP, Fuchs BD, et al. Efficacy and safety of a paired sedation and ventilator weaning protocol for mechanically ventilated patients in intensive care (awakening and breathing controlled trial): a randomised controlled trial. Lancet 2008; 371:126.

50. Wreen M. Medical futility and physician discretion. J Med Ethics 2004;30:275–8.

51. Mohindra RK. Medical futility: a conceptual model. J Med Ethics 2007;33:71–5.

52. Helft PR, Siegler M, Lantos J. The rise and fall of the futility movement. N Engl J Med 2000;343:293–6.

53. Schneiderman LJ, Jecker NS, Jonsen AR. Medical futility: its meaning and ethical implications. Ann Intern Med 1990;112:949–54.

54. Nasraway SA. Unilateral withdrawal of life-sustaining therapy: is it time? Are we ready? Crit Care Med 2001;29:215–7.

55. Luce JM. Physicians do not have a responsibility to provide futile or unreasonable care if a patient or family insists. Crit Care Med 1995;23:760–6.

56. Burns JP, Truog RD. Futility: a concept in evolution. Chest 2007;132:1987–93.

57. Schneiderman LJ, Jecker NS, Jonsen AR. Medical futility: response to critiques. Ann Intern Med 1996; 125:669–74.

58. Caplan AL. Odds and ends: trust and the debate over medical futility. Ann Intern Med 1996;125:688–9.

59. Atkinson S, Bihari D, Smithies M, et al. Identification of futility in intensive care. Lancet 1994;344:1203–6.

60. Anonymous. Withholding and withdrawing life-sustaining therapy. Ann Intern Med 1991;115: 478–85.

61. Cher DJ, Lenert LA. Method of Medicare reimbursement and the rate of potentially ineffective care of critically ill patients. [Erratum appears in JAMA 1998 Jun 17; 279(23): 1876]. JAMA 1997;278:1001–7.

62. Curtis JR, Park DR, Krone MR, et al. Use of the medical futility rationale in do-not-attempt-resuscitation orders. JAMA 1995;273:124–8.

63. Civetta JM. Futile care or caregiver frustration? A practical approach. Crit Care Med 1996;24:346–51.

64. Waisel DB, Truog RD. The cardiopulmonary resuscitation-not-indicated order: futility revisited. Ann Intern Med 1995;122:304–8.

65. Curtis JR, Patrick DL, Caldwell ES, et al. The attitudes of patients with advanced AIDS toward use of the medical futility rationale in decisions to forgo mechanical ventilation. Arch Intern Med 2000;160: 1597–601.

66. Frick S, Uehlinger DE, Zuercher Zenklusen RM. Medical futility: predicting outcome of intensive care unit patients by nurses and doctors- a prospective comparative study. Crit Care Med 2003;31: 456–61.

67. Rubenfeld GD, Crawford SW. Withdrawing life support from mechanically ventilated recipients of bone marrow transplants: a case for evidence-based guidelines. Ann Intern Med 1996;125:625–33.

68. Scales DC, Thiruchelvam D, Kiss A, et al. Intensive care outcomes in bone marrow transplant recipients: a population-based cohort analysis. Crit Care 2008;12:R77.

69. Jackson SR, Tweeddale MG, Barnett MJ, et al. Admission of bone marrow transplant recipients to the intensive care unit: outcome, survival and prognostic factors. Bone Marrow Transplant 1998; 21:697–704.

70. Becker KJ, Baxter AB, Cohen WA, et al. Withdrawal of support in intracerebral hemorrhage may lead to self-fulfilling prophecies. Neurology 2001;56: 766–72.

71. Cohen NH. Assessing futility of medical interventions-is it futile? Crit Care Med 2003;31:646–8.

72. Tonelli MR. Waking the dying: must we always attempt to involve critically ill patients in end-of-life decisions? Chest 2005;127:637–42.

73. McNicoll L, Pisani MA, Zhang Y, et al. Delirium in the intensive care unit: occurrence and clinical course in older patients. J Am Geriatr Soc 2003; 51:591–8.

74. Ely EW, Inouye SK, Bernard GR, et al. Delirium in mechanically ventilated patients: validity and reliability of the confusion assessment method for the intensive care unit (CAM-ICU). JAMA 2001; 286:2703–10.

75. Pisani MA, Redlich C, McNicoll L, et al. Underrecognition of preexisting cognitive impairment by physicians in older ICU patients. Chest 2003;124: 2267–74.

76. Cassell EJ, Leon AC, Kaufman SG. Preliminary evidence of impaired thinking in sick patients. Ann Intern Med 2001;134:1120–3.

77. Curtis JR, White DB. Practical guidance for evidence-based ICU family conferences. Chest 2008;134:835–43.

78. Berger JT, DeRenzo EG, Schwartz J. Surrogate decision making: reconciling ethical theory and clinical practice. Ann Intern Med 2008;149:48–53.

79. Torke AM, Alexander GC, Lantos J, et al. The physician-surrogate relationship. Arch Intern Med 2007; 167:1117–21.

80. White DB, Curtis JR, Wolf LE, et al. Life support for patients without a surrogate decision maker: who decides? Ann Intern Med 2007;147:34–40.

81. Puchalski CM, Zhong Z, Jacobs MM, et al. Patients who want their family and physician to make resuscitation decisions for them: observations from SUPPORT and HELP. Study to understand prognoses and preferences for outcomes and risks of treatment. Hospitalized Elderly Longitudinal Project. J Am Geriatr Soc 2000;48:S84–90.

82. Crawley LM, Marshall PA, Lo B, et al. Strategies for culturally effective end-of-life care. Ann Intern Med 2002;136:673–9.

83. Kagawa-Singer M, Blackhall LJ. Negotiating cross-cultural issues at the end of life: "you got to go where he lives." JAMA 2001;286:2993–3001.

84. Azoulay E, Pochard F, Chevret S, et al. Half the family members of intensive care unit patients do not want to share in the decision-making process: a study in 78 French intensive care units. Crit Care Med 2004;32:1832–8.

85. Coppola KM, Ditto PH, Danks JH, et al. Accuracy of primary care and hospital-based physicians' predictions of elderly outpatients' treatment preferences with and without advance directives. Arch Intern Med 2001;161:431–40.

86. Uhlmann RF, Pearlman RA, Cain KC. Physicians' and spouses' predictions of elderly patients' resuscitation preferences. J Gerontol 1988;43:M115–21.

87. Wenger NS, Oye RK, Bellamy PE, et al. Prior capacity of patients lacking decision making ability early in hospitalization: implications for advance directive administration. The SUPPORT investigators. Study to understand prognoses and preferences for outcomes and risks of treatments. J Gen Intern Med 1994;9:539–43.

88. Connecticut's living will laws. Available at: http://www.ct.gov/ag/cwp/browse.asp?a=2130&bc=0&c=19278. Accessed November 2, 2008.

89. Upadya A, Muralidharan V, Thorevska N, et al. Patient, physician, and family member understanding of living wills. Am J Respir Crit Care Med 2002;166:1430–5.

90. Morrell ED, Brown BP, Qi R, et al. The do-not-resuscitate order: associations with advance directives, physician specialty and documentation of discussion 15 years after the patient self-determination act. J Med Ethics 2008;34:642–7.

91. Teno JM, Licks S, Lynn J, et al. Do advance directives provide instructions that direct care? J Am Geriatr Soc 1997;45:508–12.

92. Perkins HS. Controlling death: the false promise of advance directives. Ann Intern Med 2007;147:51–7.

93. Ditto PH, Danks JH, Smucker WD, et al. Advance directives as acts of communication: a randomized controlled trial. Arch Intern Med 2001;161:421–30.

94. Wright AA, Zhang B, Ray A, et al. Associations between end-of-life discussions, patient mental health, medical care near death, and caregiver bereavement adjustment. JAMA 2008;300:1665–73.

95. Siegel MD, Hayes E, Vanderwerker LC, et al. Psychiatric illness in the next of kin of patients who die in the intensive care unit. Crit Care Med 2008;36:1722–8.

96. Lloyd CB, Nietert PJ, Silvestri GA. Intensive care decision making in the seriously ill and elderly. Crit Care Med 2004;32:649–54.

97. Danis M, Patrick DL, Southerland LI, et al. Patients' and families' preferences for medical intensive care. JAMA 1988;260:797–802.

98. Sulmasy DP, Terry PB, Weisman CS, et al. The accuracy of substituted judgments in patients with terminal diagnoses. [see comment]. Ann Intern Med 1998;128:621–9.

99. Danis M, Gerrity MS, Southerland LI, et al. A comparison of patient, family, and physician assessments of the value of medical intensive care. Crit Care Med 1988;16:594–600.

100. Fried TR, Bradley EH, Towle VR. Valuing the outcomes of treatment: do patients and their caregivers agree? Arch Intern Med 2003;163:2073–8.

101. Wittink MN, Morales KH, Meoni LA, et al. Stability of preferences for end-of-life treatment after 3 years of follow-up: the Johns Hopkins Precursors Study. Arch Intern Med 2008;168:2125–30.

102. Danis M, Garrett J, Harris R, et al. Stability of choices about life-sustaining treatments. Ann Intern Med 1994;120:567–73.

103. Fried TR, O'Leary J, Van Ness P, et al. Inconsistency over time in the preferences of older persons with advanced illness for life-sustaining treatment. J Am Geriatr Soc 2007;55:1007–14.

104. Lockhart LK, Ditto PH, Danks JH, et al. The stability of older adults' judgments of fates better and worse than death. Death Stud 2001;25:299–317.

105. Choudhry NK, Choudhry S, Singer PA. CPR for patients labeled DNR: the role of the limited aggressive therapy order. [See comment]. Ann Intern Med 2003;138:65–8.

106. Fried TR, Byers AL, Gallo WT, et al. Prospective study of health status preferences and changes in preferences over time in older adults. Arch Intern Med 2006;166:890–5.

107. Fried TR, Van Ness PH, Byers AL, et al. Changes in preferences for life-sustaining treatment among older persons with advanced illness. J Gen Intern Med 2007;22:495–501.

108. Finucane TE. How gravely ill becomes dying: a key to end-of-life care. JAMA 1999;282:1670–2.

109. Fried TR, Bradley EH, Towle VR, et al. Understanding the treatment preferences of seriously ill patients. [See comment]. N Engl J Med 2002;346:1061–6.

110. Lautrette A, Ciroldi M, Ksibi H, et al. End-of-life family conferences: rooted in the evidence. Crit Care Med 2006;34:S364–72.

111. Lautrette A, Darmon M, Megarbane B, et al. A communication strategy and brochure for relatives of patients dying in the ICU. [erratum appears in N Engl J Med 2007 Jul 12;357(2):203]. N Engl J Med 2007;356:469–78.

112. Lilly CM, De Meo DL, Sonna LA, et al. An intensive communication intervention for the critically ill. Am J Med 2000;109:469–75.

113. Curtis JR, Engelberg RA, Wenrich MD, et al. Missed opportunities during family conferences about end-of-life care in the intensive care unit. Am J Respir Crit Care Med 2005;171:844–9.

114. Gilligan T, Raffin TA. End-of-life discussions with patients. Timing and truth-telling. [comment]. Chest 1996;109:11–2.

115. Afessa B, Keegan MT, Mohammad Z, et al. Identifying potentially ineffective care in the sickest critically ill patients on the third ICU day. Chest 2004; 126:1905–9.

116. Back AL, Arnold RM, Quill TE. Hope for the best, and prepare for the worst. Ann Intern Med 2003; 138:439–44.

117. Larson AM, Curtis JR. Integrating palliative care for liver transplant candidates: "too well for transplant, too sick for life." JAMA 2006;295:2168–76.

118. Shanawani H, Wenrich MD, Tonelli MR, et al. Meeting physicians' responsibilities in providing end-of-life care. Chest 2008;133:775–86.

119. Beach MC, Morrison RS. The effect of do-not-resuscitate orders on physician decision-making. J Am Geriatr Soc 2002;50:2057–61.

120. Gelbman BD, Gelbman JM. Deconstructing DNR. J Med Ethics 2008;34:640–1.

121. White DB, Braddock CH 3rd, Bereknyei S, et al. Toward shared decision making at the end of life in intensive care units: opportunities for improvement. Arch Intern Med 2007;167:461–7.

122. Heyland DK, Cook DJ, Rocker GM, et al. Decision-making in the ICU: perspectives of the substitute decision-maker. Intensive Care Med 2003;29:75–82.

123. Heyland DK, Frank C, Groll D, et al. Understanding cardiopulmonary resuscitation decision making: perspectives of seriously ill hospitalized patients and family members. Chest 2006;130:419–28.

124. McDonagh JR, Elliott TB, Engelberg RA, et al. Family satisfaction with family conferences about end-of-life care in the intensive care unit: increased proportion of family speech is associated with increased satisfaction. Crit Care Med 2004;32: 1484–8.

125. Selph RB, Shiang J, Engelberg R, et al. Empathy and life support decisions in intensive care units. J Gen Intern Med 2008;23:1311–7.

126. Stapleton RD, Engelberg RA, Wenrich MD, et al. Clinician statements and family satisfaction with family conferences in the intensive care unit. Crit Care Med 2006;34:1679–85.

127. Nelson JE, Mercado AF, Camhi SL, et al. Communication about chronic critical illness. Arch Intern Med 2007;167:2509–15.

128. Tulsky JA, Chesney MA, Lo B. How do medical residents discuss resuscitation with patients? J Gen Intern Med 1995;10:436–42.

129. White DB, Engelberg RA, Wenrich MD, et al. Prognostication during physician-family discussions about limiting life support in intensive care units. [See comment]. Crit Care Med 2007;35:442–8.

130. LeClaire MM, Oakes JM, Weinert CR. Communication of prognostic information for critically ill patients. Chest 2005;128:1728–35.

131. Zahuranec DB, Brown DL, Lisabeth LD, et al. Early care limitations independently predict mortality after intracerebral hemorrhage. [See comment]. Neurology 2007;68:1651–7.

132. Rady MY, Johnson DJ. Admission to intensive care unit at the end-of-life: is it an informed decision? Panminerva Med 2004;18:705–11.

133. Diem SJ, Lantos JD, Tulsky JA. Cardiopulmonary resuscitation on television. Miracles and misinformation. N Engl J Med 1996;334:1578–82.

134. Azoulay E, Chevret S, Leleu G, et al. Half the families of intensive care unit patients experience inadequate communication with physicians. Crit Care Med 2000;28:3044–9.

135. Dunn WF, Adams SC, Adams RW. Iatrogenic delirium and coma: a "near miss." Chest 2008; 133:1217–20.

136. Murphy DJ, Burrows D, Santilli S, et al. The influence of the probability of survival on patients' preferences regarding cardiopulmonary resuscitation. N Engl J Med 1994;330:545–9.

137. Pham K, Thornton JD, Engelberg RA, et al. Alterations during medical interpretation of ICU family conferences that interfere with or enhance communication. Chest 2008;134:109–16.

138. Siegel MD. Lost in translation: family conferences for families that don't speak English. Crit Care Med, in press.

139. Norris WM, Wenrich MD, Nielsen EL, et al. Communication about end-of-life care between language-discordant patients and clinicians: insights from medical interpreters. J Palliat Med 2005;8:1016–24.

140. Lowe S. New census bureau data reveal more older workers, homeowners, non-English speakers. U.S. Census Bureau news. September 12, 2007. Available at: http://www.census.gov/Press-Release/

www/releases/archives/american_community_survey_
acs/010601.html. Accessed July 7, 2008.

141. Hudelson P. Improving patient-provider communication: insights from interpreters. Fam Pract 2005;
22:311–6.

142. Thornton JD, Pham K, Engelberg RA, et al. Families
with limited English proficiency receive less information and support in interpreted ICU family
conferences. Crit Care Med, in press.

143. Crawley L, Payne R, Bolden J, et al. Palliative and
end-of-life care in the African American community.
JAMA 2000;284:2518–21.

144. Fadiman A. The spirit catches you and you fall
down. In: First paperback edition. New York: Farrar,
Straus and Giroux; 1998.

145. Sulmasy DP. Spiritual issues in the care of dying
patients. "It's okay between me and God." JAMA
2006;296:1385–92.

146. Curtis JR, Burt RA. Point: the ethics of unilateral "do
not resuscitate" orders: the role of "informed
assent." Chest 2007;132:748–51.

147. Way J, Back AL, Curtis JR. Withdrawing life
support and resolution of conflict with families.
BMJ 2002;325:1342–5.

148. Lee DK, Swinburne AJ, Fedullo AJ, et al. Withdrawing care. Experience in a medical intensive
care unit. JAMA 1994;271:1358–61.

149. Anonymous. Medical futility in end-of-life care.
Report of the Council on Ethical and Judicial
Affairs. JAMA 1999;281:937–41.

150. Fine RL, Mayo TW. Resolution of futility by due
process: early experience with the Texas Advance
Directives Act. Ann Intern Med 2003;138:743–6.

151. Luce JM. Making decisions about the forgoing of
life-sustaining therapy. Am J Respir Crit Care
Med 1997;156:1715–8.

Index

Note: Page numbers of article titles are in **boldface** type.

Clin Chest Med 30 (2009) 195–201
doi:10.1016/S0272-5231(09)00009-4
0272-5231/09/$ – see front matter © 2009 Elsevier Inc. All rights reserved.

chestmed.theclinics.com

Printed and bound by CPI Group (UK) Ltd, Croydon, CR0 4YY

03/10/2024

01040360-0009